INFORMATICS
FOR HEALTH PROFESSIONALS

Kathleen Garver Mastrian
Dee McGonigle

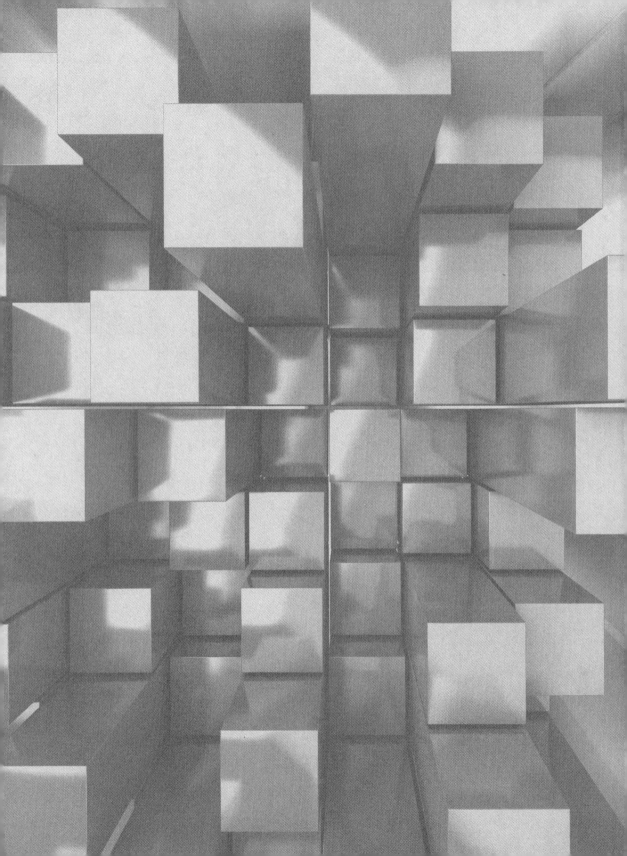

INFORMATICS

FOR HEALTH PROFESSIONALS

Kathleen Garver Mastrian, PhD, RN

Associate Professor and Program Coordinator for Nursing
Pennsylvania State University, Shenango
Senior Managing Editor, *Online Journal of Nursing Informatics (OJNI)*
Member, Health Information Management Systems Society (HIMSS)

Dee McGonigle, PhD, RN, CNE, FAAN, ANEF

Director, Virtual Learning Experiences and Professor, Graduate Program
Chamberlain College of Nursing
Fellow, American Academy of Nursing
Secretary, Expert Panel on Informatics and Technology (EPIT) for the American Academy of
Nursing Member, Serious Gaming and Virtual Environments Special Interest Group for the
Society for Simulation in Healthcare (SSH)
Fellow, NLN Academy of Nursing Education
Member, Health Information Management Systems Society (HIMSS)

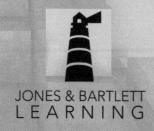

JONES & BARTLETT
LEARNING

World Headquarters
Jones & Bartlett Learning
5 Wall Street
Burlington, MA 01803
978-443-5000
info@jblearning.com
www.jblearning.com

Jones & Bartlett Learning books and products are available through most bookstores and online booksellers. To contact Jones & Bartlett Learning directly, call 800-832-0034, fax 978-443-8000, or visit our website, www.jblearning.com.

Substantial discounts on bulk quantities of Jones & Bartlett Learning publications are available to corporations, professional associations, and other qualified organizations. For details and specific discount information, contact the special sales department at Jones & Bartlett Learning via the above contact information or send an email to specialsales@jblearning.com.

15788-8

Production Credits
VP, Executive Publisher: David D. Cella
Publisher: Cathy L. Esperti
Editorial Assistant: Carter McAlister
Vendor Manager: Sara Kelly
Marketing Manager: Grace Richards
Manufacturing and Inventory Control Supervisor: Amy Bacus
Composition and Project Management: Cenveo® Publisher Services
Cover Design: Kristin Parker
Rights & Media Specialist: Jamey O'Quinn
Media Development Editor: Troy Liston
Cover Image: © Waj/Shutterstock
Printing and Binding: Edwards Brothers Malloy
Cover Printing: Edwards Brothers Malloy

Library of Congress Cataloging-in-Publication Data

Names: Mastrian, Kathleen Garver, author. | McGonigle, Dee, author.
Title: Informatics for health professionals / Kathleen Garver Mastrian, Dee McGonigle.
Description: Burlington, MA : Jones & Bartlett Learning, [2017] | Includes bibliographical references and index.
Identifiers: LCCN 2016004458 | ISBN 9781284157888 (pbk. : alk. paper)
Subjects: | MESH: Medical Informatics—methods | Knowledge | Professional Competence
Classification: LCC R858 | NLM W 26.5 | DDC 610.285—dc23
LC record available at http://lccn.loc.gov/2016004458

6048

Printed in the United States of America
20 19 18 17 16   10 9 8 7 6 5 4 3 2 1

Contents

SECTION II: CHOOSING AND USING INFORMATION SYSTEMS 109

6 Systems Development Life Cycle 113
Dee McGonigle and Kathleen Mastrian

7 Administrative Information Systems 127
Marianela Zytkowski, Susan Paschke, Dee McGonigle, and Kathleen Mastrian

SECTION IV: ADVANCED CONCEPTS IN HEALTH INFORMATICS 277

SECTION V: PRACTICE IN THE FUTURE 361

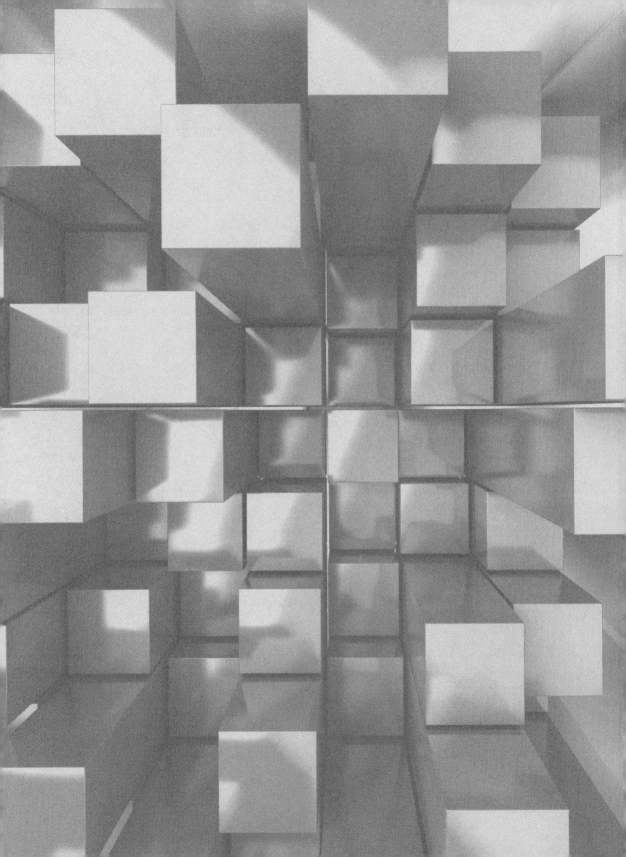

Preface

Authors' Note

This text provides an overview of health informatics from the perspective of diverse experts in the field, with a focus on health informatics and the Foundation of Knowledge model. We want our readers and students to focus on the relationship of knowledge to informatics and to embrace and maintain the caring functions essential to all of health care—messages all too often lost in the romance with technology. We hope you enjoy the text!

About this Book

The idea for this text originated with the publication of the third edition of *Nursing Informatics and the Foundation of Knowledge* (2015). We realized that other health care professionals also needed to learn about informatics and the ways that informatics supports professional practice. We know that the idea of informatics is new to many health care professionals, and we believe that all health care professionals need to be better prepared for 21st-century practice by developing a strong foundation in informatics.

According to the Association of Schools of Allied Health Professions (http://www.asahp.org/wp-content/uploads/2014/08/Health-Professions-Facts.pdf), allied health professionals represent 60% of the health workforce and are "the segment of the workforce that delivers services involving the identification, evaluation and prevention of diseases and disorders; dietary and nutrition services; and rehabilitation and health systems management" (para 1). Specifically, this text is designed to introduce dental hygienists, diagnostic medical sonographers, dietitians, medical technologists, occupational therapists, physical therapists, radiographers, respiratory therapists, and speech-language pathologists to health informatics.

Collectively, we have years of experience teaching and writing about informatics. Like most nurse informaticists, we fell into the specialty; our love affair with technology and gadgets and our willingness to be the first to try new things helped to hook us into the specialty of informatics. The rapid evolution of technology in the health care system and the role of technology in the transformation of the system initially prompted us to try to capture the essence of nursing informatics in a text. Here is a bit of background on the nursing informatics text evolution that helped to set the stage for this text.

As we were developing the first edition, we realized that we could not possibly know all there is to know about informatics and the way in which it supports practice, education, administration, and research. We also knew that our faculty roles constrained our opportunities for exposure to changes in this rapidly evolving field. Therefore, we developed a tentative outline and a working model of the theoretical framework for the text and invited participation from informatics experts and specialists around the world. We were pleased with the enthusiastic responses we received from some of those invited contributors and a few volunteers who heard about the text and asked to participate in their particular area of expertise. In this textbook, we have retained some of this valuable information from these original contributors to the first edition of the nursing informatics text.

We believe that this text provides a comprehensive elucidation of this exciting field. The theoretical underpinning of the text is the Foundation of Knowledge model. This model is introduced in its entirety in the first chapter (*Informatics, Disciplinary Science, and the Foundation of Knowledge*), which discusses disciplinary science and its relationship to health informatics. We believe that humans are organic information systems that are constantly acquiring, processing, and generating information or knowledge in both their professional and their personal lives. It is their high degree of knowledge that characterizes humans as extremely intelligent, organic machines. Individuals have the ability to manage knowledge—an ability that is learned and honed from birth. We make our way through life interacting with our environment and being inundated with information and knowledge. We experience our environment and learn by acquiring, processing, generating, and disseminating knowledge. As we interact in our environment, we acquire knowledge that we must process. This processing effort causes us to redefine and restructure our knowledge base and generate new knowledge. We then share (disseminate) this new knowledge and receive feedback from others. The dissemination and feedback initiate this cycle of knowledge over again as we acquire, process, generate, and disseminate the knowledge gained from sharing and re-exploring our own knowledge base. As others respond to our knowledge dissemination and we acquire new knowledge, we engage in rethinking and reflecting on our knowledge, processing, generating, and then disseminating anew.

The purpose of this text is to provide a set of practical and powerful tools to ensure that the reader gains an understanding of health informatics and moves from information through knowledge to wisdom. Defining the demands of health professionals and providing tools to help them survive and succeed in the Knowledge Era remains a major challenge. Exposing allied health students to the principles and tools used in health informatics helps to prepare them to meet the challenge of practicing in the Knowledge Era while striving to improve patient care at all levels.

The text provides a comprehensive framework that embraces knowledge so that readers can develop their knowledge repositories and the wisdom necessary to act on and apply that knowledge. The text is divided into five sections:

- The *Building Blocks of Health Informatics* (HI) section covers the building blocks of HI: disciplinary science, information science, computer science, cognitive science, and the ethical and legal aspects of managing information.
- The *Choosing and Using Information Systems* section explains how systems are developed, covers important functions of administrative application systems in health care, discusses the human–technology interface, provides important information on electronic security, and explains work flow and meaningful use in relation to electronic systems.
- The *Informatics Applications for Care Delivery* section covers health care delivery applications including electronic health records (EHRs), patient engagement and connected health, patient safety and quality outcomes technologies, interdisciplinary collaboration, and informatics tools for community and population health promotion.
- The *Advanced Concepts in Health Informatics* section presents subject matter on informatics tools for health professional education, data mining, translational research for generating best practices, and the exciting fields of bioinformatics and computational biology.
- The *Practice in the Future* section focuses on the future of health informatics, emphasizes the need to preserve caring and patient-centered functions in technology-laden environments, and summarizes the relationship of informatics to the Foundation of Knowledge model and organizational knowledge management.

The introduction to each section explains the relationship between the content of that section and the Foundation of Knowledge model. This text places the material within the context of knowledge acquisition, processing, generation, and dissemination. It serves health care professionals who need to understand, use, and evaluate knowledge. Throughout the text where appropriate, we have included case scenarios demonstrating why a topic is important and research briefs presented in text boxes to encourage the reader to access current research and to focus on cutting-edge innovations, meaningful use, and patient safety as appropriate to each topic.

As college professors, our major responsibility is to prepare the practitioners and leaders in the field. Our primary objective is to develop the most comprehensive and user-friendly HI text on the market to prepare health professionals for current and future practice challenges. In particular, this text provides a solid groundwork from which to integrate informatics principles into practice.

Goals of this text are as follows:

- Impart core HI principles that should be familiar to every health professional.
- Help the reader understand knowledge and how it is acquired, processed, generated, and disseminated.
- Demonstrate the value of the HI discipline as an attractive field of specialization.

The overall vision, framework, and pedagogy of this text offers benefits to readers by highlighting established principles while drawing out new ones that continue to emerge as health care and technology evolve.

Acknowledgments

We are deeply grateful to the contributors who provided this text with a richness and diversity of content that we could not have captured alone. Joan Humphrey provided social media content integrated throughout the text. We especially wish to acknowledge the superior work of Alicia Mastrian, graphic designer of the Foundation of Knowledge model, which serves as the theoretical framework on which this text is anchored. We would also like to thank Craig McGonigle for his insightful contributions to this text. We could never have completed this project without the dedicated and patient efforts of the Jones & Bartlett Learning staff, especially Cathy Esperti, Sara Peterson, and Carter McAlister. Both fielded our questions and concerns in a very professional and respectful manner.

Kathy acknowledges the loving support of her family: husband Chip, children Ben and Alicia, sisters Carol and Sue, and parents Bob and Rosalie Garver. Kathy also acknowledges those friends who understand the importance of validation, especially Katie, Lisa, Kathy, Anne, and Barbara.

Dee acknowledges the undying love, support, patience, and continued inspiration of her best friend and husband, Craig, and her son, Craig, who has also made her so very proud. She sincerely thanks her friends and family for their support and encouragement.

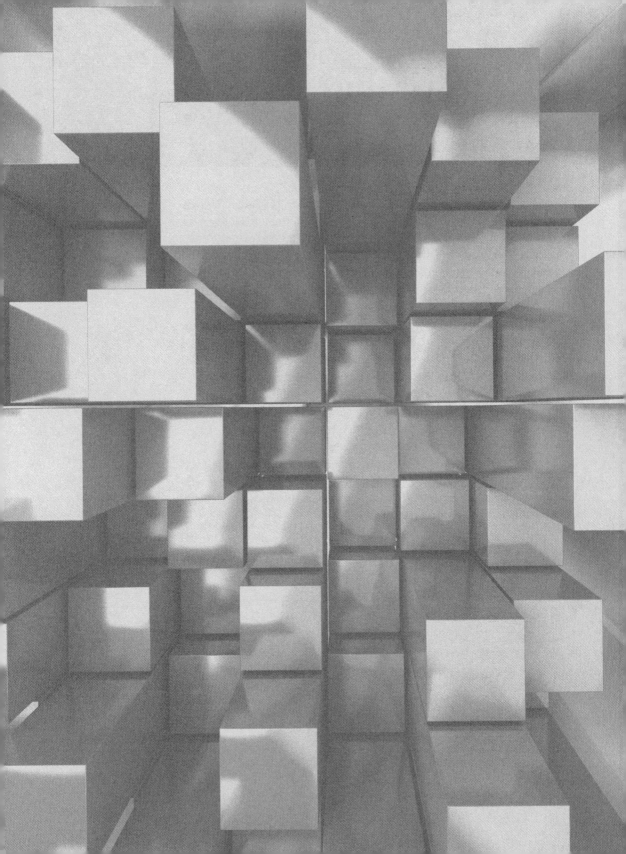

Contributors

Ida Androwich, PhD, RN, BC, FAAN
Loyola University Chicago
School of Nursing
Maywood, IL

Emily Barey, MSN, RN
Director of Nursing Informatics
Epic Systems Corporation
Madison, WI

Lisa Reeves Bertin, BS, EMBA
Pennsylvania State University
Sharon, PA

Brett Bixler, PhD
Pennsylvania State University
University Park, PA

Jennifer Bredemeyer, RN
Loyola University Chicago
School of Nursing
Skokie, IL

Steven Brewer, PhD
Assistant Professor, Administration of Justice
Pennsylvania State University
Sharon, PA

Sylvia M. DeSantis, MA
Pennsylvania State University
University Park, PA

Judith Effken, PhD, RN, FACMI
University of Arizona
College of Nursing
Tucson, AZ

Kathleen M. Gialanella, JD, RN, LLM
Law Offices
Westfield, NJ
Associate Adjunct Professor
Teachers College, Columbia University
New York, NY
Adjunct Professor
Seton Hall University, College of Nursing and School of Law
South Orange and Newark, NJ

Denise Hammel-Jones, MSN, RN-BC, CLSSBB
Greencastle Associates Consulting
Malvern, PA

Glenn Johnson, MLS
Pennsylvania State University
University Park, PA

June Kaminski, MSN, RN
Kwantlen University College
Surrey, British Columbia, Canada

Julie Kenney, MSN, RNC-OB
Clinical Analyst Advocate Health Care
Oak Brook, IL

Margaret Ross Kraft, PhD, RN
Loyola University Chicago
School of Nursing
Maywood, IL

Wendy L. Mahan, PhD, CRC, LPC
Pennsylvania State University
University Park, PA

Craig McGonigle, MBA, BSB
CEO, Mick Enterprise, Inc.
Dillon, SC

Heather McKinney, PhD
Pennsylvania State University
University Park, PA

Nickolaus Miehl, MSN, RN
Clinical Instructor and Simulation Specialist
Oregon Health and Science University Monmouth Campus
Portland, OR

Lynn M. Nagle, PhD, RN
Assistant Professor
University of Toronto
Toronto, ON, Canada

Jeff Swain
Instructional Designer
Pennsylvania State University
University Park, PA

Denise D. Tyler, MSN/MBA, RN-BC
Implementation Specialist
Healthcare Provider, Consulting
ACS, a Xerox Company
Dearborn, MI

A Visual Walkthrough

Informatics for Health Professionals drives comprehension through a variety of strategies geared toward meeting the learning needs of students while also generating enthusiasm about the topic. This interactive approach addresses diverse learning styles, making this the ideal text to ensure mastery of key concepts. The pedagogical aids that appear in most chapters include the following:

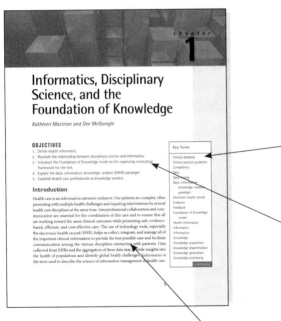

Key Terms

Found in a list at the beginning of each chapter, these terms will create an expanded vocabulary. The "www" icon directs students to the text's online resources, where they can review these terms in an interactive glossary and use flash cards to nail down their definitions. Use the access code at the front of your book to access these additional resources. If you do not have an access code, one can be purchased at http://www.jblearning.com.

Objectives

The chapter objectives provide instructors and students with a snapshot of the key information they will encounter in each chapter. They serve as a checklist to help guide and focus study. Objectives can also be found within the text's online resources.

Introductions

Found at the beginning of each chapter, chapter introductions provide an overview highlighting the importance of the chapter's topic. They also help keep students focused as they read.

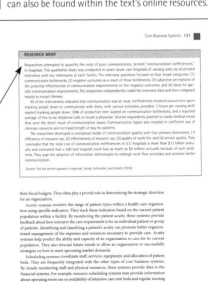

Research Briefs

These summaries encourage students to access current research in the field.

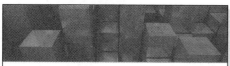

Summary

This chapter provided an overview of informatics and core informatics competencies, the DIKW paradigm, and the relationship of the paradigm to disciplinary science and established that health care professionals are knowledge workers. The Foundation of Knowledge model was introduced as the organizing conceptual framework for this text. Core informatics competencies were presented with an opportunity for self-assessment. In subsequent chapters, the reader will learn more about how informatics supports health care professionals in their many and varied roles. We suggest that in the future, health care research will make significant contributions to the development of the practice sciences for health care professionals. Technologies and translational research will abound, and clinical practices will be evidence based, thereby improving patient outcomes, decreasing safety concerns, and providing cost-effective care.

Thought-Provoking Questions

1. Describe a scenario in your discipline where you used data, information, knowledge, and wisdom.
2. Choose a clinical scenario from your recent experience and analyze it using the Foundation of Knowledge model. How did you acquire knowledge? How did you process knowledge? How did you generate knowledge? How did you disseminate knowledge? How did you use feedback, and what was the effect of the feedback on the foundation of your knowledge?
3. Complete the self-assessment of informatics competencies presented in Table 1-1 and create an action plan for achieving these competencies.

Apply Your Knowledge

This chapter introduced you to concepts related to the scientific basis of your profession and the relationship between health informatics and your discipline.

1. You are at a social event, and you are sharing a story about your education experience and your course on health informatics. A friend asks you, "What is informatics?" Answer the question by using terms and examples that a layperson will understand.
2. As the conversation continues, you share that you are excited about the allied health major you have chosen because of the scientific basis of the practice. Again, your skeptical friend asks, "What do you mean by the science of the discipline?" Answer this question by describing at least three examples of the scientific basis of practice for your discipline.

Summaries

Summaries are included at the end of each chapter to provide a concise review of the material covered, highlighting the most important points and describing what the future holds.

Thought-Provoking Questions

Students can work on these critical thinking assignments individually or in a group while reading through the text. In addition, students can delve deeper into concepts by completing these exercises online.

Apply Your Knowledge

Each chapter contains a content application scenario to promote active learning and critical thinking skills. These activities may be assigned individually to students or may be used as group activities. We believe that when used as group activity, there is better understanding and knowledge building potential. To use as a group activity, we suggest the following directions to students: Huddle with a fellow student or a team of students to read and craft responses to the application scenario. Share your responses, and compare and contrast them to craft a consensus response for the class. These activities also work well in an electronic environment with students chatting online synchronously or asynchronously in a discussion forum.

Case Studies

Case studies encourage active learning and promote critical thinking skills. Students can ask questions, analyze situations, and solve problems in a real-world context.

---

178 CHAPTER 10: Work Flow and Meaningful Use

as Virginia Mason University Medical Center, among others, have experienced significant quality and cost gains from the widespread implementation of Lean development throughout their organization.

Work Flow Analysis and Informatics Practice

The functional area of analysis identifies the specific functional qualities related to work flow analysis. Particularly, health informatics should develop techniques necessary to assess and improve human–computer interaction. Work flow analysis, however, is not relevant solely to analysis but rather is part of every functional area that the informatics support personnel engage in. Support personnel need to understand work flow and appreciate how lack of efficient work flow for health care professionals affects patient care.

A critical aspect of the informatics support role is work flow design. Health informatics is uniquely positioned to engage in the analysis and redesign of processes and tasks surrounding the use of technology. Work flow redesign is one of the fundamental skills sets that make up the discipline of this specialty. Moreover, work flow analysis should be part of every technology implementation, and the role of the informaticist within this team is to direct others in the execution of this task or to perform the task directly.

Unfortunately, many health care professionals find themselves in an informatics support capacity without sufficient preparation for a process analysis role. One area of practice that is particularly susceptible to inadequate preparation is the ability to facilitate process analysis. Work flow analysis requires careful attention to detail and the ability to moderate group discussions, organize concepts, and generate solutions. These skills can be acquired through a formal academic informatics program or through courses that teach the discipline of Six Sigma or Lean, by example. Regardless of where these skills are acquired, it is important to understand that they are now and will continue to remain a vital aspect of the informatics role.

CASE STUDY

In my experience consulting, I have seen several examples of organizations that engage in the printing of paper reports that replicate information that has been entered and is available with the electronic health record. These reports are often reviewed, signed, and acted on instead of using the electronic information. Despite the knowledge that the information contained in these reports was outdated the moment the report was printed and that the very nature of using the report for work flow is an inefficient practice, this method of clinical work flow remains prevalent in many hospitals across the United States.

There is an underlying fear that drives the decisions to mold a paper-based work flow around clinical technology. There is also a lack of the appropriate amount of integration that would otherwise allow this information to be available in an electronic form.

Denise Hammel-Jones

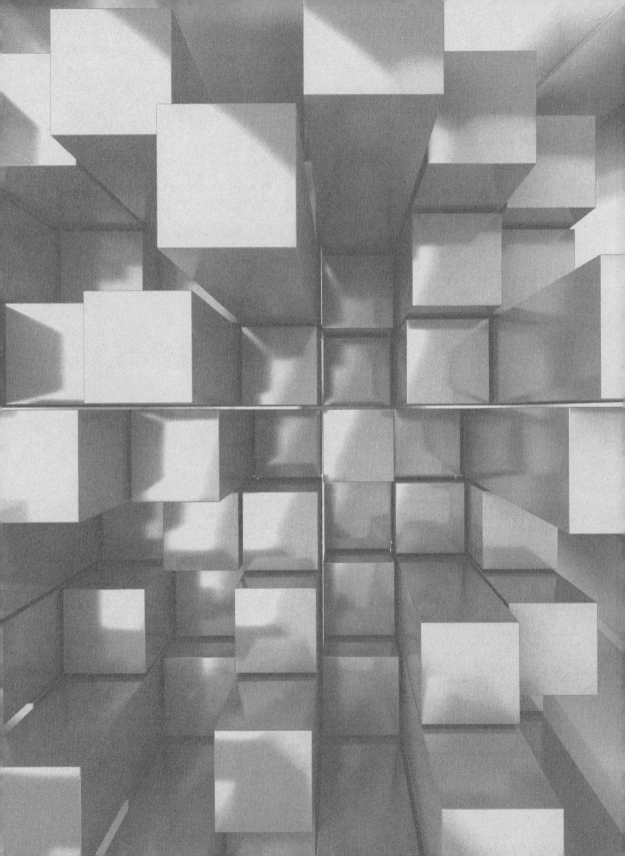

Section I

Building Blocks of Health Informatics

Health care professionals are information-dependent knowledge workers. As health care continues to evolve in an increasingly competitive information marketplace, professionals—that is, the knowledge workers—must be well prepared to make significant contributions by harnessing appropriate and timely information. Health informatics (HI), a product of the scientific synthesis of information in the practice discipline, encompasses concepts from computer science, cognitive science, information science, and disciplinary science. HI continues to evolve as more and more professionals access, use, and develop the information, computer, and cognitive sciences necessary to advance disciplinary science for the betterment of patients and the health care professions. Regardless of their future roles in the health care milieu, it is clear that health care professionals need to understand the ethical application of computer, information, and cognitive sciences to advance the health care disciplinary sciences.

To implement HI, one must view it from the perspective of both the current health care delivery system and specific, individual organizational needs while anticipating and creating future applications in both the health care system and the allied health professions. Health care professionals should be expected to discover opportunities to use HI, participate in the design of solutions, and be challenged to identify, develop, evaluate, modify, and enhance applications to improve patient care. This text is designed to provide the reader with the information and knowledge needed to meet this expectation.

Section I presents an overview of the building blocks of HI: disciplinary, information, computer, and cognitive sciences. Also included in this section is a chapter on ethical and legal applications of health care informatics. This first section lays the foundation for the remainder of the book.

The *Informatics, Disciplinary Science, and the Foundation of Knowledge* chapter describes disciplinary science and introduces the Foundation of Knowledge model as the conceptual framework for the book. In this chapter, a clinical case scenario involving a physical therapist is used to illustrate the concepts central to disciplinary science and the data, information, knowledge, wisdom paradigm central to health informatics. Core informatics competencies are identified, and a self-assessment tool for informatics competencies is also provided.

Information is a central concept and health care's most valuable resource. Information science and systems, together with computers, are constantly changing the way health care organizations conduct their business. This will continue to evolve.

To prepare for these innovations, the reader must understand fundamental information and computer concepts, covered in the *Introduction to Information, Information Science, and Information Systems* and *Computer Science and the Foundation of Knowledge Model* chapters, respectively. Information science deals with the interchange (or flow) and scaffolding (or structure) of information and involves the application of information tools for solutions to patient care and business problems in health care. To be able to use and synthesize information effectively, an individual must be able to obtain, perceive, process, synthesize, comprehend, convey, and manage the information. Computer science deals with understanding the development, design, structure, and relationship of computer hardware and software. This science offers extremely valuable tools that, if used skillfully, can facilitate the acquisition and manipulation of data and information by health care professionals, who can then synthesize these resources into an ever-evolving knowledge and wisdom base. This not only facilitates professional development and the ability to apply evidence-based practice decisions within patient care but, if the results are disseminated and shared, can also advance the profession's knowledge base. The development of knowledge tools, such as the automation of decision making and strides in artificial intelligence, has altered the understanding of knowledge and its representation. The ability to structure knowledge electronically facilitates the ability to share knowledge structures and enhance collective knowledge.

As discussed in the *Introduction to Cognitive Science and Cognitive Informatics* chapter, cognitive science deals with how the human mind functions. This science encompasses how people think, understand, remember, synthesize, and access stored information and knowledge. The nature of knowledge, including how it is developed, used, modified, and shared, provides the basis for continued learning and intellectual growth.

The *Ethical and Legal Aspects of Health Informatics* chapter focuses on ethical issues associated with managing private information with technology and provides a framework for analyzing ethical issues and supporting ethical decision making. In addition, this chapter provides insights into the rules of the Health Insurance Portability and Accountability Act and an overview of the rules associated with technology implementation as defined by the HITECH Act. The information provided in this text reflects current rules that were in effect at the time of publication. The reader should follow the rules development and evolution of informatics legislation at the U.S. Department of Health and Human Services website (http://www.hhs.gov) to obtain the most current information related to health information management.

The material within this book is placed within the context of the Foundation of Knowledge model (shown in **Figure I-1** and periodically throughout the book but more fully introduced and explained in the *Informatics, Disciplinary Science, and the Foundation of Knowledge* chapter). The Foundation of Knowledge model is used throughout the text to illustrate how knowledge is used to meet the needs of health care delivery systems, organizations, patients, and health care professionals. It is through interaction with these building blocks—the theories, architecture, and tools—that one acquires the bits and pieces of data necessary, processes these into information, and generates and disseminates the resulting knowledge. Through this dynamic exchange, which includes feedback, individuals continue the interaction and use of these sciences to input or acquire, process, and output or disseminate generated knowledge. Humans experience their environment and learn by acquiring, processing, generating, and disseminating knowledge. When they then share (disseminate) this new knowledge and receive feedback on the knowledge they have shared, the feedback initiates the cycle of knowledge all over again. As individuals acquire, process, generate, and disseminate knowledge, they are motivated to share, rethink, and explore their own knowledge base. This complex process is captured in the Foundation of Knowledge model. Throughout the chapters in the *Building Blocks of Health Informatics* section, readers are challenged to think about how the model can help them to understand the ways in which they acquire, process, generate, disseminate, and then receive feedback on their new knowledge of the building blocks of HI. Health care professionals, as knowledge workers, must be able to understand the evolving specialty of HI to harness and use the tools available for managing the vast amount of health care data and information central to their practice. It is essential that HI capabilities be appreciated, promoted, expanded, and advanced to facilitate the work of the health care professionals, improve patient care, and enhance the science of the professions.

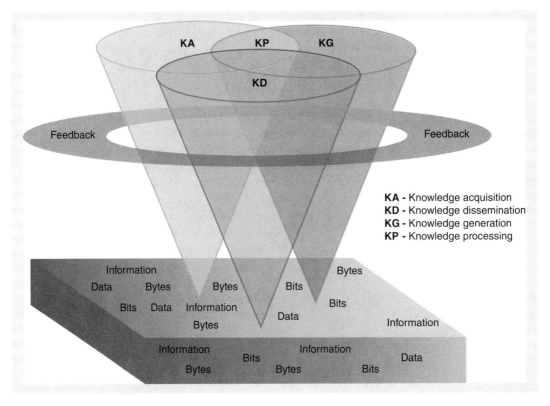

Figure I-1 Foundation of Knowledge Model
Source: Designed by Alicia Mastrian.

Informatics, Disciplinary Science, and the Foundation of Knowledge

Kathleen Mastrian and Dee McGonigle

OBJECTIVES

1. Define health informatics.
2. Illustrate the relationship between disciplinary science and informatics.
3. Introduce the Foundation of Knowledge model as the organizing conceptual framework for the text.
4. Explain the data, information, knowledge, wisdom (DIKW) paradigm.
5. Establish health care professionals as knowledge workers.

Introduction

Health care is an information intensive endeavor. Our patients are complex, often presenting with multiple health challenges and requiring interventions by several health care disciplines at the same time. Interprofessional collaboration and communication are essential for the coordination of this care and to ensure that all are working toward the same clinical outcomes while promoting safe, evidence-based, efficient, and cost-effective care. The use of technology tools, especially the **electronic health record** (EHR), helps us collect, integrate, and manage all of the important clinical information to provide the best possible care and facilitate communication among the various disciplines interacting with patients. Data collected from EHRs and the aggregation of these data may provide insights into the health of populations and identify global health challenges. **Informatics** is the term used to describe the science of information management in health care.

Key Terms

Clinical database
Clinical practice guideline
Competency
Data
Data mining
Data–information–
knowledge–wisdom
paradigm
Electronic health record
Evidence
Feedback
Foundation of Knowledge
model
Health informatics
Informatics
Information
Knowledge
Knowledge acquisition
Knowledge dissemination
Knowledge generation
Knowledge processing

(continues)

<table>
<tr><td>

Key Terms (continued)

Knowledge worker
Relational database
Wisdom

</td></tr>
</table>

All health care workers, regardless of discipline, need a basic understanding of informatics principles. That is, how are data, information, and knowledge used in the discipline, and how does this understanding promote wisdom in practice? All health care workers need a core skill set related to the use of computers, EHRs, various health care technologies, and an understanding of how knowledge is generated in their respective disciplines. The study of informatics provides these insights.

We will use the more general term **health informatics** throughout the text, as many of the principles and concepts we are discussing are applicable across disciplines. When you are thinking about your specific field, it is appropriate to substitute its name for the more general term *health*. For example, dental informatics, physical therapy informatics, respiratory therapy informatics, and nutrition or dietary informatics are all acceptable terms. In this text, we define health informatics as the combination of principles from the disciplinary science, computer science, information science, and cognitive science. The more traditional definitions of informatics do not include cognitive science, but we believe that the principles of cognitive science provide important insights in the understanding of informatics, especially when one is exploring knowledge structures in a discipline. In this chapter, we will explore the core elements of informatics—the **data–information–knowledge–wisdom (DIKW) paradigm** and the foundation of disciplinary knowledge using the **Foundation of Knowledge model**, the organizing conceptual framework of this text. We will also introduce the core informatics competencies needed by all health care professionals to practice in the information-intensive 21st-century health care environments. Various chapters and sections of the text will then expand on the core informatics competencies as a way of helping you attain them.

The DIKW Paradigm

Let's begin this exploration of the DIKW paradigm using the following patient scenario:

> *Tom H. is a physical therapist who works in a metropolitan hospital providing physical therapy services to a wide variety of patients. Today, Tom is evaluating the mobility of a 90-year-old man with multiple health challenges—aortic stenosis, atrial fibrillation, hypertension controlled with medication, and arthritis— who was admitted to the hospital for treatment of gross hematuria. The patient lives at home with his wife, who reports progressive weakness and reluctance to ambulate. The urologist wrote the consult for physical therapy to help the patient meet his goal of continuing to live at home. Tom first reviews the EHR to learn the key diagnoses, the patient's blood count, and the latest set of vital signs before approaching the patient. The clinical decision support system (CDSS) of the EHR also lists the patient as a fall risk. After interviewing the patient and checking the oxygen saturation level with a pulse oximeter, Tom prepares to assess the patient's ambulation. Tom asks the patient to sit up first and pause, then carefully assists him to a standing position. Tom notices that the patient's walker is not adjusted properly for his height, so Tom makes the adjustment before they begin to walk.*

Pause to consider Tom's actions so far and how they relate to the DIKW paradigm. Tom relied on the **data** and **information** that he acquired during his review of the EHR and the patient interview and assessment to deliver appropriate care to his patient. Tom also used technology (a pulse oximeter) to assist with and support the delivery of care. What is not immediately apparent (and, some would argue, is transparent, done without conscious thought) is that Tom reached into his **knowledge** base of previous learning and experiences to direct his care so that he could act with transparent **wisdom**. Tom knew that since the patient had multiple cardiovascular issues, orthostatic hypotension was a real possibility, so he asked the patient to sit up on the edge of the bed and pause before attempting to stand. He wants to measure the effect of exertion on the patient's oxygen saturation, so he obtains a baseline using the oximeter. Tom also noticed that the walker was not adjusted to the correct height. While all of these actions appear almost automatic, they are the result of Tom's learning and previous experiences as well as evidence generated over many years of clinical research.

> Tom and the patient begin their walk. Tom notices that the patient walks slowly and carefully with an appropriate gait and uses the walker effectively. After about 30 steps, the patient's breathing becomes a bit more labored, and he slows down even more. Tom suggests turning around to head back to the room. Tom notices that the patient is starting to sweat and that his breathing is becoming more labored. He helps the patient into bed and checks the oxygen saturation once again, finding that it is has dropped to 92% from 99%. Tom elevates the head of the bed, checks the patient's blood pressure and pulse, and signals for the nurse to initiate oxygen therapy. Tom will use the EHR to communicate his findings to others involved with the patient's care.

Tom clearly applied his knowledge from physical therapy science and some of the basic sciences, such as anatomy, physiology, psychology, and chemistry, as he determined the patient's immediate needs and the reasons for his weakness and lack of stamina. Tom understands that the patient's already compromised cardiovascular system (medical diagnoses of hypertension, atrial fibrillation, and aortic stenosis) has been further stressed by the blood loss and the low blood counts that he read about in the EHR. He gathered data and then analyzed and interpreted those data to form a conclusion—the essence of science. Tom will use the EHR to communicate his findings, concerns, and recommendations for a graduated exercise program designed to increase the patient's stamina and strength. While this scenario is specific to physical therapy, other allied health disciplines rely on the DIKW paradigm to direct their interventions. Can you think of a patient scenario specific to your discipline?

The steps of using information, applying knowledge to a problem, and acting with wisdom form the basis of the science of health professional practice. Information is composed of data that were processed using knowledge. For information to be valuable, it must be accessible, accurate, timely, complete, cost effective, flexible, reliable, relevant, simple, verifiable, and secure. Knowledge is the awareness and understanding of a set of information and ways that information can be made useful to support a specific task or arrive at a decision. In the case scenario, Tom used accessible, accurate, timely, relevant, and verifiable data and information. He compared those data and information to the patient and to his knowledge base and previous experiences to determine which data and information were relevant to the current case. By applying his previous knowledge to data, he converted those data into information and information into new knowledge—that is, an understanding of which interventions were appropriate in this case. Thus, information is data made functional through the application of knowledge.

Humans acquire data and information in bits and pieces and then transform the information into knowledge. The information-processing functions of the brain are frequently compared to those of a computer and vice versa (an idea discussed further in Chapter 4). Humans can be thought of as organic information systems that are constantly acquiring, processing, and generating information or knowledge in their professional and personal lives. We have an amazing ability to manage knowledge. This ability is learned and honed from birth as individuals make their way through life interacting with the environment and being inundated with data and information. Each person experiences the environment and learns by acquiring, processing, generating, and disseminating knowledge.

Tom, for example, acquired knowledge in his physical therapy education program and continues to build his foundation of knowledge by engaging in such activities as reading research and theory articles, attending continuing education programs, consulting with expert colleagues, and using **clinical databases** and **clinical practice guidelines**. As he interacts in the environment, he acquires knowledge that must be processed. This processing effort causes him to redefine and restructure his knowledge base and generate new knowledge. Tom can then share (disseminate) this new knowledge with colleagues, and he may receive **feedback** on the knowledge that he shares. This dissemination and feedback builds the knowledge foundation anew as Tom acquires, processes, generates, and disseminates new knowledge as a result of his interactions. As others respond to his **knowledge dissemination** and he acquires yet more knowledge, he is engaged to rethink, reflect on, and reexplore his **knowledge acquisition**, leading to further processing, generating, and then disseminating knowledge. This ongoing process is captured in the Foundation of Knowledge model, which is used as an organizing framework for this text.

The Foundation of Knowledge Model

In order to simplify the understanding of the Foundation of Knowledge model, it may be helpful to think back on an early learning experience. Recall the first time you got behind the wheel of a car. There was so much to remember and do and so much to pay attention to, especially if you wanted to avoid an accident. You had to think about how to start the car, adjust the mirrors, fasten the seat belt, and shift the car into gear. You had to take in data and information from friends and family members who tried to "tell" you how to drive. They disseminated knowledge and you acquired it, and they most likely provided lots of feedback about your driving. As you drove down the street, you also noticed multiple bits of data in the environment, such as stop signs, traffic signals, turn signals, speed limit signs, and so on, and tried to interpret these environmental data into usable information for the current situation. You had to pay attention to lots of things at the same time in order to drive safely. As your confidence grew with experience, you were able to drive more effectively and generated new knowledge about driving that became part of your personal knowledge structure. After lots of driving experiences, the process of driving became transparent and seamless. Think about this example in relation to a skill that you have acquired or are acquiring in your health profession education. How does or did your learning experience mirror the components of the Foundation of Knowledge model?

Let's explore the model in more detail. At its base, the model contains bits, bytes (computer terms for chunks of information), data, and information in a random representation (**Figure 1-1**). Growing out of the base are separate cones of light that expand as they reflect upward; these cones represent knowledge acquisition, **knowledge generation**, and knowledge dissemination. At the intersection of the cones and forming a new cone is **knowledge processing**. Encircling and cutting through the knowledge cones is feedback that acts on and may transform any or all aspects of knowledge represented by the cones. One should imagine the model as a dynamic figure in which the cones of light and the feedback rotate and interact rather than remain static. Knowledge acquisition, knowledge generation, knowledge dissemination, knowledge processing, and feedback are constantly evolving for health care professionals. The transparent effect of the cones is deliberate and is intended to suggest that as knowledge grows and expands, its use becomes more transparent—a person uses this knowledge during practice without even being consciously aware of which aspect of knowledge is being used at any given moment.

Experienced practitioners, thinking back to their novice years, may recall feeling like their head was filled with bits of data and information that did not form any type of cohesive whole. As the model depicts, the processing of knowledge begins a bit later (imagine a time line applied vertically) with early experiences on the bottom and expertise growing as the processing of knowledge ensues. Early on in the education experience, conscious attention is focused mainly on knowledge acquisition, and students depend on their instructors and others to process, generate, and disseminate knowledge. As students become more comfortable with the science of their discipline, they begin to take over some of the other Foundation of Knowledge functions. However, to keep up with the explosion of information in health care, they must continue to rely on the knowledge generation of expert theorists and researchers and the dissemination of their work. There must be a conscious commitment to lifelong learning and the use of knowledge in practice in order to be a successful practitioner in any health care field.

The Foundation of Knowledge model permeates this text, reflecting the understanding that knowledge is a powerful tool and that health care workers focus on information as a key building block of knowledge. The application of the model is described in

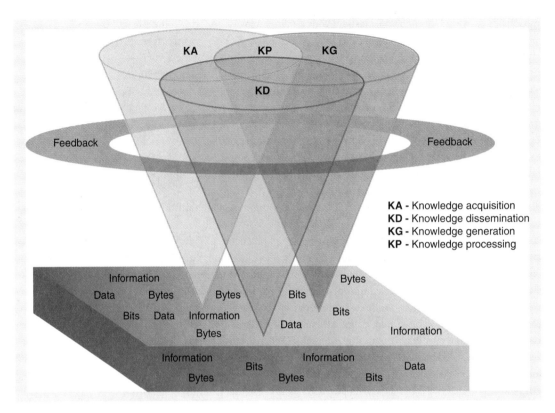

Figure 1-1 Foundation of Knowledge Model
Source: Designed by Alicia Mastrian.

each section of the text to help the reader understand and appreciate the foundation of knowledge in disciplinary science and see how it applies to health informatics. All of the various health practice roles (clinical practice, administration, education, research, and informatics) involve the science of the discipline. Health care professionals are **knowledge workers**. Knowledge workers are those who work with information and generate information and knowledge as a product. Health care professionals are knowledge acquirers, providing convenient and efficient means of capturing and storing knowledge. They are knowledge users, meaning individuals or groups who benefit from valuable, viable knowledge. Health care professionals are knowledge engineers, designing, developing, implementing, and maintaining knowledge. They are knowledge managers, capturing and processing collective expertise and distributing it where it can create the largest benefit. Finally, they are knowledge developers and generators, changing and evolving knowledge based on the tasks at hand and the information available.

In the case scenario, at first glance one might label Tom as a knowledge worker, a knowledge acquirer, and a knowledge user. However, stopping here might sell Tom short in his practice of physical therapy science. Although he acquired and used knowledge to help him achieve his work, he also processed the data and information he collected to develop a science-based approach to the patient and a plan of care. The knowledge stores that Tom used to develop and glean knowledge from valuable information are generative (having the ability to originate and produce or generate) in nature. For example, Tom may have learned something new about his patient's culture from the patient or his wife that he will file away in the knowledge repository of his mind to be used in another similar situation. As he compares this new cultural information to what he already knows, he may gain insight into the effect of culture on a patient's response to illness. In this sense, Tom is a knowledge generator. If he shares this newly acquired knowledge with another practitioner and as he records his observations and his conclusions, he is then disseminating knowledge. Tom also uses feedback from the various technologies he has applied to monitor his patient's status. In addition, he may rely on feedback from laboratory reports or even other practitioners to help him rethink, revise, and apply the knowledge about this patient that he is generating.

To have ongoing value, knowledge must be viable. Knowledge viability refers to applications (most technology based) that offer easily accessible, accurate, and timely information obtained from a variety of resources and methods and presented in a manner so as to provide the necessary elements to generate new knowledge. In the case scenario, Tom may have felt the need to consult an electronic database or a clinical guidelines repository that he has downloaded on his tablet or that reside in the EHR or networked computer system to assist him in the development of a comprehensive plan for his patient. In this way, Tom uses technology and **evidence** to support and inform his practice. Remember also in this scenario that an alert appeared in the patient's EHR informing Tom of the fall-risk status of the patient. Clinical information technologies that support and inform professional practice, administration, education, and research are an important part of informatics and are covered in detail in the latter sections of this text.

This text provides a framework that embraces knowledge so that readers can develop the wisdom necessary to apply what they have learned. Wisdom is the application of knowledge to an appropriate situation. Wisdom uses knowledge and experience to heighten common sense and insight to exercise sound judgment in practical matters. Wisdom is developed through knowledge, experience, insight, and reflection. Wisdom is sometimes thought of as the highest form of common sense, resulting from accumulated knowledge or erudition (deep, thorough learning) or enlightenment (education that results in understanding and the dissemination of knowledge). It is the ability to apply valuable and viable knowledge, experience, understanding, and insight while being prudent and sensible. Knowledge and wisdom are not synonymous: Knowledge abounds with others' thoughts and information, whereas wisdom is focused on one's own mind and the synthesis of experience, insight, understanding, and knowledge.

Some health care professional roles might be viewed as focused more on some aspects than on other aspects of the foundation of knowledge. For example, one might argue that educators are primarily knowledge disseminators and that researchers are knowledge generators. Although the more frequent output of their efforts can certainly be viewed in this way, it is important to realize that health care professionals use all of the aspects of the Foundation of Knowledge model regardless of their area of practice. For educators to be effective, they must be in the habit of constantly building and rebuilding their foundation of knowledge about the discipline in which they are teaching. In addition, as they develop and implement curricular innovations, they must evaluate the effectiveness of those changes. In some cases, they use formal research techniques to achieve this goal and, therefore, generate knowledge about the best and most effective teaching strategies. Similarly, researchers must acquire and process new knowledge as they design and conduct their research studies. All health care professionals have the opportunity to be involved in the formal dissemination of knowledge via their participation in professional conferences, either as presenters or as attendees. In addition, some disseminate knowledge by formal publication of their ideas. In the cases of conference presentation and publication, these professionals may receive feedback that stimulates rethinking about the knowledge they have generated and disseminated, in turn prompting them to acquire and process data and information anew.

All health care professionals, regardless of their practice arena, must use informatics and technology to inform and support that practice. The case scenario discussed Tom's use of a monitoring device that provides feedback on the physiologic status of the patient. It was also suggested that Tom might consult a clinical database or a practice guideline residing on a tablet or a clinical agency network as he develops an appropriate plan of action for his physical therapy interventions. Perhaps the clinical information system (CIS) in the agency supports the collection of aggregated data about patients in a **relational database**, providing an opportunity for **data mining** by administrators or researchers. Data mining provides opportunities to explore large amounts of data to look for patterns in the data as a way of evaluating or informing practice. As more health care facilities and professional practices embrace the use of EHRs, opportunities for data mining will increase. We will discuss data mining in more detail in a later chapter.

We have established that health care professionals are knowledge workers and that all must use informatics and technology to inform and support practice. This text is designed to include the necessary content to prepare health care professionals for practice in the ever-changing and technology-laden health care environments. So what do health care professionals need to know about informatics, and what informatics skills and competencies are necessary for safe, effective practice?

Core Informatics Competencies

A **competency** demonstrates proficiency. According to Hunter, McGonigle, and Hebda (2013), "At its most basic level, competency denotes having the knowledge, skills, and ability to perform or do a specific task, act, or job" (p. 71). Based on this definition, an informatics competency would be the knowledge, skills, and ability to perform specific informatics tasks. Knowing the competencies we are expected to meet allows us to understand our strengths and weaknesses. It helps us assess where we are and where we need to go with our education and skill development.

Several national and international groups have worked to identify core informatics competencies for health care professionals. In 2008, the American Health Information Management Association (AHIMA) and the American Medical Informatics Association (AMIA) convened a task force to identify basic informatics competencies for all health care professionals who work with EHRs. The task force emphasized that

> *new graduates in any healthcare profession need a skill set adaptable to computer technologies and EHRs to support work processes and information access experienced in the course of daily workflow. Employees at all levels and job types within today's healthcare workplace need a new set of skills and knowledge to embrace and effectively utilize computer technologies and electronic information. Part of the challenge is ensuring these workers function in a broad continuum of care and effective use of health information and electronic information systems. (p. 5)*

The joint AHIMA–AMIA Task Force identified five domains for informatics competencies for all health care workers (**Figure 1-2**):

I. Health information literacy and skills
II. Health informatics skills using the EHR
III. Privacy and confidentiality of health information
IV. Health information/data technical security
V. Basic computer literacy skills (p. 6)

AHIMA also worked in collaboration with the Health Professions Network and the Employment and Training Administration to create a graphic depiction of competencies necessary for EHR interaction (AHIMA & Health Professions Network, n.d.). The electronic health records competency model is divided into six levels—personal effectiveness competencies, academic competencies, workplace competencies, industry-wide technical competencies, industry-sector technical competencies, and a management competencies level shared with occupation-specific requirements. Although beyond the scope of this discussion, it is important to realize the extent of work in the competency development arena.

Clearly, the degree of interaction with EHRs will vary somewhat from profession to profession; however, we can say with confidence that health care technologies will continue to evolve and that everyone in the health field must be prepared to embrace and interact with new technologies. We believe that everyone, regardless of health care discipline, needs to acquire core health informatics skills for 21st-century practice.

Table 1-1 provides you with an opportunity to assess your core informatics skills and competencies. The list of competencies is derived from several sources—the Academy of Nutrition and Dietetics (2012) Delphi study of nutrition informatics competencies

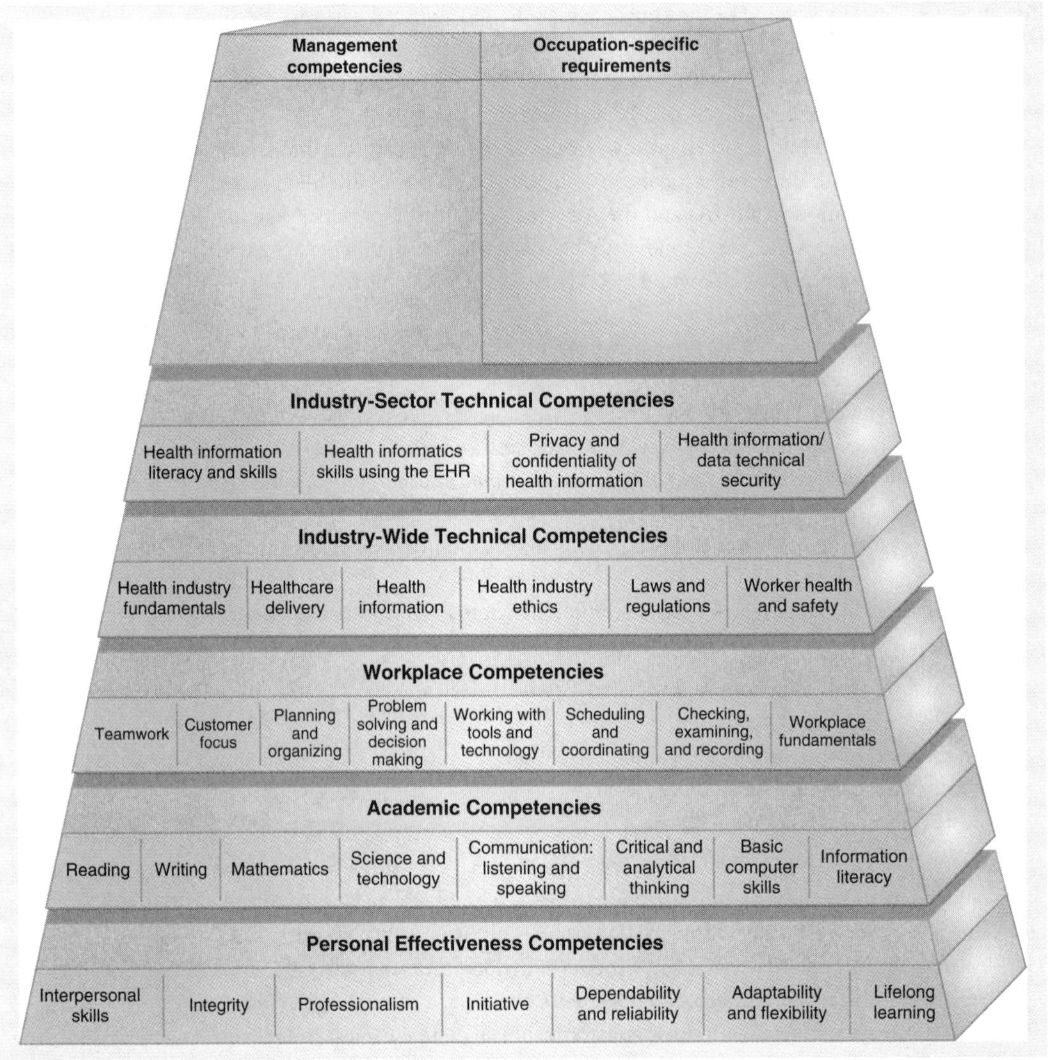

Figure 1-2 Electronic Health Records Competency Model

(Ayres, Greer-Carney, McShane, Miller, & Turner, 2012), the AHIMA–AMIA (2008) Task Force for the development of EHR competencies, the Competency Model Clearinghouse (n.d.-a, n.d.-b), and the authors' long-term experiences teaching nursing informatics. The subsequent chapters in this text provide information to help you gain these valuable informatics competencies and skills.

TABLE 1-1   SELF-ASSESSMENT OF CORE INFORMATICS COMPETENCIES

Please rate each of the following core informatics competencies on the following scale by assigning the number in the rating block that best describes your level of competency:

1. Unaware; no experience
2. Basic awareness
3. Some experience
4. Moderately competent
5. Proficient

Health Information Literacy and Skills	1–5
Recognize a need for information	
Select specific types of information resources appropriate to information needs	
Effectively use a browser to search for information	
Assess the credibility of information—authority, accuracy, timeliness, and value in fulfilling need	
Differentiate between data, information, and knowledge	
Differentiate between scholarly and popular sources of information	
Locate and retrieve information from a variety of credible electronic sources	

Health Informatics Skills using the EHR	
Understand the relationship between the organization's mission and meaningful use of the EHR	
Differentiate between types of health records—paper, EHR, and personal health records	
Understand expectations for EHR documentation and adhere to institution polices, requirements of accreditation agencies, and professional standards of the discipline	
Use various electronic tools to update the EHR, including portable computing devices, word processing, spreadsheet, database, and desktop presentation applications	
Locate information specific to your practice in the EHR	
Know and adhere to the standard terminologies for the discipline	
Identify and adhere to discipline-specific classification health-related terminologies for coding of procedures	
Use health record data collection tools appropriately—drop-down menus and checklists	
Use text notes appropriately to amplify and clarify information not easily documented in pre-prepared menus	
Access reference material available in the EHR for clinical decision support	
Use remote access tools for documentation in the EHR, such as workstation on wheels (WOW), tablets, smartphones, smart room technology, telehealth tools, etc.	
Use health record tools and software applications to create trended data reports to measure patient outcomes	
Ensure accuracy of documentation in the health record	
Ensure data quality and recognize and correct inaccurate data in the EHR	
Use the EHR to its fullest extent to exchange information with other providers, coordinate care, avoid duplication of services, promote safe practice, and increase patient satisfaction	

(continues)

TABLE 1-1   SELF-ASSESSMENT OF CORE INFORMATICS COMPETENCIES (continued)
Resolve minor technological problems associated with using an EHR
Know who to contact for help with using or troubleshooting the EHR
Understand basic principles of work flow and the impact of technology
Define work-arounds and identify how they may create safety issues
Provide feedback on system usability to improve work flow
Privacy and Security of Health Information
Know key aspects of national laws and organizational policies governing privacy and security of health information
Know and adhere to institutional policies and procedures for signing in and using the EHR
Know principles of authentication for access to EHRs
Follow security and privacy policies and procedures to the use of networks, including intranets and the Internet
Create strong passwords and safeguard them to prevent unauthorized access by others
Define protected health information
Identify what constitutes authorized use of protected health information
Understand confidentiality and what constitutes a breach of confidentiality
Differentiate between confidentiality and anonymity
Know how to secure devices used to collect private health information
Describe procedures for preventing unauthorized use of the EHR
Understand how the use of all electronic devices leaves a trail that can be audited for unauthorized use
Know institutional procedures for reporting data breaches
Understand potential information security issues associated with the use of personal electronic devices in the workplace
Know where to find general policies related to electronic security and specific policies related to personal devices
Describe potential issues related to the use of social media by health care professionals
Describe the consequences of inappropriate use of personal health information (disciplinary measures, fines, and prison penalties)
Computer Literacy Skills
Understand and efficiently use basic computer hardware (e.g., PCs and printers) and software (e.g., word processing and spreadsheet software) to perform tasks
Understand common computer terms
Describe common functions and capabilities of a computer
Use word processing programs to create, edit, save, and retrieve document files
Save a document in an alternative file format or zip a series of documents for efficient transmission
Efficiently scan, save, and share documents
Possess file management skills to organize files—name appropriately, use folders, etc.

TABLE 1-1 SELF-ASSESSMENT OF CORE INFORMATICS COMPETENCIES (continued)
Use basic reference materials and tools (thesaurus, grammar, and spell-checker) to ensure accuracy
Format documents according to discipline specific style—American Psychological Association, Modern Language Association, etc.
Effectively use the Internet and web-based tools to manage basic workplace tasks (e.g., timekeeping, maintaining employee records, and shared calendars)
Compose professional e-mails to communicate business-related information to coworkers, colleagues, and customers
Create and send e-mails, respond appropriately, and attach files to e-mails
Use CC and BCC functions appropriately
Describe principles of netiquette
Use a computer as an education tool—download podcast, participate in webinar, or join a community of practice
Provide information and support for patient education using gaming, smartphone apps, and computer-based tools
Use spreadsheet software to enter, manipulate, edit, and format text and numerical data
Effectively create, save, and print worksheets, charts, and graphs
Use presentation software effectively
Understand and use firewalls and software to protect devices from viruses, spam, and cookies

The self-assessment tool presented here represents information on core informatics competencies pulled from several different health professions. You may want to look specifically at your professional organization's website to see how informatics competencies are discussed. Remember that this is only the beginning; new technologies will continue to emerge and evolve. Possessing basic informatics competency will serve you well, as many of these basic skills are translatable and provide a strong platform for learning more complex technology skills in the future.

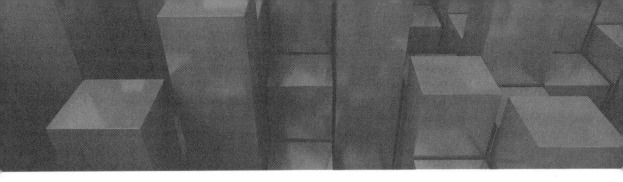

Summary

This chapter provided an overview of informatics and core informatics competencies, the DIKW paradigm, and the relationship of the paradigm to disciplinary science and established that health care professionals are knowledge workers. The Foundation of Knowledge model was introduced as the organizing conceptual framework for this text. Core informatics competencies were presented with an opportunity for self-assessment. In subsequent chapters, the reader will learn more about how informatics supports health care professionals in their many and varied roles. We suggest that in the future, health care research will make significant contributions to the development of the practice sciences for health care professionals. Technologies and translational research will abound, and clinical practices will be evidence based, thereby improving patient outcomes, decreasing safety concerns, and providing cost-effective care.

Thought-Provoking Questions

1. Describe a scenario in your discipline where you used data, information, knowledge, and wisdom.
2. Choose a clinical scenario from your recent experience and analyze it using the Foundation of Knowledge model. How did you acquire knowledge? How did you process knowledge? How did you generate knowledge? How did you disseminate knowledge? How did you use feedback, and what was the effect of the feedback on the foundation of your knowledge?
3. Complete the self-assessment of informatics competencies presented in Table 1-1 and create an action plan for achieving these competencies.

Apply Your Knowledge

This chapter introduced you to concepts related to the scientific basis of your profession and the relationship between health informatics and your discipline.

1. You are at a social event, and you are sharing a story about your education experience and your course on health informatics. A friend asks you, "What is informatics?" Answer the question by using terms and examples that a layperson will understand.
2. As the conversation continues, you share that you are excited about the allied health major you have chosen because of the scientific basis of the practice. Again, your skeptical friend asks, "What do you mean by the science of the discipline?" Answer this question by describing at least three examples of the scientific basis of practice for your discipline.

References

American Health Information Management Association and American Medical Informatics Association. (2008). Health information management and informatics core competencies for individuals working with electronic health records. http://library.ahima.org/xpedio/groups/public/documents/ahima/bok1_040723.pdf

American Health Information Management Association and Health Professions Network. (n.d.). Health: Electronic health records competency model. http://www.careeronestop.org/CompetencyModel/competency-models/electronic-health-records.aspx

Ayres, E., Greer-Carney, J., McShane, P., Miller, A., & Turner, P. (2012). Nutrition informatics competencies across all levels of practice: A national Delphi study. *Journal of the Academy of Nutrition and Dietetics, 112*(12), 2042–2053.

Competency Model Clearinghouse. (n.d.-a). Basic computer skills. http://www.careeronestop.org/competencymodel/blockModel.aspx?tier_id=2&block_id=819&EHR=Y

Competency Model Clearinghouse. (n.d.-b). Health informatics skills using the EHR. http://www.careeronestop.org/CompetencyModel/blockModel.aspx?tier_id=5&block_id=836&EHR=Y

Hunter, K., McGonigle, D., & Hebda, T. (2013). TIGER-based measurement of nursing informatics competencies: The development and implementation of an online tool for self-assessment. *Journal of Nursing Education and Practice, 3*(12), 70–80. doi: 10.5430/jnep.v3n12p70

Introduction to Information, Information Science, and Information Systems

Dee McGonigle, Kathleen Mastrian, and Craig McGonigle

OBJECTIVES

1. Reflect on the progression from data to information to knowledge.
2. Describe the term *information*.
3. Assess how information is acquired.
4. Explore the characteristics of quality information.
5. Describe an information system.
6. Explore data acquisition or input and processing or retrieval, analysis, and synthesis of data.
7. Assess output or reports, documents, summaries, alerts, and outcomes.
8. Describe information dissemination and feedback.
9. Define information science.
10. Assess how information is processed.
11. Explore how knowledge is generated in information science.

Introduction

This chapter explores information, information systems (IS), and information science. The key word here, of course, is *information*. Health care professionals are **knowledge workers**, and they deal with information on a daily basis. Many concerns and issues arise with health care information, such as ownership, access, disclosure, exchange, security, privacy, disposal, and dissemination. With

Key Terms
Acquisition
Alert
Analysis
Chief information officer
Chief technical officer
Chief technology officer
Cloud computing
Cognitive science
Communication science
Computer-based   information system
Computer science
Consolidated Health   Informatics
Data
Dissemination
Document
Electronic health record
(continues)

the gauntlet of developing **electronic health records** (EHR) having been laid down, public and private sector stakeholders have been collaborating on a wide-ranging variety of health care information solutions. These initiatives include **Health Level 7** (HL7), the eGov initiative of **Consolidated Health Informatics'** (CHI's), the **National Health Information Infrastructure** (NHII), the **Nationwide Health Information Network** (NHIN), **Next-Generation Internet** (NGI), **Internet2**, and iHealth record. There are also **health information exchange** (HIE) systems, such as Connecting for Health, the eHealth initiative, the **Federal Health Information Exchange** (FHIE), the **Indiana Health Information Exchange** (IHIE), the **Massachusetts Health Data Consortium** (MHDC), the **New England Health EDI Network** (NEHEN), the State of New Mexico **Rapid Syndromic Validation Project** (RSVP), the Southeast Michigan e-Prescribing Initiative, and the Tennessee Volunteer eHealth Initiative (Goldstein, Groen, Ponkshe, & Wine, 2007). The most recent federal government initiative, the HITECH Act, set 2014 as the deadline for implementing electronic health records, yet clinics, private practices, and hospitals continue to struggle with the implementation and/or use of their electronic health records (for an overview of HIPAA and HITECH legislation, see Chapter 5).

It is evident from the previous brief listing that there is a need to remedy health care **information technology** concerns, challenges, and issues faced today. One of the main issues deals with how health care information is managed to make it meaningful. It is important to understand how people obtain, manipulate, use, share, and dispose of this information. This chapter deals with the information piece of this complex puzzle.

Information

Suppose someone states the number 99.5. What does that mean? It could be a radio station or a score on a test. Now suppose someone says that Ms. Howsunny's temperature is 99.5°F—what does that convey? It is then known that 99.5 is a person's temperature. The data (99.5) were processed to the information that 99.5° is a specific person's temperature. **Data** are raw facts. Information is processed data that have meaning. Health care professionals constantly process data and information to provide the best possible care for their patients.

Many types of data exist, such as alphabetic, numeric, audio, image, and video data. Alphabetic data refer to letters, numeric data refer to numbers, and alphanumeric data combine both letters and numbers. This includes all text and the numeric outputs of digital monitors. Some of the alphanumeric data encountered by health care professionals are in the form of patients' names, identification numbers, or medical record numbers. Audio data refer to sounds, noises, or tones, such as monitor alerts or alarms, taped or recorded messages, and other sounds. Image data include graphics and pictures, such as graphic monitor displays or recorded electrocardiograms, radiographs, magnetic resonance imaging outputs, and computed tomography (CT) scans. Video data refer to animations, moving pictures, or moving graphics, such as a physical therapist's video of a patient. Using these data, one may review the ultrasound of a pregnant patient, examine a patient's echocardiogram, watch an animated video for professional development, or learn how to operate a new technology tool, such as a pump or a monitoring system. The data we gather, such as heart and lung sounds or X-rays, help us produce information. For example, if a patient's X-rays show a fracture, it is interpreted into information, such as spiral, compound, or hairline. This information is then processed into knowledge, and a treatment plan is formulated based on the health care professional's wisdom.

The integrity and quality of the data rather than the form are what matter. Integrity refers to whole, complete, correct, and consistent data. Data integrity can be compromised through human error; viruses, worms, or other computer bugs; hardware failures or crashes; transmission errors; or hackers entering the system. Information technologies help to decrease these errors by putting into place safeguards, such as backing up files on a routine basis, error detection for transmissions, and user **interfaces** that help people enter the data correctly. High-quality data are relevant and accurately represent their corresponding concepts. Data are dirty when a database contains errors, such as duplicate, incomplete, or outdated records. One author (D.M.) found 50 cases of tongue cancer in a database she examined for data quality. When the records were tracked down and analyzed and the dirty data removed, only one case of tongue cancer remained. In this situation, the data for the same person had been entered erroneously 49 times. The major problem was with the patient's identification number and name: The number was changed, or his name was misspelled repeatedly. If researchers had just taken the number of cases in that defined population as 50, they would have concluded that tongue cancer was an epidemic, resulting in flawed information that is not meaningful. As this example demonstrates, it is imperative that data be clean if the goal is quality information. The data that are processed into information must be of high quality and integrity to create meaning to inform our practice.

To be valuable and meaningful, information must be of good quality. Its value relates directly to how the information informs decision making. Characteristics of valuable, quality information include accessibility, security, timeliness, accuracy, relevancy, completeness, flexibility, reliability, objectivity, utility, transparency, verifiability, and reproducibility.

Accessibility is a must; the right user must be able to obtain the right information at the right time and in the right format to meet his or her needs. Getting meaningful information to the right user at the right time is as vital as generating the information in the first place. The right user refers to an authorized user who has the right to obtain the data and information he or she is seeking. Security is a major challenge because unauthorized users must be blocked while the authorized user is provided with open, easy access (see Chapter 9).

Timely information means that the information is available when it is needed for the right purpose and at the right time. Knowing who won the lottery last week does not help one to know if the person won it today. Accurate information means that there are no errors in the data and information. Relevant information is a subjective descriptor in that the user must have information that is relevant or applicable to his or her needs. If a health care provider is trying to decide whether a patient needs insulin and only the patient's CT scan information is available, this information is not relevant for that current need. However, if one needs information about the CT scan, the information is relevant.

Complete information contains all of the necessary essential data. If the health care provider needs to contact the only relative listed for the patient and his or her contact information is listed but the approval for that person to be a contact is missing, this information is considered incomplete. Flexible information means that the information can be used for a variety of purposes. Information concerning the inventory of supplies in a clinic, for example, can be used by health care personnel who need to know if an item is available for use. The manager of the clinic accesses this information to help decide which supplies need to be ordered, to determine which items are used most frequently, and to do an economic assessment of any waste.

Reliable information comes from reliable or clean data gathered by authoritative and credible sources. Objective information is as close to the truth as one can get; it is not subjective or biased but rather is factual and impartial. If someone states something, it must be determined whether that person is reliable and whether what he or she is stating is objective or tainted by his or her own perspective.

Utility refers to the ability to provide the right information at the right time to the right person for the right purpose. Transparency allows users to apply their intellect to accomplish their tasks while the tools housing the information disappear. Verifiable information means that one can check to verify or prove that the information is correct. Reproducibility refers to the ability to produce the same information again.

Information is acquired either by actively looking for it or by having it conveyed by the environment. All of the senses (vision, hearing, touch, smell, and taste) are used to gather input from the surrounding world, and as technologies mature, more and more **input** will be obtained through the senses. Currently, people receive information from computers (output) through vision, hearing, or touch (input), and the response (output) to the computer (input) is the interface with technology. Gesture recognition is increasing, and interfaces that incorporate it will change the way people become informed. Many people access the Internet on a daily basis seeking information or imparting information. Individuals are constantly becoming informed, discovering, or learning; becoming re-informed, rediscovering, or relearning; and purging what has been acquired. The information acquired through these processes is added to the knowledge base. **Knowledge** is the awareness and understanding of a set of information and ways that information can be made useful to support a specific task or arrive at a decision. This knowledge building is an ongoing process engaged in while a person is conscious and going about his or her normal daily activities.

Information Science

Information science has evolved over the last 50 some years as a field of scientific inquiry and professional practice. It can be thought of as the science of information, studying the application and usage of information and knowledge in organizations and the interface or interaction between people, organizations, and IS. This extensive, interdisciplinary science integrates features from **cognitive science, communication science, computer science, library science**, and the **social sciences**. Information science is concerned primarily with the input, processing, output, and feedback of data and information through technology integration with a focus on comprehending the perspective of the **stakeholders** involved and then applying information technology as needed. It is systemically based, dealing with the big picture rather than individual pieces of technology.

Information science can also be related to determinism. Specifically, it is a response to technologic determinism—the belief that technology develops by its own laws, that it realizes its own potential, limited only by the material resources available, and must therefore be regarded as an autonomous system controlling and ultimately permeating all other subsystems of society (Web Dictionary of Cybernetics and Systems, 2007, para. 1).

This approach sets the tone for the study of information as it applies to itself, the people, the technology, and the varied sciences that are contextually related depending on the needs of the setting or organization; what is important is the interface between the stakeholders and their systems and the ways they generate, use, and locate information. According to Cornell University (2010), "Information Science brings together faculty, students and researchers who share an interest in combining computer science with the social sciences of how people and society interact with information" (para. 1). Information science is an interdisciplinary, people-oriented field that explores and enhances the interchange of information to transform society, communication science, computer science, cognitive science, library science, and the social sciences. Society is dominated by the need for information, and knowledge and information science focuses on systems and individual users by fostering user-centered approaches that enhance society's information capabilities, effectively and efficiently linking people, information, and technology. This impacts the configuration and mix of organizations and influences the nature of work—namely, how knowledge workers interact with and produce meaningful information and knowledge.

Information Processing

Information science enables the processing of information. This processing links people and technology. Humans are organic information systems, constantly acquiring, processing, and generating information or knowledge in their professional and personal lives. This high degree of knowledge, in fact, characterizes humans as extremely intelligent organic machines. The premise of this text revolves around this concept, and the text is organized on the basis of the Foundation of Knowledge model: knowledge **acquisition**, knowledge processing, knowledge generation, and knowledge dissemination.

Information is data that are processed using knowledge. For information to be valuable or meaningful, it must be accessible, accurate, timely, complete, cost effective, flexible, reliable, relevant, simple, verifiable, and secure. Knowledge is the awareness and understanding of an information set and ways that information can be made useful to support a specific task or arrive at a decision. As an example, if an architect were going to design a building, part of the knowledge necessary for developing a new building would be understanding how the building will be used, what size of building is needed compared to the available building space, and how many people will have or need access to this building. Therefore, the work of choosing or rejecting facts based on their significance or relevance to a particular task, such as designing a building, is also based on a type of knowledge used in the process of converting data into information.

Information can then be considered data made functional through the application of knowledge. The knowledge used to develop and glean knowledge from valuable information is generative (having the ability to originate and produce or generate) in nature. Knowledge must also be viable. Knowledge viability refers to applications that offer easily accessible, accurate, and timely information obtained from a variety of resources and methods and presented in a manner so as to provide the necessary elements to generate knowledge.

Information science and computational tools are extremely important in enabling the processing of data, information, and knowledge in health care. In this environment, the hardware, software, networking, algorithms, and human organic ISs work together to create meaningful information and generate knowledge. The links between information processing and scientific discovery are paramount. However, without the ability to generate practical results that can be disseminated, the processing of data, information, and knowledge is for naught. It is the ability of machines (inorganic ISs) to support and facilitate the functioning of people (human organic ISs) that refines, enhances, and evolves practice by generating knowledge. This knowledge represents five rights: the right information, accessible by the right people in the right settings, applied the right way at the right time.

An important and ongoing process is the struggle to integrate new knowledge and old knowledge so as to enhance wisdom. Wisdom is the ability to act appropriately; it assumes actions directed by one's own wisdom. Wisdom uses knowledge and experience to heighten common sense and insight to exercise sound judgment in practical matters. It is developed through knowledge, experience, insight, and reflection. Wisdom is sometimes thought of as the highest form of common sense, resulting from accumulated knowledge or erudition (deep, thorough learning) or enlightenment (education that results in understanding and the dissemination of knowledge). It is the ability to apply valuable and viable knowledge, experience, understanding, and insight while being prudent and sensible. Knowledge and wisdom are not synonymous because knowledge abounds with others' thoughts and information, whereas wisdom is focused on one's own mind and the synthesis of one's own experience, insight, understanding, and knowledge.

If clinicians are inundated with data without the ability to process it, the situation results in too much data and too little wisdom. Consequently, it is crucial that clinicians have viable ISs at their fingertips to facilitate the acquisition, sharing, and use of knowledge while maturing wisdom; this process leads to empowerment.

Information Science and the Foundation of Knowledge

Information science is a multidisciplinary science that encompasses aspects of computer science, cognitive science, social science, communication science, and library science to deal with obtaining, gathering, organizing, manipulating, managing, storing, retrieving, recapturing, disposing of, distributing, and broadcasting information. Information science studies everything that deals with information and can be defined as the study of ISs. This science originated as a subdiscipline of computer science as practitioners sought to understand and rationalize the management of technology within organizations. It has since matured into a major field of management and is now an important area of research in management studies. Moreover, information science has expanded its scope to examine the human–computer interaction, interfacing, and interaction of people, ISs, and corporations. It is taught at all major universities and business schools worldwide.

Modern-day organizations have become intensely aware of the fact that information and knowledge are potent resources that must be cultivated and honed to meet their needs. Thus, information science or the study of ISs—that is, the application and usage of knowledge—focuses on why and how technology can be put to best use to serve the information flow within an organization.

Information science impacts information interfaces, influencing how people interact with information and subsequently develop and use knowledge. The information a person acquires is added to his or her knowledge base. Knowledge is the awareness and understanding of an information set and ways that information can be made useful to support a specific task or arrive at a decision.

Health care organizations are affected by and rely on the evolution of information science to enhance the recording and processing of routine and intimate information while facilitating human-to-human and human-to-systems communications, delivery of health care products, dissemination of information, and enhancement of the organization's business transactions. Unfortunately, the benefits and enhancements of information science technologies have also brought to light new risks, such as glitches and loss of information and hackers who can steal identities and information. Solid leadership, guidance, and vision are vital to the maintenance of cost-effective business performance and cutting-edge, safe information technologies for the organization. This field studies all facets of the building and use of information. The emergence of information science and its impact on information have also influenced how people acquire and use knowledge.

Information science has already had a tremendous impact on society and will undoubtedly expand its sphere of influence further as it continues to evolve and innovate human activities at all levels. What visionaries only dreamed of is now possible and part of reality. The future has yet to fully unfold in this important arena.

Introduction to Information Systems

Consider the following scenario: You have just been hired by a large health care facility. You enter the personnel office and are told that you must learn a new language to work on the unit where you have been assigned. This language is used just on this unit. If you had been assigned to a different unit, you would have to learn another language that is specific to that unit and so on. Because of the differences in various units' languages, interdepartmental sharing and information exchange (known as interoperability) are severely hindered.

This scenario might seem far-fetched, but it is actually how workers once operated in health care—in silos. There was a system for the laboratory, one for finance, one for clinical departments, and so on. As health care organizations have come to appreciate the importance of communication, tracking, and research, however, they have developed integrated **information systems** that can handle the needs of the entire organization.

Information and information technology have become major resources for all types of organizations, and health care is no exception (see **Box 2-1**). Information technologies help to shape a health care organization, in conjunction with personnel, money, materials, and equipment. Many health care facilities have hired **chief information officers** (CIOs) or **chief technical officers** (CTOs), also known as **chief technology officers**. The CIO is involved with the information technology infrastructure, and this role is sometimes expanded to include the position of chief knowledge officer. The CTO is focused on organizationally based scientific and technical issues and is responsible for technological research and development as part of the organization's products and services. The CTO and CIO must be visionary leaders for the organization because so much of the business of health care relies on solid infrastructures that generate potent and timely information and knowledge. The CTO and CIO are sometimes interchangeable positions, but in some organizations the CTO reports to the CIO. These positions will become critical roles as companies continue to shift from being product oriented to knowledge oriented and as they begin emphasizing the production process itself rather than the product. In health care, ISs must be able to handle the volume of data and information necessary to generate the needed information and knowledge for best practices because the goal is to provide the highest quality of patient care.

Information Systems

Information systems can be manually based, but for the purposes of this text, the term refers to **computer-based information systems** (CBISs). According to Jessup and Valacich (2008), computer-based ISs "are combinations of hardware, software and telecommunications networks that people build and use to collect, create, and distribute useful data, typically in organizational settings" (p. 10). Along the same lines, ISs are also defined as a collection of interconnected elements that gather, process, store and distribute data and information while providing a feedback structure to meet an objective

(Stair & Reynolds, 2016). ISs are designed for specific purposes within organizations. They are only as functional as the decision-making capabilities, problem-solving skills, and programming potency built in and the quality of the data and information input into them (see Chapter 6). The capability of the IS to disseminate, provide feedback, and adjust the data and information based on these dynamic processes is what sets them apart. The IS should be a user-friendly entity that provides the right information at the right time and in the right place.

BOX 2-1   EXAMPLES OF INFORMATION SYSTEMS

An IS acquires data or inputs; processes data through the retrieval, **analysis**, or **synthesis** of those data; disseminates or outputs information in the form of reports, documents, summaries, alerts, prompts, or outcomes; and provides for responses or feedback. Input or data acquisition is the activity of collecting and acquiring raw data. Input devices include combinations of hardware, software, and **telecommunications**, including keyboards, light pens, touchscreens, mice or other pointing devices, automatic scanners, and machines that can read magnetic ink characters or lettering. To watch a pay-per-view movie, for example, the viewer must first input the chosen movie, verify the purchase, and have a payment method approved by the vendor. The IS must acquire this information before the viewer can receive the movie.

Processing—the retrieval, analysis, or synthesis of data—refers to the alteration and transformation of the data into helpful or useful information and outputs. The processing of data includes storing it for future use; comparing the data, making calculations, or applying formulas; and taking selective actions. Processing devices consist of combinations of hardware, software, and telecommunications and include processing chips where the central processing unit and main memory are housed. Some of these chips are quite ingenious. According to Schupak (2005), the bunny chip could save the pharmaceutical industry money while sparing "millions of furry creatures, with a chip that mimics a living organism" (para. 1). The HμREL Corporation has developed environments or biologic ISs that reside on chips and actually mimic the functioning of the human body. Researchers can use these environments to test for both the harmful and beneficial effects of drugs, including those that are considered experimental and that could be harmful if used in human and animal testing. Such chips also allow researchers to monitor a drug's toxicity in the liver and other organs.

One patented HμREL microfluidic "biochip" comprises an arrangement of separate but fluidically interconnected "organ" or "tissue" compartments. Each compartment contains a culture of living cells drawn from or engineered to mimic the primary functions of the respective organ or tissue of a living animal. Microfluidic channels permit a culture medium that serves as a "blood surrogate" to recirculate just as in a living system, driven by a microfluidic pump. The geometry and fluidics of the device are fashioned to simulate the values of certain related physiologic parameters found in the living creature. Drug candidates or other substrates of interest are added to the culture medium and allowed to recirculate through the device. The effects of drug compounds and their metabolites on the cells within each respective organ compartment are then detected by measuring or monitoring key physiologic events. The cell types used may be derived from either standard cell culture lines or primary tissues (HμREL Corporation, 2010, paras. 2–3). As new technologies such as the HμREL chips continue to evolve, more and more robust ISs that can handle a variety of biological and clinical applications will be seen.

Returning to the movie rental example, the IS must verify the data entered by the viewer and then process the request by following the steps necessary to provide access to the movie that was ordered. This processing must

(continues)

BOX 2-1 **EXAMPLES OF INFORMATION SYSTEMS (continued)**

be instantaneous in today's world, where everyone wants everything *now*. After the data are processed, they are stored. In this case, the rental must also be processed so that the vendor receives payment for the movie, whether electronically, via a credit card or checking account withdrawal, or by generating a bill for payment.

Output or **dissemination** produces helpful or useful information that can be in the form of reports, documents, summaries, alerts, or outcomes. **Reports** are designed to inform and are generally tailored to the context of a given situation or user or user group. Reports may include charts, figures, tables, graphics, pictures, hyperlinks, references, or other documentation necessary to meet the needs of the user. **Documents** represent information that can be printed, saved, e-mailed or otherwise shared, or displayed. **Summaries** are condensed versions of the original designed to highlight the major points. **Alerts** are warnings, feedback, or additional information necessary to assist the user in interacting with the system. **Outcomes** are the expected results of input and processing. **Output** devices are combinations of hardware, software, and telecommunications and include sound and speech synthesis outputs, printers, and monitors.

Continuing with the movie rental example, the IS must be able to provide the consumer with the movie ordered when it is wanted and somehow notify the purchaser that he or she has, indeed, purchased the movie and is granted access. The IS must also be able to generate payment either electronically or by generating a bill while storing the transactional record for future use.

Feedback or responses are reactions to the inputting, processing, and outputs. In ISs, feedback refers to information from the system that is used to make modifications in the input, processing actions, or outputs. In the movie rental example, what if the consumer accidentally entered the same movie order three times but really wanted to order the movie only once? The IS would determine that more than one movie order is out of range for the same movie order at the same time and provide feedback. Such feedback is used to verify and correct the input. If undetected, the viewer's error would result in an erroneous bill and decreased customer satisfaction while creating more work for the vendor, which would have to engage in additional transactions with the customer to resolve this problem. The *Nursing Informatics Practice Applications: Care Delivery* section of this text provides detailed descriptions of clinical ISs that operate on these same principles to support health care delivery.

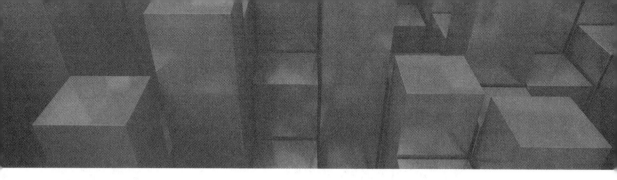

Summary

Information systems deal with the development, use, and management of an organization's information technology infrastructure. An IS acquires data or inputs; processes data through the retrieval, analysis, or synthesis of those data; disseminates or outputs in the form of reports, documents, summaries, alerts, or outcomes; and provides for responses or feedback. Quality decision-making and problem-solving skills are vital to the development of effective, valuable ISs. Today's organizations now recognize that their most precious asset is their information, as represented by their employees, experience, competence or know-how, and innovative or novel approaches, all of which are dependent on a robust information network that encompasses the information technology infrastructure.

In an ideal world, all ISs would be fluid in their ability to adapt to any and all users' needs. They would be Internet oriented and global, where resources are available to everyone. Think of **cloud computing**—it is just the beginning point from which ISs will expand and grow in their ability to provide meaningful information to their users. As technologies advance, so will the skills and capabilities to comprehend and realize what ISs can become.

It is important to continue to develop and refine functional, robust, visionary ISs that meet the current meaningful information needs while evolving systems that are even better prepared to handle future information and knowledge needs of the health care industry.

Thought-Provoking Questions

1. How do you acquire information? Choose 2 hours out of your busy day and try to notice all of the information that you receive from your environment. Keep diaries indicating where the information came from and how you knew it was information and not data.
2. Reflect on an IS with which you are familiar, such as the automatic banking machine. How does this IS function? What are the advantages of using this system (i.e., why not use a bank teller instead)? What are the disadvantages? Are there enhancements that you would add to this system?
3. In health care, think about a typical day of practice and describe the setting. How many times do you interact with ISs? What are the ISs that you interact with, and how do you access them? Are they at the patient's side, handheld, or station based? How does their location and ease of access impact patient care?
4. Briefly describe an organization and discuss how our need for information and knowledge impacts the configuration and interaction of that organization with other organizations. Also discuss how the need for information and knowledge influences the nature of

work or how knowledge workers interact with and produce information and knowledge in this organization.

5. If you could meet only four of the rights discussed in this chapter, which one would you omit and why? Also, provide your rationale for each right you chose to meet.

Apply Your Knowledge

Consider the following example of the relationship between data, information knowledge, and wisdom provided by Bellinger, Castro, and Mills (2004, para. 6).

Data represent a fact or statement of event without relation to other things.

Example: It is raining.

Information embodies the understanding of a relationship of some sort, possibly cause and effect.

Example: The temperature dropped 15 degrees, and then it started raining.

Knowledge represents a pattern that connects and generally provides a high level of predictability as to what is described or what will happen next.

Example: If the humidity is very high and the temperature drops substantially, the atmosphere is often unlikely to be able to hold the moisture so it rains.

Wisdom embodies more of an understanding of fundamental principles embodied within the knowledge that are essentially the basis for the knowledge being what it is. Wisdom is essentially systemic.

Example: It rains because it rains. And this encompasses an understanding of all the interactions that happen between raining, evaporation, air currents, temperature gradients, changes, and raining.

Select an example of data from your profession, and follow it through the DIKW paradigm as above.

References

Bellinger, G., Castro, D., & Mills, A. (2004). Data, information, knowledge, and wisdom. http://www.systems-thinking.org/dikw/dikw.htm

Cornell University. (2010). Information science. http://www.infosci.cornell.edu

Goldstein, D., Groen, P., Ponkshe, S., & Wine, M. (2007). *Medical informatics 20/20*. Sudbury, MA: Jones and Bartlett.

HμREL Corporation. (2010). Human-relevant: HμREL. Technology overview. http://www.hurelcorp.com/overview.php

Jessup, L., & Valacich, J. (2008). *Information systems today* (3rd ed.). Upper Saddle River, NJ: Pearson Prentice Hall.

Schupak, A. (2005). Technology: The bunny chip. http://members.forbes.com/forbes/2005/0815/053.html

Stair, R., & Reynolds, G. (2016). *Principles of information systems* (12th ed.). Boston: Cengage Learning.

Web Dictionary of Cybernetics and Systems. (2007). Technological determinism. http://pespmc1.vub.ac.be/ASC/TECHNO_DETER.html

Computer Science and the Foundation of Knowledge Model

June Kaminski, Dee McGonigle, Kathleen Mastrian, and Craig McGonigle

OBJECTIVES

1. Describe the essential components of computer systems, including both hardware and software.
2. Recognize the rapid evolution of computer systems and the benefit of keeping up to date with current trends and developments.
3. Analyze how computer systems function as tools for managing information and generating knowledge.
4. Define the concept of human–technology interfaces.
5. Articulate how computers can support collaboration, networking, and information exchange.

Introduction

In this chapter, the discipline of computer science is introduced through a focus on computers and the hardware and software that make up these evolving systems. **Computer science** offers extremely valuable tools that, if used skillfully, can facilitate the **acquisition** and manipulation of data and **information** by health care professionals, who can then synthesize these into an evolving knowledge and **wisdom** base. This process can facilitate **professional development** and the ability to apply evidence-based practice decisions within your practice and, if the results are disseminated and shared, can also advance the professional knowledge base.

This chapter begins with a look at common computer hardware, followed by a brief overview of operating, productivity, creativity, and communication

Key Terms
Acquisition
Application programming
interface
Applications
Arithmetic logic unit
Basic input/output
system
Binary system
Bit
Bus
Byte
Cache memory
Central processing unit
Communication software
Compact disk–read-only
memory
Compact disk–recordable
Compact disk–rewritable
Compatibility
Computer
Computer science
(continues)

software. It concludes with a glimpse at how computer systems help to shape knowledge and collaboration and an introduction to human–technology interface dynamics.

The Computer as a Tool for Managing Information and Generating Knowledge

Throughout history, various milestones have signaled discoveries, inventions, or philosophic shifts that spurred a surge in **knowledge** and understanding within the human race. The advent of the computer is one such milestone, which has sparked an intellectual metamorphosis whose boundaries have yet to be fully understood. Computer **technology** has ushered in what has been called the **Information Age**, an age when data, information, and knowledge are both accessible and able to be manipulated by more people than ever before in history. How can a mere machine lead to such a revolutionary state of knowledge potential? To begin to answer this question, it is best to examine the basic structure and components of computer systems.

Essentially, a **computer** is an electronic information-processing machine that serves as a tool with which to manipulate data and information. The easiest way to begin to understand computers is to realize they are input–output systems. These unique machines accept data input via a variety of devices, process data through logical and arithmetic rendering, store the data in memory components, and output data and information to the user.

Since the advent of the first electronic computer in the mid-1940s, computers have evolved to become essential tools in every walk of life, including the health professions. The complexity of computers has increased dramatically over the years and will continue to do so. "Computing has changed the world more than any other invention of the past hundred years, and has come to pervade nearly all human endeavors. Yet, we are just at the beginning of the computing revolution; today's computing offers just a glimpse of the potential impact of computers" (Evans, 2010, p. 3). Major computer manufacturers and researchers, such as Intel, have identified the need to design computers to mask this growing complexity. The sophistication of computers is evolving at amazing speed, yet ease of use or **user-friendly** aspects are also increasing accordingly. This is achieved by honing hardware and software capabilities until they work seamlessly together to ensure user-friendly, intuitive tools for users of all levels of expertise. **Box 3-1** provides information about computing surfaces, an evolving technology.

According to Intel Corporation's technology research team, the goal is "technology that just works." To conceal complexity, Intel Research is looking at a number of solutions by doing the following:

- "Relating user mental models with complex systems and technology to improve the use and adaptation of systems across devices and contexts.

BOX 3-1   MICROSOFT SURFACE TENSION? iTABLE

Dee McGonigle

Do not get too attached to your mouse and keyboard because they will be outdated soon if Microsoft and PQ Labs have their way. Microsoft has introduced the **Microsoft Surface**, and PQ Labs is building custom iTables, according to Kumparak (2009). Have you ever thought of digital information you can touch and grab? Microsoft and PQ Labs are leading us into the next generation of computing, known as surface or table computing.

Surface or table computing consists of a multitouch, multiuser interface that allows one to "grab" digital information and then collaborate, share, and store that information, without using a mouse or keyboard—just the hands and fingers, and such devices as a digital camera and **personal digital assistant** (PDA). This interface generally rests on top of a table and is so advanced that it can actually sense objects, touch, and gestures from many users (Microsoft, 2008).

Imagine entering a restaurant and interacting with the menu through the surface of the table where you sit. Once you have completed your order, you can begin computing by using the capabilities built into the surface or using your own device, such as a PDA. You can set the PDA on the surface and download images, graphics, and text to the surface. You can even communicate with others using full audio and video while waiting for your order. When you have finished eating, you simply set your credit card on the surface, and it is automatically charged; you pick up your credit card and leave. This is certainly a different kind of eating experience—but one that will become common for the next generation of users.

You might be wondering when this new age of computing will be touched by typical users. In fact, it is already used in Las Vegas as well as selected casinos, banks, restaurants, and hotels throughout the United States and Canada.

You should seek to explore this new interface, which will forever change how we interact and compute. Think of the ramifications for health care.

REFERENCES

Kumparak, G. (2009). Look out, Microsoft Surface: The iTable might just trump you in every way. http://www.crunchgear.com/2009/01/10/look-out-microsoft-surface-the-itable-mightjust-trump-you-in-every-way

Microsoft. (2008). Microsoft Surface: General questions. http://www.microsoft.com/SURFACE/about_faqs/faqs.aspx

Key Terms (continued)
Microprocessor
Microsoft Surface
Modem
Monitor
Motherboard
Mouse
MPEG-1 Audio Layer-3
Networks
Nonsynchronous
Office suite
Open-source software
Operating system
Palm computers
Parallel port
Peripheral component interconnection
Personal computer
Personal digital assistant
Plug and play
Port
Portability
Portable operating system interface for Unix
Power supply
Presentation
Processing
Productivity software
Professional development
Programmable read-only memory
Publishing
QWERTY
Random-access memory
Read-only memory
Security
Serial port
Small Computer System Interface
Software
Sound card
Spreadsheet
Supercomputers
(continues)

- Enabling devices to explore their environment to discover other devices and capabilities, and then form integrated 'teams' that self-organize for higher functionality and performance.
- Better control of failure modes, graceful **degradation**, and self-healing across ensembles of devices.
- Zero-knowledge applications and interoperation." (Intel Corporation, 2008, para. 2).

Key Terms (continued)
Synchronous dynamic random-access memory
Technology
Terabyte
Throughput
Touchscreen
Universal serial bus
User-friendly
User interface
Video adapter card
Virtual memory
Wearable technology
Wisdom
Word processing
World Wide Web
Yottabyte
Zettabyte

One example of this type of complexity masked in simplicity is the evolution of "**plug and play**" computer add-ons, where a peripheral, such as an iPod or game console, can be simply plugged into a serial or other **port** and instantly used.

Computers are universal machines because they are general-purpose, symbol-manipulating devices that can perform any task represented in specific programs. For example, they can be used to draw an image, calculate statistics, write an essay, or record your patient data. In a nutshell, computers can be used for data and information storage, retrieval, analysis, generation, and transformation.

Most computers are based on scientist John Von Neumann's model of a processor–memory–input–output architecture. In this model, the logic unit and control unit are parts of the processor, the **memory** is the storage region, and the input and output segments are provided by the various computer devices, such as the keyboard, mouse, monitor, and printer. Recent developments have provided alternative configurations to the Von Neumann model—for example, the parallel computing model, where multiple processors are set up to work together. Nevertheless, today's computer systems share the same basic configurations and components inherent in the earliest computers.

Computer Components

Hardware

Computer **hardware** refers to the actual physical body of the computer and its components. Several key components in the average computer work together to shape a complex yet highly usable machine that serves as a tool for knowledge management, communication, and creativity.

Protection: The Casing

The most noticeable component of any computer is the outer case. **Desktop** personal computers have either a desktop case, which lies flat, horizontally on a desk, and often with the computer monitor positioned on top of it, or a tower case, which stands vertically and usually sits beside the monitor or on a lower shelf or the floor. Most cases come equipped with a case fan, which is extremely critical for keeping the computer components cool when in use. **Laptop** computers combine the casing in a flat rectangular casing that is attached to the hinged or foldable monitor. **Palm computers** and personal digital assistants also have a protective outer plastic and metal case with an embedded liquid crystal display screen.

Central Processing Unit

Sometimes conceptualized as the "brain" of the computer, the **central processing unit** (CPU) is the computer component that actually **executes**, calculates, and processes the binary computer code (which consists of various configurations of 0s and 1s), instigated by the **operating system** (OS) and other **applications** on the computer. The CPU serves as the command center that directs the actions of all other computer components, and it manages both incoming and outgoing data that are processed across components. Common CPUs include the Pentium, K6, PowerPC, and Sparc models.

The CPU contains specific mechanical units, including registers, **arithmetic logic units** (ALUs), a floating point unit, control circuitry, and cache memory. Together, these inner components form the computer's central processor. Registers consist of data-storing circuits whose contents are processed by the adjacent arithmetic and logic units or the floating point unit. **Cache memory** is extremely quick memory that holds whatever data and code are being used at any one time. The CPU uses the cache to store in-process data so that it can be quickly retrieved as needed. The CPU is protected by a heat sink, a copper or aluminum metal block that cools the processor (often with the help of a fan) to prevent overheating.

In the past, the speed and power of a CPU were measured in units of **megahertz** (MHz) and was written as a value in MHz (e.g., 400 MHz, meaning that the **microprocessor** ran at 400 MHz, executing 400 million cycles per second). Today, it is more common to see the speed measured in **gigahertz** (GHz) (1 GHz is equal to 1,000 MHz); thus, a CPU that operates at 4 GHz is 1,000 times faster than an older one that operates at 4 MHz. The more cycles a processor can complete per second, the faster computer programs can run.

In recent years, processor manufacturers, such as Intel, have moved to multicore microprocessors, which are chips that combine two or more processors. In fact, multiple microprocessors have become a standard in both personal and professional-level computers. "Minicomputers, which were traditionally made from off-the-shelf logic or from gate arrays, have been replaced by servers made using microprocessors. **Mainframes** have been almost replaced with multiprocessors consisting of small numbers of off-the-shelf microprocessors. Even high-end **supercomputers** are being built with collections of microprocessors" (Hennessy & Patterson, 2006, p. 3).

Motherboard

The **motherboard** has been called the "central nervous system" of the computer. It is a key foundational component because all other components are connected to it in some way (either directly via local sockets, attached directly to it, or connected via cables). This includes **universal serial bus** (USB) controllers, Ethernet network controllers, integrated graphics controllers, and so forth. The essential structures of the motherboard include the major chip set, super input/output chip, basic input/output system read-only memory (ROM), **bus** communications pathways, and a variety of sockets that allow components to plug into the board. The chip set (often a pair of chips) determines the computer's CPU type and memory. It also houses the north bridge and south bridge controllers that allow the buses to transfer data from one to another.

Power Supply

The **power supply** is a critical component of any computer because it provides the essential electrical energy needed to allow a computer to operate. The power supply unit converts the 120-volt AC main power (provided via the power cable from the wall socket into which the computer is plugged) into low-voltage DC power. Computers depend on a reliable, steady supply of DC power to function properly. The more devices and programs used on a computer, the larger the power supply should be to avoid damage and malfunctioning. Power supplies normally range from 160 to 700 watts, with an average of 300 to 400 watts. Most contemporary power supply units come equipped with at least one fan to cool the unit under heavy use. The power supply is controlled by pressing the on and off switch as well as the reset switch (which restarts the system) of a computer.

Laptop and other portable computing machines, such as electronic readers and tablet computers, are equipped with a rechargeable battery power supply and the standard plug-in variety.

Hard Disk

This component is so named because of the rigid hard disks that reside in it, which are mounted to a spindle that is spun by a motor when in use. Drive heads (most computers have two or more heads) produce a magnetic field through their transducers that magnetizes the disk surface as a voltage is applied to the disk. The **hard disk** acts as a permanent data storage area that holds **gigabytes** (GB) or even **terabytes** (TB) worth of data, information, documents, and programs saved on the computer, even when the computer is shut off. Disk drives are not infallible, however, so backing up important data is imperative.

The computer writes binary data to the hard drive by magnetizing small areas of its surface. Each drive head is connected to an actuator that moves along the disk to hover over any point on the disk surface as it spins. The parts of the hard disk are encased in a sealed unit. The hard drive is managed by a disk controller, which is a circuit board that controls the motor and actuator arm assembly. The **hard drive** produces the voltage waveform that contacts the heads to write and read data and handles communications with the motherboard. It is usually located within the computer's hard outer casing. Some people also attach a second hard drive externally to increase available memory or to back up data.

Main Memory or Random-Access Memory

Random-access memory (RAM) is considered to be volatile memory because it is a temporary storage system that allows the processor to access program codes and data while working on a task. The contents of RAM are lost once the system is rebooted or shut off or loses power.

The memory is actually situated on small chip boards, which sport rows of pins along the bottom edge and are plugged into the motherboard of the computer. These memory chips contain complex arrays of tiny memory circuits that can be either set by the CPU during write operations (puts them into storage) or read by the CPU during data retrieval. The circuits store the data in binary form as either a low (on) voltage stage, expressed as a 0, or a high (off) voltage stage, expressed as a 1. All of the work being done on a computer resides in RAM until it is saved onto the hard drive or other storage drive. Computers generally come with 2 GB of RAM or more, and some offer more RAM via **graphics cards** and other expansion cards.

A certain portion of the RAM, called the **main memory**, serves the hard disk and facilitates interactions between the hard disk and central processor. Main memory is provided by **dynamic random-access memory** (DRAM) and is attached to the processor using specific addresses and data buses.

Synchronous dynamic random-access memory (SDRAM) (also known as static dynamic RAM) is "much faster than conventional (**nonsynchronous**) memory because it can synchronize itself with a microprocessor's bus" (Null & Lobor, 2006, p. 8).

Read-Only Memory

Read-only memory (ROM) is essential permanent or semipermanent nonvolatile memory that stores saved data and is critical in the working of the computer's OS and other activities. ROM is stored primarily in the motherboard, but it may also be available through the graphics card, other expansion cards, and peripherals. In recent years, rewritable ROM chips that may include other forms of ROM, such as **programmable read-only memory** (PROM), erasable ROM, **electronically erasable programmable read-only memory** (EEPROM), and a **flash memory** (a variation of electronically erasable programmable ROM), have become available.

Basic Input/Output System

The **basic input/output system** (BIOS) is a specific type of ROM used by the computer when it first boots up to establish basic communication between the processor, motherboard, and other components. Often called boot firmware, it controls the computer from the time the machine is switched on until the primary OS (e.g., Windows, Mac OS X, or Linux) takes over. The **firmware** initializes the hardware and boots (loads and executes) the primary OS.

Virtual Memory

Virtual memory is a special type of memory is stored on the hard disk to provide temporary data storage so data can be swapped in and out of the RAM as needed. This capability is particularly handy when working with large data-intensive programs, such as games and multimedia.

Integrated Drive Electronics Controller

The **integrated drive electronics** (IDE) controller component is the primary interface for the hard drive, **compact disk–read-only memory** (CD-ROM), or **digital video disk** (DVD) drive, and the floppy disk drive (found largely on pre-2010 computers).

Peripheral Component Interconnection Bus

This component is important for connecting additional plug-in components to the computer. It uses a series of slots on the motherboard to allow **peripheral component interconnection** card plug-in.

Small Computer System Interface

The **Small Computer System Interface** (SCSI) component provides the means to attach additional devices, such as scanners and extra hard drives, to the computer.

DVD/CD Drive

The CD-ROM drive reads and records data to portable CDs using a laser diode to emit an infrared light beam that reflects onto a track on the CD using a mirror positioned by a motor. The light reflected on the disk is directed by a system of lenses to a photodetector that converts the light pulses into an electrical signal; this signal is then decoded by the drive electronics to the motherboard. Both **compact disk–recordable** (CD-R) and **compact disk–rewritable** (CD-RW) drives are common. The same principle applies to **digital video disk–recordable** (DVD-R) and **digital video disk–rewritable** (DVD-RW) drives. A DVD drive can do everything a CD drive can do, plus it can play the content of disks and, if it is a recordable unit, can record data on blank DVDs.

Flash or USB Drive

This portable memory device uses electronically erasable programmable ROM to provide fast permanent memory.

Modem

A **modem** is a component that can be situated either externally (external modem) or internally (internal modem) relative to the computer and enables Internet connectivity via a cable connection through network adapters situated within the computer apparatus.

Connection Ports

All computers have connection ports made to fit different types of plug-in devices. These ports include a monitor cable port, keyboard and mouse ports, a network cable port, microphone/speaker/auxiliary input ports, USB ports, and printer ports (SCSI or parallel). These ports allow data to move to and from the computer via peripheral or storage devices. Specific ports include the following:

- **Parallel**: connects to a printer
- **Serial**: connects to an external modem
- **USB**: connects to myriad plug-in devices, such as portable flash drives, digital cameras, **MPEG-1 Audio Layer-3** (MP3) players, graphics tablets, and light pens, using a plug-and-play connection (the ability to add devices automatically)

- FireWire (IEEE 1394): often used to connect digital-video devices to the computer
- Ethernet: connects networking apparatus, such as Internet and modem cables

Graphics Card

Most computers come equipped with a graphics accelerator card slotted in the micro-processor of a computer to process image data and output those data to the monitor. These in situ graphic cards provide satisfactory graphics quality for two-dimensional art and general text and numerical data. However, if a user intends to create or view three-dimensional images or is an active game user, one or more graphics enhancement cards are often installed.

Video Adapter Cards

Video adapter cards provide video memory, a video processor, and a digital-to-ana-log converter that works with the CPU to output higher-quality video images to the monitor.

Sound Card

The **sound card** converts digital data into an analog signal that is then output to the computer's speakers or headphones. The reverse is also accomplished by inputting a signal from a microphone or other audio recording equipment, which then converts the analog signal to a digital signal.

Bit

A **bit** is the smallest possible chunk of data memory used in computer processing and is depicted as either a 1 or a 0. Bits make up the **binary system** of the computer.

Byte

A **byte** is a chunk of memory that consists of 8 bits; it is considered to be the best way to indicate computer memory or storage capacity. In modern computers, bytes are described in units of **megabytes** (MB); GB, where 1 GB equals 1,000 MB; or TB, where 1 TB equals 1 trillion bytes or 1,000 GB. **Box 3-2** discusses storage capacities.

Software

Software comprises the application programs developed to facilitate various user func-tions, such as writing, artwork, organizing meetings, surfing the Internet, communi-cating with others, and so forth. For the purposes of this overview, the various types of software have been divided into four categories: (1) OS software, (2) productivity software, (3) **creativity software**, and (4) communication software.

User-friendliness is a critical condition for effective software adoption. "End user performance is likely to be facilitated by [the degree of] user friendliness of software packages" (Mahmood, 2003, p. 71). The easier and more intuitive a software package seems to be to a user influences that user's perception of how clear the package is to

BOX 3-2 STORAGE CAPACITIES

Dee McGonigle and Kathleen Mastrian
Storage and memory capacities are evolving. In the past few decades, there have been great leaps in data storage. It all begins with the bit, the basic unit of data storage, composed of 0s and 1s, also known as binary digits (bit). A byte is generally considered to be equal to 8 bits. The files on a computer are stored as binary files. The software that is used translates these binary files into words, numbers, pictures, images, or video. Using this binary code in the binary numbering system, measurement is counted by factors of 2, such as 1, 2, 4, 8, 16, 32, 64, and 128. These multiples of the binary system in computer usage are also prefixed based on the metric system. Therefore, a kilobyte (KB) is actually 2 to the 10th power (210), or 1,024 bytes, but is typically considered to be 1,000 bytes. This is why one sees 1,024 or multiples of that number instead of an even 1,000 mentioned at times in relation to kilobytes.

In the early 1980s, kilobytes were the norm as far as computer capacity went, and 128 KB machines were launched for personal use. Subsequent decades, however, have seen advanced computing power and storage capacity. As capabilities soared, so did the ability to save and store what was used and created. Megabytes (MB) emerged as a common unit of measure; a megabyte is 1,048,576 bytes but is considered to be roughly equivalent to 1 million bytes. The next leap in computer capacity was one that some people could not even imagine: gigabytes (GB). A gigabyte is 1,073,741,824 bytes but is generally rounded to 1 billion bytes. Some computing experts are very concerned that valuable bytes are lost when these measurements are rounded, whereas hard drive manufacturers use the decimal system so their capacity is expressed as an even 1 billion bytes per gigabyte.

The next advancements in computer capacity are moving into the range of terabytes (TB), petabytes (PB), exabytes (EB), zettabytes (ZB), and yottabytes (YB). These terms storage capacity are defined as follows:

TB: 1,000 GB
PB: 1,000,000 GB
EB: 1,000 PB
ZB: 1,000 EB
YB: 1,000 ZB

To put all of this in perspective, Williams (n.d., para. 5) writes about the data powers of 10:

2 KB: a typewritten page
2 MB: a high-resolution photograph
10 MB: a minute of high-fidelity sound or a digital chest X-ray
50 MB: a digital mammogram
1 GB: a symphony in high-fidelity sound or a movie at TV quality
1 TB: all the X-ray films in a large technologically advanced hospital
2 PB: the contents of all U.S. academic research libraries
5 EB: all words ever spoken by human beings

We have not even addressed ZB and YB. Stay tuned.

REFERENCE

Williams, R. (n.d.). Data powers of ten. http://ict.stmargaretsacademy.org.uk/computing/hardware/dataquan/d_p_ten2.html

understand and to use. The rapid evolution of hardware mentioned previously has been equally matched by the phenomenal development in software over the past three or four decades.

Commercial Software

Several large commercial software companies, such as Apple, Microsoft, IBM, and Adobe, dominate the market for software and have done so since the advent of the **personal computer**. Licensed software has evolved over time; hence, most products have a long version history. Many software packages, such as office suites, are expensive to purchase; in turn, there is a "digital divide" as far as access and affordability go across societal spheres, especially when viewed from a global perspective.

Open-Source Software

The **open-source software** movement began several years ago but recently has become a powerful movement that is changing the software production and consumer market. In addition to commercially available software, a growing number of open-source software packages are being developed in all four of the categories addressed in this chapter. The open-source movement was begun by developers who wished to offer their creations to others for the good of the community and encouraged them to do the same. Users who modify or contribute to the evolution of open-source software are obligated to share their new code, but essentially the software is free to all. Both Open Office and KOffice are examples of open-source productivity software.

OS Software

The OS is the most important software on any computer. It is the very first program to load on computer start-up and is fundamental for the operation of all other software and the computer hardware. Examples of commonly used OSs include the Microsoft Windows family, Linux, Mac OS X, and Unix. The OS manages both the hardware and the software and provides a reliable, consistent interface for the software applications to work with the computer's hardware. An OS must be both powerful and flexible to adapt to the myriad types of software available, which are made by a variety of development companies. New versions of the major OSs are equipped to deal with multiple users and handle multitasking with ease. For example, a user can work on a word processing document while listening for an "e-mail received" signal, have an **Internet browser** window open to look for references on the Internet as needed, listen to music in the CD drive, and download a file—all at the same time.

OS tasks can be described in terms of six basic processes:

- Memory management
- Device management

- Processor management
- Storage management
- Application interface
- **User interface** (usually a **graphical user interface** [GUI])

OSs should be convenient to use, easy to learn, reliable, safe, and fast. They should also be easy to design, implement, and maintain and should be flexible, reliable, error free, and efficient. For example, Silbershatz, Baer Galvin, and Gagne (2013) described how "Microsoft's design goals for Windows included security, reliability, Windows and POSIX application compatibility, high performance, extensibility, portability, and international support" (p. 831). The following goals were established by Microsoft:

- **Portability**: The OS can be moved from one hardware architecture to another with few changes needed.
- **Security**: The OS incorporates hardware protection for virtual memory and software protection mechanisms for OS resources, including encryption and digital signature capabilities.
- **Portable operating system interface for Unix (POSIX) compliance**: Applications designed to follow the POSIX (IEEE 1003.1) standard can be compiled to run on Windows without changing the source code. Windows XP had higher compatibility with the applications that ran on earlier versions of Windows, such as Windows 95.
- Multiprocessor support: The OS is designed for symmetrical multiprocessing.
- **Extensibility**: This capability is provided by using a layered architecture with a protected executive layer for basic system services, several server subsystems that operate in user mode, and a modular structure that allows additional environmental subsystems to be added without affecting the executive layer.
- International support: The Windows OS supports different locales via the national language support application programming interface (API).
- **Compatibility with MS-DOS and MS-Windows applications.**

Productivity Software

Productivity software, such as **office suites**, is the type of software most commonly used both in the workplace and on personal computers. Several software companies produce these multiple-program software, which usually bundles together **word processing, spreadsheets, databases, presentation**, Web development, and **e-mail** programs.

The intent of office suites is generally to provide all of the basic programs that office or knowledge workers need to do their work. The bundled programs within the suite are organized to be compatible with one another, are designed to look similar to one another for ease of use, and provide a powerful array of tools for data manipulation, information gathering, and knowledge generation. Some office suites add other programs, such as database creation software, mathematical editors, drawing, and desktop

TABLE 3-1 OFFICE SUITE SOFTWARE FEATURES AND EXAMPLES		
OFFICE SUITE SOFTWARE		
Program	**Application**	**Examples**
Word processing	Composition, editing, formatting, and producing text documents	Microsoft Word, Open Office Writer, KOffice KWord, Corel WordPerfect or Corel Write, Apple Pages
Spreadsheets	Grid-based documents in ledger format; organizes numbers and text; calculates statistical formulae	Microsoft Excel, Open Office Calc, KOffice Kspread, Corel Quattro Pro, Apple Numbers
Presentations	Slideshow software, usually used for business or classroom presentations using text, images, graphs, media	Microsoft Power Point, Open Office Impress, KOffice KPresenter, Corel Show, Apple Keynote
Databases	Database creation for text and numbers	Microsoft Access (in elite packages), Open Office Base, KOffice Kexi, Corel Calculate, Corel Paradox
E-mail	Integrated e-mail program to send and receive electronic mail	Microsoft Outlook, Corel WordPerfect Mail, Mozilla Thunderbird
Drawing	Graphics and diagram drawing	Open Office Draw, Corel Presentation Graphics, KOffice Kivio, Karbon, Krita
Math formulas	Inserts math equations in word processing and presentation work	Open Office Math, KOffice KFormula
Desktop publishing	Page layouts and publication-ready documents	Microsoft Publisher (in elite packages), Apple Pages

publishing programs. **Table 3-1** summarizes the programs included in five of the most popular office suites: Microsoft Office, Open Office, KOffice, Corel WordPerfect Suite, and Apple iWork (for Macintosh computers). Of these five, Open Office (for Windows, Linux, Solaris, Mac OS X, FreeBSD, and HP-UX OSs) and KOffice (for Linux environments but also being developed for Windows and Mac OS X platforms) are open-source, free software.

Creative Software

Creative software includes programs that allow users to draw, paint, render, record music and sound, and incorporate digital video and other multimedia in professional aesthetic ways to share and convey information and knowledge (**Table 3-2**).

Communication Software

Networking and **communication software** enable users to dialogue, share, and network with other users via the exchange of e-mail or **instant messages**, by accessing

TABLE 3-2   CREATIVE SOFTWARE FEATURES AND EXAMPLES

CREATIVE SOFTWARE	
Program and Application	**Software Examples**
Raster graphics programs Draw, paint, render, manipulate and edit images, fonts, and photographs to create pixel-based (dot points) digital art and graphics	Adobe Photoshop and Fireworks, Ulead PhotoImpact, Corel Draw, Painter, and Paint Shop Pro, GIMP (open source), KOffice's Krita (open source)
Vector graphics programs Mathematically rendered, geometric modeling is applied through shapes, curves, lines, points and manipulated for shape, color, size. Ideal for printing and three-dimensional (3D) modeling	Adobe Flash, Freehand, and Illustrator, CorelDraw and Designer, Open Office Draw (open source), Mirosoft Visio, Xara Xtreme, KOffice Karbon14 (open source)
Desktop publishing programs Page layout and publishing preparation for printed and web documents, such as magazines, journals, books, newsletters, brochures	Adobe InDesign, Corel PageMaker, Microsoft Publisher, Scribus (open source), QuarkXPress, Apple Pages (note that many of the graphics programs can also be used for DTP)
Web design programs Create, edit, update webpages using specific codes, such as XML, CSS, HTML, and JAVA	Adobe Dreamweaver, Coffee Cup, Microsoft FrontPage, Nvu (open source), W3C's Amaya (open source)
Multimedia programs Combines text, audio, images, animation, and video into interactive content for electronic presentation	Adobe Flash, Microsoft Movie Maker, Apple QuickTime and FinalCut Studio, Corel VideoStudio, Ulead VideoStudio, Real Studio, CamStudio (open source), Audacity (open source)

the World Wide Web, or by engaging in virtual meetings using **conferencing software** (**Table 3-3**).

Acquisition of Data and Information: Input Components

Input devices include the keyboard, mouse, joysticks (typically used for playing computer games), game controllers or pads; Web cameras (webcams), stylus (often used with tablets or personal digital assistants), image scanners for copying a digital image of a document or picture, or other plug-and-play input devices, such as digital cameras, digital video recorders (camcorders), MP3 players, electronic musical instruments, and physiologic monitors (**Figure 3-1**). These devices are the origin or medium used to input text, visual, audio, or multimedia data into the computer system for viewing, listening, manipulating, creating, or editing. The two primary input devices on a computer are the keyboard and mouse.

Keyboard

Computer **keyboards** are very similar to the typewriter keyboards of earlier days and usually serve as the prime input device that enables the user to type words, numbers,

TABLE 3-3   COMMUNICATION SOFTWARE FEATURES AND EXAMPLES

COMMUNICATION SOFTWARE

E-mail client
Allows user to read, edit, forward, and send email messages to other users via an Internet connection. The software can be resident on the computer or accessed via the World Wide Web

Resident programs
Microsoft Outlook and Outlook Express, Eudora, Pegasus, Mozilla Thunderbird, Lotus Notes
Web-based programs
Gmail, Yahoo Mail, Hotmail

Internet browsers
Enables user to access, browse, download, upload, and interact with text, audio, video, and other Web-based documents

Mozilla Firefox, Microsoft Internet Explorer, Google Chrome, Apple Safari, Opera, Microbrowser (for mobile access)

Instant messaging (IM)
Real-time text messaging between users, can attach images, videos, and other documents via personal computer, cell phone, hand-held devices

MSN Instant Messenger, Microsoft Live Messenger, Yahoo Messenger, Apple iChat

Conferencing
Enables user to communicate in a virtual meeting room setting to share work, discussions, planning, using an intranet or Internet environment; can exhibit files, video, screen shots of content

Adobe Acrobat Connect, Microsoft Live Meeting or Meeting Space, GotoMeeting, Meeting Bridge, Free Conference, RainDance, WebEx

and commands into the computer's programs. Standard computer keyboards have 101 keys and are organized to facilitate Latin-based languages using a **QWERTY** layout (so named because these letters appear on the first six keys in the first row of letters).

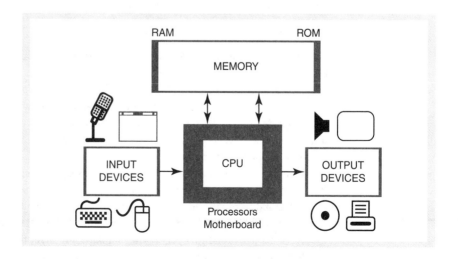

Figure 3-1
Computer System

Certain keys are used as command keys, particularly the control (Ctrl), alternate (Alt), delete (Del), and shift keys, all of which can be used to activate useful commands. The escape (Esc) key allows the user instantly to exit a process or program. The F keys, numbered F1 through F12, are function keys. They are used in different ways by particular programs. If a program instructs users to press the F8 key, they would do so by pressing F8. The print screen (PrtScn) key sends a graphical picture or screenshot of a computer screen to the clipboard. This copied screenshot can then be pasted in any graphic program that can work with bitmap files.

Mouse

The **mouse** is the second most commonly used input device. It is manipulated by the user's hand to point, click, and move objects around on the computer screen. A mouse can come in a number of different configurations, including a standard mechanical trackball serial mouse, bus mouse, PS/2 mouse, USB-connected mouse, optical lens mouse, cordless mouse, and optomechanical mouse.

Processing of Data and Information: Throughput/ Processing Components

All of the hardware discussed earlier in this chapter is involved in the **throughput** or **processing** of input data and in the preparation of output data and information. Specific software is used, depending on the application and data involved. One key hardware component, the computer monitor, is a unique example of a visible throughput component—it is the part of the computer that users focus on the most when they are working on a computer. Input data can be visualized and accessed by manipulating the mouse and keyboard input devices, but it is the monitor that receives the user's attention. The monitor is critical for the efficient rendering during this part of the cycle because it facilitates user access and control of the data and information.

Monitor

The **monitor** is the visual display that serves as the landscape for all interactions between user and machine. It typically resembles a television screen and comes in various sizes (usually ranging from 15 to 21 inches) and configurations. Monitors either are based on cathode ray tubes (the conventional monitor with a large section behind the screen) or are thinner, flat-screen liquid crystal display devices. Some computer monitors also have a **touchscreen** that can serve as an input device when the user touches specific areas of the screen.

Monitors vary in their refresh rate (usually measured in megahertz) and dot pitch. Both of these characteristics are important for user comfort. The faster the refresh rate, the cleaner and clearer the image on the screen because the monitor refreshes the screen contents more frequently. For example, a monitor with a 100 MHz refresh rate refreshes the screen contents 100 times per second. Similarly, the larger the dot pitch factor, the smaller the dots that make up the screen image, which provides a more detailed display on the monitor and also facilitates clarity and ease of viewing.

If equipped with a touchscreen, a monitor can also serve as an input device when activated by a stylus or finger pressure. Some users might also consider the monitor to be an output device because access to input and stored documents is often performed via the screen (e.g., reading a document that is stored on the computer or viewable from the Internet).

Dissemination: Output Components

Output devices carry data in a usable form through exit devices in or attached to a computer. Common forms of output include printed documents, audio or video files, physiologic summaries, scan results, and saved files on portable disk drives, such as a CD, DVD, flash drive, or external hard drive. Output devices literally put data and information at the user's fingertips, which can then be used to develop knowledge and even wisdom. The most commonly used output devices include printers, speakers, and portable disk drives.

Printer

Printers are external components that can be attached to a computer using a printer cord that is secured into the computer's printer port. Printers enable users to print a hard paper copy of documents that are housed on the computer.

The most common printer types are the ink-jet and laser printers. Ink-jet printers are more economical to use and offer quite good quality; they apply ink to paper using a jet-spray mechanism. Laser printers produce publisher-ready quality printing if combined with good-quality paper but cost more in terms of printing supplies. Both types of printers can print in black and white or in color.

Speakers

All computers have some sort of speaker setup, usually small speakers embedded in the monitor, in the case, or, if a laptop, close to the keyboard. Often, external speakers are added to a computer system using speaker connectors; these devices provide enhanced sound and a more enjoyable listening experience.

What is the Relationship of Computer Science to Knowledge?

Scholars and researchers are just beginning to understand the effects that computer systems, architecture, applications, and processes have on the potential for knowledge acquisition and development. Users who have access to contemporary computers equipped with full Internet access have resources at their fingertips that were only dreamed of before the 21st century. Entire library collections are accessible, with many documents available in full printable form. Users are also able to contribute to the development of knowledge through the use of productivity, creativity, and communication software. In addition, using the World Wide Web interface, users are able to disseminate knowledge on a grand scale with other users.

This deluge of information available via computers must be mastered and organized by the user if knowledge is to emerge. Discernment and the ability to critique and filter this information must also be present to facilitate the further development of wisdom.

The development of an understanding of computer science principles as they apply to technology used in your practice can facilitate optimal usage of the technology for knowledge development in the profession. The maxim that "knowledge is power" and that the skillful use of computers lies at the heart of this power is a presumption: Once health care professionals become comfortable with the various technologies, they can shape them, refine them, and apply them in new and different ways, just as they have always adapted earlier equipment and technologies. Health care professionals must harness the power of data and information through the use of computer technologies to build knowledge and gain wisdom.

How Does the Computer Support Collaboration and Information Exchange?

Computers can be linked to other computers through networking software and hardware to promote communication, information exchange, work sharing, and collaboration. Such **networks** can be local or organizationally based, with computers joined together into a local area network or organized on a wider area scope (e.g., a city or district) using a metropolitan area network or encompassing computers at an even greater distance (e.g., a whole country or continent or the Internet itself) using a wide area network configuration (Sarkar, 2006). Network interface cards are used to connect a computer and its modem to a network.

Networks within health care can manifest in several different configurations, including client-focused networks, such as in telehealth, e-health, and client support networks; work-related networks, including virtual work and virtual social networks; and learning and research networks, as in communities of practice. These trends are still in their infancy in most work environments (and most health care professionals' personal lives), but they are predicted to grow dramatically in the future:

> As the Net generation grows in influence, the trend will be toward networks, not hierarchies; toward open collaboration rather than authority; toward consensus rather than arbitrary edict. The communication support provided by networks and information systems will also alter patterns of social interaction within a healthcare organization. This technology provides a medium for greater accessibility to shared information and support for rich interpersonal exchange and collaboration across departmental boundaries. (Richards, 2001, p. 10)

Virtual social networks are another form of professional network that have expanded phenomenally since the advent of the Internet and other computer software and hardware:

> Electronic media do more than just expand access to vast bodies of information. They also serve as a convenient vehicle for building virtual social networks for

creating shared knowledge through collaborative learning and problem solving. Cross pollination of ideas through worldwide connectivity can boost creativity synergistically in the co-construction of knowledge. (Bandura, 2002, p. 4)

Health care–related virtual social networks provide a cyberspace for specific health care professionals to make contacts, share information and ideas, and build a sense of community. Social communication software is used to provide a dynamic virtual environment, and often virtual social networks provide communicative capabilities through posting tools, such as blogs, forums, and wikis; e-mail for sharing ideas on a smaller scale; collaborative areas for interaction, creating, and building digital artifacts or planning projects; navigation tools for moving through the virtual network landscape; and profiles to provide a space for each member to disclose personal information with others. Health care professionals who have to engage in shift work often find that virtual social networks can provide a sense of connection with other professionals that is available around the clock. Because time is often a factor in any social interchange, virtual communication offers an alternative for practicing health care professionals, who can access information and engage in interchanges at any time of day. With active participation, the interchanges and shared information and ideas of the network can culminate in valuable social and cultural capital, available to all members of that network. Often, health care professional virtual social networks are created for the purpose of exchanging ideas on practice issues and best practices; to become more knowledgeable about new trends, research, and innovations in health care; or to participate in advocacy, activist, and educational initiatives.

Through the use of portable disk devices, such as flash drives, CDs, and DVDs, people can share information, documents, and communications by exchanging files. Since the advent of the Internet in the mid-1980s, the World Wide Web has evolved to become a viable and user-friendly way for people to collaborate and exchange information, projects, and other knowledge-based files, such as websites, e-mail, social networking applications, and webinar logs. **Box 3-3** provides information on Web 2.0, the latest iteration of the World Wide Web.

What is the Human–Technology Interface?

In the context of using a computer system, the human–technology interface is facilitated by the input and output devices discussed previously in this chapter. Specifically, the keyboard, mouse, monitor, laser pen, joystick, stylus, game pads and controls, and other USB or plug-and-play devices, such as MP3 players, digital cameras, digital camcorders, musical instruments, and handheld smaller computers, such as PDAs, are all viable devices for interfacing with a computer.

The GUI associated with the OS of a computer provides the onscreen environment for direct interaction between the user and the computer. The typical GUI provided by Windows or Mac OS X utilizes a user-friendly desktop metaphor interface that is made up of the input and output devices and icons that represent files, programs, actions, and processes. These interface icons can be activated by clicking the mouse buttons to

BOX 3-3   WEB 2.0 TOOLS

Dee McGonigle, Kathleen Mastrian, and Wendy Mahan

Web 2.0—the name given to the new World Wide Web tools—enables users to collaborate, network socially, and disseminate knowledge with other users on a scale that was once not even comprehensible. These programs promote data and information exchange, feedback, and knowledge development and dissemination.

To facilitate a selective review of the Web 2.0 tools available, they have been categorized into three areas here: (1) tools for creating and sharing information, (2) tools for collaborating, and (3) tools for communicating. Examples of tools for creating and sharing information include blogs, podcasts, Flickr, YouTube, Hellodeo, Jing, Screencast-o-matic, Facebook, MySpace, and MakeBeliefsComix. Examples of tools for collaborating with others include Google Docs, Zoho, wikis, Del.icio.us, and Gliffy. Finally, some tools for communicating with others include Adobe Connect, Vyew, Skype, Twitter, and instant messaging.

The application of the creating and sharing information tools has led to an explosion of social networking on the Web. YouTube has promoted the "broadcast yourself" proliferation. Anyone can launch a video onto YouTube that is shared with others over the Web. Similarly, Flickr allows users to upload and tag personal photos to share either privately or publicly. Both Facebook and MySpace promote socializing on the Web. Facebook is a social utility, and MySpace is a place for friends, according to the descriptions found on these websites. Other tools let users create and share recorded messages, diagrams, screen captures, and even custom comic strips.

Collaborating over the Web has become easier. Indeed, it is a way of life for many people. Google Docs and Zoho allow users to create online and share and collaborate in realtime. Wikis are server-based software programs that enable users to generate and edit webpage content using any browser. Del.icio.us is a social bookmarking manager that uses tags to identify or describe the bookmarks that can be shared with others.

Communicating with others includes audio- and videoconferencing in realtime. Adobe Connect is a comprehensive Web communications solution. Although a fee-based service, it does provide a free trial. Users should read all of the documentation on Adobe's site before downloading, installing, and using this software. Vyew is free, always-on collaboration plus live webinars. Skype allows users to make calls in audio only or with video. Users can download Skype for free, but, depending on the type of calls made, fees or charges could be assessed. Individuals should read through all of the information before downloading, installing, and using this software. Twitter allows participants to answer the question "What are you doing?" with messages containing 140 or fewer characters. Although Twitter can be used to keep the friends in a person's network updated on daily activities, it can also be used for other purposes, such as asking questions or expressing thoughts. In addition, Twitter can be accessed by cell phones, so users can stay in touch on the go.

Along with all of the advantages and intellectual harvesting capabilities from the use of these tools come serious security issues. Wagner (2007) warns the user to "bear in mind before you jump in that you're giving information to a third-party company to store" (para. 5). He also states that "you should talk to your company's legal and compliance offices to be sure you're obeying the law and regulations with regard to managing company's information" (para. 5). One suggestion that Wagner offers is that if you do not want to involve a third party, "wikis provide a good alternative for organizations looking to maintain control of their own software. Organizations can install wiki software on their own, internal servers" (para. 6).

This new wave of Web-based tools facilitates the ability to interact, exchange, collaborate, communicate, and share in ways that have only begun to be realized. As the tools and their innovative uses continue to expand, users need to stay vigilant to handle the associated security challenges. These Web 2.0 tools are providing a new cyber-playground that is limited only by users' own imaginations and intelligence. We encourage you to explore these tools. Refer to this text's companion website (http://go.jblearning.com/mcgonigle) for more information.

BOX 3-3 WEB 2.0 TOOLS (continued)

REFERENCE

Wagner, M. (2007). Nine easy Web-based collaborative tools. http://www.forbes.com/2007/02/26/google-microsoft-bluetie -enttech-cx_mw_0226smallbizresource.html

perform various actions, such as to provide information, execute functions, open and manipulate folders (directories), select options, and so forth.

Although these aspects of a computer system may be taken for granted, they are critical in facilitating a sense of comfort and competency in users of the system. This environment is particularly critical in health care when computers are used in the context of care. One question that arises is, Do health care professionals control these information technology tools, or do the tools shape the activities, decisions, and attention of the health care professionals as users of technology? Both possibilities can be answered in the affirmative to some extent, but the former is the safest situation for health care (for an expanded discussion of this issue, see Chapter 19). If the health care professional needs to focus on the software or hardware because of difficult-to-use programs, confusing GUI schema, or sheer complexity in the programming, the health care professional's provision of care will suffer. It is critical that any software and hardware used in the practice milieu be expertly designed to facilitate care in a user-friendly, intuitive way. This is one reason that all health care professional practice areas are developing informatics experts, to be placed in positions of authority where they can facilitate the adoption of computer systems within health care environments. It is essential that the activities of the health care professionals are reflected well within the software that is used in the specific care setting. If health care professionals are knowledgeable about computers and related technologies, they will be able to provide meaningful data and information about how computer systems best work within their particular care areas.

In an ideal world, health care professionals would be able to use and interact with computer technologies effectively to enhance patient care. They would understand computer science and know how to harness its capabilities to benefit the profession and ultimately their patients.

Looking to the Future

The current trends toward **wearable technology**, smaller and faster handheld and portable computer systems, and high-quality video and voice-activated inventions will further facilitate the use of computers in all areas of health care practice and professional development. The field of computer science will continue to contribute to the evolving art and science of health care informatics. New trends promise to bring wide-sweeping and (it is hoped) positive changes to health care. Computers and other technologies have the potential to support a more patient-oriented or patient-centered health care system in which patients truly become active participants in their own health care planning and decisions. Mobile health technology, telehealth, sophisticated electronic health records, and next-generation technology are predicted to contribute to high-quality care and consultation within health care settings, including patients' homes and communities.

Computers are becoming more powerful yet more compact, which will contribute to the development of expanding technological initiatives. Some of these initiatives are described here. These innovations are some of the many computer and technological applications being used and developed. As health care professionals gain proficiency in capitalizing on the creative, time-saving, and interactive capabilities emerging from information technology research, the field of health care informatics will grow in similar proportions.

Voice-Activated Communicators

Voice-activated communicators are being used and new iterations developed by a variety of companies, including Vocera Communications. Vocera (2015) developed the Vocera B3000n Communication Badge that

> is a lightweight, voice-controlled, wearable device that enables instant two-way or one to many conversations using intuitive and simple commands. The Vocera Badge is widely used by mobile workers who need wearable devices that provide the convenience and expedience of being able to respond to calls without pressing a button (i.e. sterile operating rooms, nuclear power plants, hotel staff, security personnel). (para. 1)

These new technologies will permit health care professionals to use wireless, hands-free devices to communicate with one another and to record data. This technology is becoming a user-friendly and cost-effective way to increase clinical productivity.

Game and Simulation Technology

Game and simulation technology is offering realistic, innovative ways to teach content in general, including health care informatics concepts and skills. The same technology that powers video games is being used to create dynamic educational interfaces to help students learn about pathophysiology, care guidelines, and a host of other topics. Such applications are also very valuable for client education and health promotion materials. The "serious games" industry is growing since video game producers are now looking beyond mere entertainment to address public and private policy, management, and leadership issues and topics, including those related to health care. For example, the Games for Health Project, initiated by the Robert Wood Johnson Foundation (2015), is working on developing best practices to support innovation in health care training, messaging, and illness management. The Serious Games & VE Arcade & Showcase is presented at the annual meetings of the Society for Simulation in Healthcare (2015) (http://www.ssih.org) and is continuing to flourish with numerous products available to demonstrate.

Virtual Reality

Virtual reality is another technological breakthrough that is and will continue to influence health care education and professional development. Virtual reality is a three-dimensional, computer-generated "world" where a person (with the right equipment) can move about and interact as if he or she were actually in the visualized location. The person's senses are immersed in this virtual reality world using special gadgetry, such as head-mounted displays, data gloves, joysticks, and other hand tools. The equipment and special technology provides a sense of presence that is lacking in multimedia and other complex programs. According to Smith (2015), "It's crazy but true: Virtual reality will be a real thing in people's homes by this time next year" (para. 1). There are numerous products available. Virtual Realities (2015) stated that they provide "head mounted displays, head trackers, motion trackers, data gloves, 3D controllers, haptic devices, stereoscopic 3D displays, VR domes and virtual reality software. Virtual realities products are used by government, educational, industrial, medical and entertainment markets worldwide" (para. 1). Oculus VR (2015) developed Rift, which is the next generation of virtual reality products, and they are currently distributing the developer kits. HTC (2015) manufactures consumer electronics and developed the Vive headset. Smith believes that the Vive headset will be on the market soon, followed by Oculus Rift headsets and Sony's Morpheus headset for their PlayStation 4.

Mobile Devices

Mobile devices will be used more by health care professionals both at the point of care and in planning, documenting, interacting with the interprofessional health care team, and research. They will be using such powerful wearable technologies as nano-based diagnostic sensors in their personal lives, just as their patients do. Health care professionals will also be generating their own data streams and receiving data from the wearable and mobile devices their patients use. Silbershatz et al. (2013) stated that Apple IOS and Google Android are "currently dominating mobile computing" (p. 37). Perry (2015) stated that it is "estimated more than 177 million wearable devices will be in use by 2018" (para. 5). Cisco (2014) reported that "by the year 2020, the majority of Generation X and Y professionals believe that smartphones and wearable devices will be the workforce's most important 'connected' device—while the laptop remains the workplace device of choice" (para. 1). Data are truly at our fingertips.

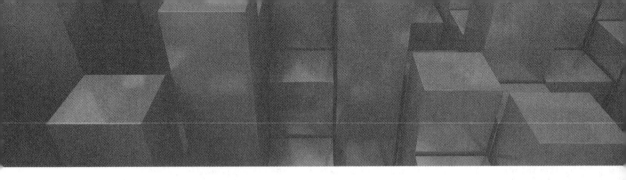

Summary

The field of computer science is one of the fastest-growing disciplines. Astonishing innovations in computer hardware, software, and architecture have occurred over the past few decades, and there are no indications that this trend will come to a halt anytime soon. Computers have increased in speed, accuracy, and efficiency yet now cost less and have reduced physical size compared to their forebears. These trends are predicted to continue. Current computer hardware and software serve as vital and valuable tools for both health care professionals and patients to engage in onscreen and online activities that provide rich access to data and information. Productivity, creativity, and communication software tools also enable health care professionals to work with computers to further foster knowledge acquisition and development. Wide access to vast stores of information and knowledge shared by others facilitates the emergence of wisdom in users, which can then be applied to health care in meaningful and creative ways. It is imperative that health care professionals become discerning yet skillful users of computer technology to apply the principles of health care informatics to practice and to contribute to their profession's ever-growing body of knowledge.

Working Wisdom

Since the beginning of their professions, health care professionals have applied their ingenuity, resourcefulness, and professional awareness of what works to adapt technology and objects to support patient care, usually with the intention of promoting efficiency but also in support of patient comfort and healing. This resourcefulness could also be applied effectively to the adaptation of information technology within the care environment to ensure that the technology truly does serve patients and the interprofessional health care team.

Consider this question: "How can you develop competency in using the various computer hardware and software not only to promote efficient patient care and to develop yourself professionally but also to further the development of your profession's body of knowledge?"

Thought-Provoking Questions

1. How can knowledge of computer hardware and software help health care professionals participate in information technology adoption decisions in the practice area?
2. How can new computer software help health care professionals engage in professional development, collaboration, and knowledge dissemination activities at their own pace and leisure?

Apply Your Knowledge

You are a member of the health care professional/information technology council. The council has been charged by the administration with researching the configuration of various portable computer devices. Each member of the council is expected to select and examine one portable computer device. Search the Internet and select a portable computer device to evaluate. This may be any type of portable computer device, including (but not limited to) a laptop, a notebook, and a tablet.

1. Identify the specific computer device, the model you are evaluating, and the URL for the device description providing the information for your responses to the questions.
2. What processor does it have?
   a. What is a processor?
   b. Why is it important?
   c. How much speed does this processor have?
3. How much RAM does it have?
   a. What is RAM?
   b. Why is it important to know this feature and the available options when choosing this device for multimedia purposes?
   c. What type of RAM does it have?
4. What is the size of the hard drive?
   a. What is a hard drive?
   b. Why is it important to know this feature?
5. What is the difference between system and application software?
   a. Identify and describe one system software that for this device.
   b. Identify and describe one application software for this device.

Additional Resources

BBC Absolute Beginner's Guide to Using Your Computer: A WebWise Guide. http://www.bbc.co.uk/webwise/abbeg/abbeg.shtml

BBC's Computer Tutor: The BBC's Guide to Using a Computer. http://www.bbc.co.uk/webwise/topics/your-computer

Laptop Buying Guide: 8 Essential Tips http://blog.laptopmag.com/laptop-buying-guide

Nursing Informatics and the Foundation of Knowledge http://go.jblearning.com/mcgonigle

Society for Simulation in Healthcare http://www.ssih.org

References

Bandura, A. (2002). Growing primacy of human agency in adaptation and change in the electronic era. *European Psychologist, 7*(1), 2–16.

Cisco. (2014). Working from Mars with an Internet brain implant: Cisco study shows how technology will shape the "Future of Work." http://newsroom.cisco.com/press-release-content?type=webcontent&articleId=1528226

Evans, D. (2010). Introduction to computing: Explorations in language, logic, and machines. http://www.computingbook.org

Hennessy, J., & Patterson, D. (2006). *Computer architecture: A quantitative approach* (4th ed.). San Francisco: Morgan Kaufmann.

HTC. (2015). HTC's VR vision. Finally, the future. http://www.htcvr.com

Intel Corporation. (2008). Concealing complexity. Technology and research. http://techresearch.intel.com/articles/Exploratory/1430.htm

Mahmood, M. (2003). *Advanced topics in end user computing.* Hershey, PA: Idea Group.

Null, L., & Lobor, J. (2006). *The essentials of computer organization and architecture* (2nd ed.). Sudbury, MA: Jones and Bartlett.

Oculus VR. (2015) Step into the Rift. https://www.oculus.com/en-us/rift

Perry, L. (2015). Evolving millennial connections using wearables. http://blogs.cisco.com/tag/wearable-technology

Richards, J. A. (2001). Nursing in a digital age. *Nursing Economic$, 19*(1), 6–12.

Robert Wood Johnson Foundation. (2015). Games for health. http://gamesforhealth.org/about

Sarkar, N. (2006). *Tools for teaching computer networking and hardware concepts.* Hershey, PA: Idea Group.

Silbershatz, A., Baer Galvin, P., & Gagne, G. (2013). *Operating system concepts* (9th ed.). Hoboken, NJ: John Wiley & Sons. http://sist.sysu.edu.cn/~isscwli/OSRef/Abraham%20Silberschatz-Operating%20System%20Concepts%20(9th,2012.12).pdf

Smith, D. (2015). 3 virtual reality products will dominate our living rooms by this time next year. http://www.businessinsider.com/virtual-reality-is-getting-real-2015-5

Society for Simulation in Healthcare. (2015). International Meeting for Simulation in Healthcare (IMSH). http://www.ssih.org/Events/IMSH-2016

Virtual Realities. (2015). Worldwide distributor of virtual reality. https://www.vrealities.com

Vocera. (2015). Vocera badge. http://www.vocera.com/product/vocera-badge

Introduction to Cognitive Science and Cognitive Informatics

Dee McGonigle and Kathleen Mastrian

OBJECTIVES

1. Describe cognitive science.
2. Assess how the human mind processes and generates information and knowledge.
3. Explore cognitive informatics.
4. Examine artificial intelligence and its relationship to cognitive science and computer science.

Introduction

Cognitive science is the fourth of four basic building blocks used to understand informatics. Section I began by examining disciplinary science, information science, and computer science and considering how each relates to and helps one understand the concept of informatics. This chapter explores the building blocks of cognitive science, **cognitive informatics** (CI), and **artificial intelligence** (AI).

Throughout the centuries, cognitive science has intrigued philosophers and educators alike. Beginning in Greece, the ancient philosophers sought to comprehend how the **mind** works and what the nature of **knowledge** is. This age-old quest to unravel the processes inherent in the working **brain** has been undertaken by some of the greatest minds in history. However, it was only about 50 years ago that computer operations and actions were linked to cognitive science, meaning theories of the mind, intellect, or brain. This association led to the expansion of cognitive science to examine the complete array of cognitive processes, from lower-level perceptions to higher-level critical thinking, logical analysis, and reasoning.

Key Terms
Artificial intelligence
Brain
Cognitive informatics
Cognitive science
Computer science
Connectionism
Decision making
Empiricism
Epistemology
Human mental workload
Intelligence
Intuition
Knowledge
Logic
Memory
Mind
Neuroscience
Perception
Problem solving
Psychology
Rationalism
Reasoning
Wisdom

The focus of this chapter is the impact of cognitive science on health informatics (HI). This section provides the reader with an introduction and overview of cognitive science, the nature of knowledge, wisdom, and AI as they apply to the Foundation of Knowledge model and HI. The applications to HI include problem solving, decision support systems, usability issues, user-centered interfaces and systems, and the development and use of terminologies.

Cognitive Science

The interdisciplinary field of cognitive science studies the mind, intelligence, and behavior from an information-processing perspective. According to Wikipedia (2013), "The term cognitive science was coined by Christopher Longuet-Higgins in his 1973 commentary on the Lighthill report, which concerned the then-current state of artificial intelligence research" (para. 36). The Cognitive Science Society and the *Cognitive Science Journal* date back to 1980 (Cognitive Science Society, 2005). Their interdisciplinary base arises from psychology, philosophy, neuroscience, computer science, linguistics, biology, and physics; covers memory, attention, perception, reasoning, language, mental ability, and computational models of cognitive processes; and explores the nature of the mind, knowledge representation, language, problem solving, decision making, and the social factors influencing the design and use of technology. Simply put, cognitive science is the study of the mind and how information is processed in the mind. As described in the *Stanford Encyclopedia of Philosophy* (2010),

> The central hypothesis of cognitive science is that thinking can best be understood in terms of representational structures in the mind and computational procedures that operate on those structures. While there is much disagreement about the nature of the representations and computations that constitute thinking, the central hypothesis is general enough to encompass the current range of thinking in cognitive science, including connectionist theories which model thinking using artificial neural networks. (para. 9)

Connectionism is a component of cognitive science that uses computer modeling through artificial neural networks to explain human intellectual abilities. Neural networks can be thought of as interconnected simple processing devices or simplified models of the brain and nervous system that consist of a considerable number of elements or units (analogs of neurons) linked together in a pattern of connections (analogs of synapses). A neural network that models the entire nervous system would have three types of units: (1) input units (analogs of sensory neurons), which receive information to be processed; (2) hidden units (analogs to all of the other neurons, not sensory or motor), which work in between input and output units; and (3) output units (analogs of motor neurons), where the outcomes or results of the processing are found.

Connectionism is rooted in how computation occurs in the brain and nervous system or biologic neural networks. On their own, single neurons have minimal computational capacity. When interconnected with other neurons, however, they have immense computational power. The connectionism system or model learns by modifying the connections linking the neurons. Artificial neural networks are unique computer programs designed to model or simulate their biologic analogs, the neurons of the brain. The mind is frequently compared to a computer, and experts in computer science strive to understand how the mind processes data and information. In contrast, experts in cognitive science model human thinking using artificial networks provided by computers—an endeavor sometimes referred to as AI. How does the mind process all of the inputs received? Which items and in which ways are things stored or placed into memory, accessed, augmented, changed, reconfigured, and restored? Cognitive science provides the scaffolding for the analysis and modeling of complicated, multifaceted human performance and has a tremendous effect on the issues impacting informatics.

The end user is the focus of this activity because the concern is with enhancing the performance in the workplace; in health care, the end user could be the actual clinician in the clinical setting, and cognitive science can enhance the integration and implementation of the technologies being designed to facilitate this knowledge worker with the ultimate goal of improving patient care delivery. Technologies change rapidly, and this evolution must be harnessed for the clinician at the bedside. To do this at all levels of clinical practice, one must understand the nature of knowledge, the information and knowledge needed, and the means by which the health care professional processes this information and knowledge in the situational context.

Sources of Knowledge

Just as philosophers have questioned the nature of knowledge, so they have also strived to determine how knowledge arises because the origins of knowledge can help one understand its nature. How do people come to know what they know about themselves, others, and their world? There are many viewpoints on this issue, both scientific and nonscientific.

According to Holt (2006), "There are two competing traditions concerning the ultimate source of our knowledge: **empiricism** and **rationalism**" (para. 3). Empiricism is based on knowledge being derived from experiences or senses, whereas rationalism contends that "some of our knowledge is derived from reason alone and that reason plays an important role in the acquisition of all of our knowledge" (para. 5). Empiricists do not recognize innate knowledge, whereas rationalists believe that reason is more essential in the acquisition of knowledge than the senses.

Three sources of knowledge have been identified: (1) instinct, (2) reason, and (3) intuition. Instinct is when one reacts without reason, such as when a car is heading toward a pedestrian and he jumps out of the way without thinking. Instinct is found in both humans and animals, whereas reason and intuition are found only in humans. Reason "collects facts, generalizes, reasons out from cause to effect, from effect to cause, from premises to conclusions, from propositions to proofs" (Sivananda, 2004, para. 4). **Intuition** is a way of acquiring knowledge that cannot be obtained by inference, deduction, observation, reason, analysis, or experience. Intuition was described by Aristotle as "a leap of understanding, a grasping of a larger concept unreachable by other intellectual means, yet fundamentally an intellectual process" (Shallcross & Sisk, 1999, para. 4).

Some believe that knowledge is acquired through perception and logic. **Perception** is the process of acquiring knowledge about the environment or situation by obtaining, interpreting, selecting, and organizing sensory information from seeing, hearing, touching, tasting, and smelling. **Logic** is a "science that deals with the principles and criteria of validity of inference and demonstration: the science of the formal principles of **reasoning**" (*Merriam-Webster Online Dictionary*, 2007, para. 1). Acquiring knowledge through logic requires reasoned action to make valid inferences.

The sources of knowledge provide a variety of inputs, throughputs, and outputs through which knowledge is processed. No matter how one believes knowledge is acquired, it is important to be able to explain or describe those beliefs, communicate those thoughts, enhance shared understanding, and discover the nature of knowledge.

Nature of Knowledge

Epistemology is the study of the nature and origin of knowledge—that is, what it means to know. Everyone has a conception of what it means to know based on their own perceptions, education, and experiences; knowledge is a part of life that continues to grow with the person. Thus, a definition of knowledge is somewhat difficult to agree on because it reflects the viewpoints, beliefs, and understandings of the person or group defining it. Some people believe that knowledge is part of a sequential learning process resembling a pyramid, with data on the bottom, rising to information, then knowledge, and finally wisdom. Others believe that knowledge emerges from interactions and experience with the environment, and still others think that it is religiously or culturally bound. Knowledge acquisition is thought to be an internal process derived through thinking and cognition or an external process from senses, observations, studies, and interactions. Descartes's important premise "called 'the way of ideas' represents the attempt in epistemology to provide a foundation for our knowledge of the external world (as well as our knowledge of the past and of other minds) in the mental experiences of the individual" (*Encyclopedia Britannica*, 2007, para. 4).

For the purpose of this text, knowledge is defined as the awareness and understanding of a set of information and ways that information can be made useful to support a specific task or arrive at a decision. It abounds with others' thoughts and information or consists of information that is synthesized so that relationships are identified and formalized.

How Knowledge and Wisdom are used in Decision Making

The reason for collecting and building data, information, and knowledge is to be able to make informed, judicious, prudent, and intelligent decisions. When one considers the nature of knowledge and its applications, one must also examine the concept of wisdom. **Wisdom** has been defined in numerous ways:

- Knowledge applied in a practical way or translated into actions
- The use of knowledge and experience to heighten common sense and insight to exercise sound judgment in practical matters
- The highest form of common sense resulting from accumulated knowledge or erudition (deep, thorough learning) or enlightenment (education that results in understanding and the dissemination of knowledge)
- The ability to apply valuable and viable knowledge, experience, understanding, and insight while being prudent and sensible
- Focused on our own minds
- The synthesis of our experience, insight, understanding, and knowledge
- The appropriate use of knowledge to solve human problems

In essence, wisdom entails knowing when and how to apply knowledge. The decision-making process revolves around knowledge and wisdom. It is through efforts to understand the nature of knowledge and its evolution to wisdom that one can conceive of, build, and implement informatics tools that enhance and mimic the mind's processes to facilitate **decision making** and job performance.

Cognitive Informatics

Wang (2003) describes CI as an emerging transdisciplinary field of study that bridges the gap in understanding regarding how information is processed in the mind and in the computer. Computing and informatics theories can be applied to help elucidate the information processing of the brain, and cognitive and neurologic sciences can likewise be applied to build better and more efficient computer processing systems. Wang suggests that the common issue among the human knowledge sciences is the drive to develop an understanding of natural intelligence and human problem solving.

The Pacific Northwest National Laboratory (PNNL), an organization operated on behalf of the U.S. Department of Energy, suggests that the disciplines of neuroscience, linguistics, AI, and psychology constitute this field. PNNL (2008) defines CI as "the multidisciplinary study of cognition and information sciences, which investigates human information processing mechanisms and processes and their engineering applications in computing" (para. 1). CI helps to bridge this gap by systematically exploring the mechanisms of the brain and mind and exploring specifically how information is acquired, represented, remembered, retrieved, generated, and communicated. This dawning of understanding can then be applied and modeled in AI situations, resulting in more efficient computing applications. Wang explains further:

> Cognitive informatics attempts to solve problems in two connected areas in a bidirectional and multidisciplinary approach. In one direction, CI uses informatics and computing techniques to investigate cognitive science problems, such as memory, learning, and reasoning; in the other direction, CI uses cognitive theories to investigate the problems in informatics, computing, and software engineering. (p. 120)

Principles of CI and an understanding of how humans interact with computers can be used to build systems that better meet the needs of users. Longo (2015) discusses **human mental workload** (MWL) as a key component in effective system design. He states, "At a low level of MWL, people may often experience annoyance and frustration when processing information. On the other hand, a high level can also be both problematic and even dangerous, as it leads to confusion, decreases performance in information processing and increases the chances of errors and mistakes" (p. 758).

Cognitive Informatics and Health Care Practice

According to Mastrian (2008), the recognition of the potential application of principles of cognitive science to informatics is relatively new. We refer briefly to nursing informatics (NI) here because the nursing profession is an early adopter of informatics. The traditional and widely accepted definition of NI advanced by Graves and Corcoran (1989) is that NI is a combination of nursing science, computer science, and information science used to describe the processes nurses use to manage data, information, and knowledge in clinical practice. Turley (1996) proposed the addition of cognitive science to this mix, as nurse scientists are seen to strive to capture and explain the influence of the human brain on data, information, and knowledge processing and to elucidate how these factors in turn affect clinical practice decision making. The need to include cognitive sciences is imperative as researchers attempt to model and support clinical practice decision making in complex computer programs.

In 2003, Wang proposed the term *cognitive informatics* to signify the branch of information and computer sciences that investigates and explains information processing in the human brain. The science of CI grew out of interest in AI as computer scientists developed computer programs that mimic the information processing and knowledge generation functions of the human brain. CI bridges the gap between artificial and natural intelligence and enhances the understanding of how information is acquired, processed, stored, and retrieved so that these functions can be modeled in computer software.

What does this have to do with clinical practice? At its very core, clinical practice requires **problem solving** and decision making. Health care professionals help people manage their responses to illnesses and identify ways that they can maintain or restore their health. During the care delivery process, health care professionals must first recognize that there is a problem to be solved, identify the nature of the problem, pull information from knowledge stores that is relevant to the problem, decide on a plan of action, implement the plan, and evaluate the effectiveness of the interventions. When a professional has practiced the science of his or her discipline for some time, he or she tends to do these processes automatically; it is instinctively known what needs to be done to intervene in the problem. What happens, however, if the health care professional faces a situation or problem for which he or she has no experience on which to draw? The ever-increasing acuity and complexity of patient situations, coupled with the explosion of information in health care, has fueled the development of decision support software embedded in the electronic health record. This software models the human and natural decision-making processes of professionals in an artificial program. Such systems can help decision makers consider the consequences of different courses of action before implementing the action. They also provide stores of information that the user may not be aware of and can use to choose the best course of action and ultimately make a better decision in unfamiliar circumstances.

Decision support programs continue to evolve as research in the fields of cognitive science, AI, and CI is continuously generated and then applied to the development of these systems. Health care professionals must embrace—not resist—these advances as support and enhancement of the practice of their disciplinary science.

What is Artificial Intelligence?

The field of AI deals with the conception, development, and implementation of informatics tools based on intelligent technologies. This field captures the complex processes of human thought and intelligence.

Herbert Simon believes that the field of AI could have two functions: "One is to use the power of computers to augment human thinking, just as we use motors to augment human or horse power. The other is to use a computer's artificial intelligence to understand how humans think in a humanoid way" (Association for the Advancement of Artificial Intelligence [AAAI], 2007a, para. 1). According to the AAAI (2007b), AI is the "scientific understanding of the mechanisms underlying thought and intelligent behavior and their embodiment in machines" (para. 2).

John McCarthy, one of the men credited with founding the field of AI in the 1950s, stated that AI "is the science and engineering of making intelligent machines, especially intelligent computer programs. It is related to the similar task of using computers to understand human intelligence, but AI does not have to confine itself to methods that are biologically observable" (AAAI, 2007b, para. 4).

Lamont (2007) interviewed Ray Kurzweil, a visionary who defined AI as "the ability to perform a task that is normally performed by natural intelligence, particularly human natural intelligence. We have in fact artificial intelligence that can perform many tasks that used to require—and could only be done by—human intelligence" (para. 6). The intelligence factor is extremely important in AI and has been defined by McCarthy as "the computational part of the ability to achieve goals in the world. Varying kinds and degrees of intelligence occur in people, many animals, and some machines" (AAAI, 2007b, para. 4).

The challenge of this field rests in capturing, mimicking, and creating the complex processes of the mind in informatics tools, including software, hardware, and other machine technologies, with the goal that the tool be able to initiate and generate its own mechanical thought processing. The brain's processing is highly intricate and complicated. This complexity is reflected in Cohn's (2006) comment that "artificial intelligence is 50 years old this summer, and while computers can beat the world's best chess players, we still can't get them to think like a 4-year-old" (para. 1). AI uses cognitive science and computer science to replicate and generate human intelligence. This field will continue to evolve and produce artificially intelligent tools to enhance the personal and professional lives of health care professionals.

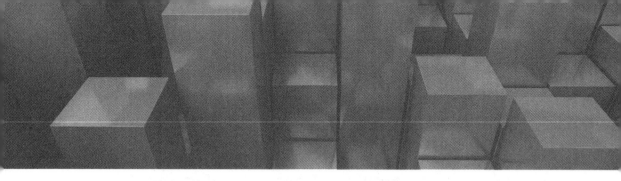

Summary

Cognitive science is the interdisciplinary field that studies the mind, intelligence, and behavior from an information-processing perspective. CI is a field of study that bridges the gap in understanding regarding how information is processed in the mind and in the computer. Computing and informatics theories can be applied to help elucidate the information processing of the brain, and cognitive and neurologic sciences can likewise be applied to build better and more efficient computer processing systems.

AI is the field that deals with the conception, development, and implementation of informatics tools based on intelligent technologies. This field captures the complex processes of human thought and intelligence. AI uses cognitive science and computer science to replicate and generate human intelligence.

The sources of knowledge, nature of knowledge, and rapidly changing technologies must be harnessed by clinicians to enhance their patient care delivery. Therefore, we must understand the nature of knowledge, the information and knowledge needed, and the means by which health care professionals process this information and knowledge in their own situational context. The reason for collecting and building data, information, and knowledge is to be able to build wisdom—that is, the ability to apply valuable and viable knowledge, experience, understanding, and insight while being prudent and sensible. Wisdom is focused on our own minds, the synthesis of our experience, insight, understanding, and knowledge. Health care professionals must use their wisdom and make informed, judicious, prudent, and intelligent decisions while providing care to patients, families, and communities. Cognitive science, CI, and AI will continue to evolve to help build knowledge and wisdom.

Thought-Provoking Questions

1. How would you describe CI? Reflect on a plan of care that you have developed for a patient. How could CI be used to create tools to help with or support this important work?
2. Think of a clinical setting with which you are familiar and envision how AI tools might be applied in this setting. Are there any current tools in use? Which current or emerging tools would enhance practice in this setting and why?
3. Use your creative mind to think of a tool of the future based on CI that would support your disciplinary practice.

Apply Your Knowledge

Two occupational therapist assistants, Mary, age 23, and Ann, age 48, are working together in a rehabilitation unit of a local hospital. The hospital has recently merged with a larger medical system and has initiated computer-based critical pathways as a progressive phase toward an expanded interdisciplinary electronic health record to be used with the planned patient smart rooms. All professionals on the rehabilitation unit have received training with the mobile device application—a critical pathway decision-making and documentation system—and the administration is planning a mock go-live on the rehabilitation unit today. All professionals on the unit are carrying mobile devices to be used for patient assessment and documentation.

Mary is excited about the mock go-live. She immediately begins working with her mobile device when completing her clinical assessments. Ann feels increasingly anxious as the morning progresses. Even though she has access to paper-based crosswalks of clinical documentation available in each patient room and at the nurse's station to guide her with documentation, Ann is having a difficult time concentrating and realizes she is getting behind in her patient care. During break, Mary is anxious to discuss the changes and the efficiency with which she can complete her patient care interventions and her documentation. She does not have a chance to say anything because Ann immediately begins complaining about her day. Ann is angry and complains bitterly about the lack of caring for patients by administration and the diverting of much-needed patient care funds to technology-focused purchases that have nothing to do with patients. She continues to complain about her lack of desire to learn all of this new technology.

At the end of the day, Mary goes home and tells her significant other that she may start looking for a new job outside of the hospital. The negativity in her work environment and the aversion to change is difficult to deal with on an ongoing basis.

At the end of the day, Ann goes home late from work after finally completing her work and tells her significant other that she may get out of health care. "Health care is not what it used to be," she explains. "Nobody cares about the patient."

Discuss and reflect on the following information from Chapters 1 to 4:

1. Mary and Ann represent two different generations. Identify the generation that each represents and discuss how this influences each professional's reaction to the introduction of technology/computers in patient care.
2. Describe the implications for practice in this setting, based on the reactions of both individuals. (Think about how technology may disrupt the typical clinical experience trajectory for these therapists.)
3. Discuss this scenario in relation to informatics competencies and CI.
4. If you were in this situation as Mary or Ann, what recommendations would you have for the administrators in an attempt to retain you and increase your satisfaction in the current work setting?

References

Association for the Advancement of Artificial Intelligence. (2007a). AI overview. http://www.aaai
.org/AITopics/html/overview.html

Association for the Advancement of Artificial Intelligence. (2007b). Cognitive science. http://
www.aaai.org/aitopics/pmwiki/pmwiki.php/AITopics/CognitiveScience

Cognitive Science Society. (2005). CSJ archive. http://www.cogsci.rpi.edu/CSJarchive/1980v04
/index.html

Cohn, D. (2006). AI reaches the golden years. http://www.wired.com/news/technology/0,71389-0
.html

Encyclopedia Britannica. (2007). Epistemology. http://www.britannica.com/eb/article-247960
/epistemology

Graves, J., & Corcoran, S. (1989). The study of nursing informatics. *Image: Journal of Nursing
Scholarship, 21*(4), 227–230.

Holt, T. (2006). Sources of knowledge. http://www.theoryofknowledge.info/sourcesofknowledge
.html

Lamont, I. (2007). The grill: Ray Kurzweil talks about "augmented reality" and the singularity. http://www.computerworld.com/action/article.do?command=viewArticleBasic&
articleId=306176

Longo, L. (2015). A defeasible reasoning framework for human mental workload representation and assessment. *Behaviour and Information Technology, 34*(8), 758–786. doi:
10.1080/0144929X.2015.1015166

Mastrian, K. (2008, February). Invited editorial: Cognitive informatics and nursing practice.
Online Journal of Nursing Informatics, 12(1). http://ojni.org/12_1/kathy.html

Merriam-Webster Online Dictionary. (2007). Logic. http://www.merriam-webster.com
/dictionary/logic

Pacific Northwest National Laboratory, U.S. Department of Energy. (2008). Cognitive informatics. http://www.pnl.gov/coginformatics

Shallcross, D. J., & Sisk, D. A. (1999). What is intuition? In T. Arnold (Ed.), *Hyponoesis glossary:
Intuition.* http://www.hyponoesis.org/Glossary/Definition/Intuition

Sivananda, S. (2004). Four sources of knowledge. http://www.dlshq.org/messages/knowledge.htm

Stanford Encyclopedia of Philosophy. (2010). Cognitive science. http://plato.stanford.edu/entries
/cognitive-science

Turley, J. (1996). Toward a model for nursing informatics. *Image: Journal of Nursing Scholarship,
28*(4), 309–313.

Wang, Y. (2003). Cognitive informatics: A new transdisciplinary research field. *Brain and Mind,
4*(2), 115–127.

Wikipedia. (2013). Cognitive science. http://en.wikipedia.org/wiki/Cognitive_science

Ethical and Legal Aspects of Health Informatics

Kathleen Mastrian, Dee McGonigle,
and Kathleen M. Gialanella

OBJECTIVES

1. Recognize ethical issues in health informatics.
2. Examine ethical implications of health informatics.
3. Evaluate professional responsibilities for the ethical use of health informatics technology.
4. Explore the ethical model for ethical decision making.
5. Describe the purposes of the Health Information Technology for Economic and Clinical Health (HITECH) Act of 2009.
6. Explore how the HITECH Act is enhancing the security and privacy protections of the Health Insurance Portability and Accountability Act (HIPAA) of 1996.
7. Determine how the HITECH Act and its impact on HIPAA apply to your practice.

Introduction

Those who followed the actual events of *Apollo 13* or who were entertained by the movie of the same name (Howard, 1995) watched the astronauts strive against all odds to bring their crippled spaceship back to Earth. The speed of their travel was incomprehensible to most viewers, and the task of bringing the spaceship back to Earth seemed nearly impossible. They were experiencing a crisis never imagined by the experts at NASA, and they made up their survival plan moment by moment. What brought them back to Earth safely? Surely, credit must be given to the technology and the spaceship's ability to withstand the trauma it experienced. Most amazing, however, were the traditional nontechnological tools, skills, and supplies

Key Terms
Access
Agency for Healthcare Research and Quality
Alternative actions
American National Standards Institute
American Recovery and Reinvestment Act
Antiprinciplism
Application (app)
Autonomy
Beneficence
Bioethics
Bioinformatics
Care ethics
Casuist approach
Centers for Medicare and Medicaid Services
Certified EHR technology
Civil monetary penalties
Compliance
(continues)

that were used in new and different ways to stabilize the spacecraft's environment and keep the astronauts safe while traveling toward their uncertain future.

This sense of constancy in the midst of change serves to stabilize experience in many different life events and contributes to the survival during crisis and change. This rhythmic process is also vital to the health care system's stability and survival in the presence of the rapidly changing events and challenges associated with the Knowledge Age. No one can dispute the fact that the Knowledge Age is changing health care in ways that will not be fully recognized and understood for years. The change is paradigmatic, and every expert who addresses this change reminds health care professionals of the need to go with the flow of rapid change or be left behind.

As with any paradigm shift, a new way of viewing the world brings with it some of the enduring values of the previous worldview. For example, as health care journeys into the brave new world of digital communications, it brings some familiar tools and skills recognized in the form of **values**, such as privacy, **confidentiality**, autonomy, and nonmaleficence. Although these basic values remain unchanged, the standards for living out these values will take on new meaning as health professionals confront new and different moral dilemmas brought on by the adoption of technological tools for information management and knowledge development. Ethical decision-making frameworks will remain constant, but the context for examining these moral issues or ethical dilemmas will become increasingly complex.

This chapter highlights some familiar ethical concepts to consider on the challenging journey into the increasingly complex future of health care informatics. Ethics and bioethics are briefly defined, and the evolution of ethical approaches from the Hippocratic ethic era to principlism to the current anti-principlism movement of ethical **decision making** is examined. New and challenging ethical dilemmas are surfacing in the venture into the unfolding era of health care informatics.

This chapter also covers key aspects of laws specific to health informatics. We provide an overview of the Health Information Technology for Economic and Clinical Health Act (HITECH) Act, including the Medicare and Medicaid **health information technology** (HIT) provisions of the law. Health care professionals need to be familiar with the goals and purposes of this law, know how it enhances the security and privacy protections of the **Health Insurance Portability and Accountability Act** (HIPAA) of 1996, and appreciate how it otherwise affects practice in the emerging age of **electronic health records** (EHRs). Readers are challenged to think constantly and carefully about practice ethics and the legal aspects of protecting health information.

Ethics

Ethics is a process of systematically examining varying viewpoints related to moral questions of right and wrong. **Ethicists** have defined the term in a variety of ways, with each reflecting a basic theoretical philosophic perspective.

Beauchamp and Childress (1994) refer to ethics as a generic term for various ways of understanding and examining the moral life. Ethical approaches to this examination may be normative, presenting standards of right or **good** action; descriptive, reporting what people believe and how they act; or explorative, analyzing the concepts and methods of ethics.

Husted and Husted (1995) emphasize a practice-based ethics, stating that "ethics examines the ways men and women can exercise their power in order to bring about human benefit—the ways in which one can act in order to bring about the conditions of happiness" (p. 3).

Velasquez, Andre, Shanks, and Myer (1987) posed the question "What is ethics?" and answered it with the following two-part response: "First, ethics refers to well-based standards of right and wrong that prescribe what humans ought to do, usually in terms of **rights**, obligations, benefits to society, fairness, or specific virtues" (para. 10). "Secondly, ethics refers to the study and development of one's ethical standards" (para. 11).

Regardless of the theoretical definition, common characteristics regarding ethics are its dialectical, goal-oriented approach to answering questions that have the potential for multiple acceptable answers.

Bioethics

Bioethics is defined as the study and formulation of health care ethics. Bioethics takes on relevant ethical problems experienced by health care providers in the provision of care to individuals and groups. Husted and Husted (1995) stated the fundamental background of bioethics that forms its essential nature:

1. The nature and needs of humans as living, thinking beings
2. The purpose and function of the health care system in a human society
3. An increased cultural awareness of human beings' essential moral status (p. 7)

Bioethics emerged in the 1970s as health care began to change its focus from a mechanistic approach of treating disease to a more holistic approach of treating people with illnesses. As technology advanced, recognition and acknowledgment of the rights and the needs of individuals and groups receiving this high-tech care also increased.

In today's technologically savvy health care environment, patients are being prescribed **applications** (apps) for their **smartphones** instead of medications in some clinical practices. Patients' smartphones are being used to interact with them in new ways and to monitor and assess their health in some cases. With apps and add-ons, for example, a provider can see the patient's ECG immediately, or the patient can monitor his or her ECG and send it to the provider as necessary. A sensor attached to the patient's mobile device could monitor blood glucose levels and many other physiologic and psychologic parameters. New health apps are developed and released every day.

Key Terms (continued)

Office of the National
   Coordinator for
   Health Information
   Technology
Open Systems
   Interconnection
Operations
Patient-centered care
Payment
Policy
Principlism
Privacy
Protected health
   information
Qualified electronic
   health record
Rights
Sarbanes-Oxley Act
Security
Self-control
Smartphones
Social media
Standard
Standards-developing
   organizations
Treatment
Truth
Uncertainty
Values
Veracity
Virtue
Virtue ethics
Wisdom

We are just beginning to realize the vast potential of these mobile devices—and the threats they sometimes pose. **Google Glass**, for example, can take photos and videos (Stern, 2013) without anyone knowing that this is occurring; in the health care environment, such a technological advancement can violate patients' privacy and confidentiality. Add these evolving developments to health care providers' engagement in social media use with their patients, and it becomes clear that personal and ethical dilemmas abound for health care professionals in the new über-connected world.

Ethical Dilemmas and Morals

Ethical dilemmas arise when moral issues raise questions that cannot be answered with a simple, clearly defined rule, fact, or authoritative view. **Morals** refer to social convention about right and wrong human conduct that is so widely shared that it forms a stable (although usually incomplete) communal consensus (Beauchamp & Childress, 1994). **Moral dilemmas** arise with **uncertainty**, as is the case when some evidence a person is confronted with indicates an action is morally right and other evidence indicates that this action is morally wrong. Uncertainty is stressful and, in the face of inconclusive evidence on both sides of the dilemma, causes the person to question what he or she should do. Sometimes the individual concludes that based on his or her moral beliefs, he or she cannot act. Uncertainty also arises from unanticipated effects or unforeseeable behavioral responses to actions or the lack of action. Adding uncertainty to the situational factors and personal beliefs that must be considered creates a need for an ethical decision-making model to help one choose the best action.

Ethical Decision Making

Ethical decision making refers to the process of making informed choices about ethical dilemmas based on a set of standards differentiating right from wrong. This type of decision making reflects an understanding of the principles and standards of ethical decision making, as well as the philosophic approaches to ethical decision making, and it requires a systematic framework for addressing the complex and often controversial moral questions.

As the high-speed era of digital communications evolves, the rights and the needs of individuals and groups will be of the utmost concern to all health care professionals. The changing meaning of communication, for example, will bring with it new concerns among health care professionals about protecting patients' rights of confidentiality, privacy, and autonomy. Systematic and flexible ethical decision-making abilities will be essential for all health care professionals.

Notably, the concept of nonmaleficence ("do no **harm**") will be broadened to include those individuals and groups whom one may never see in person but with whom one will enter into a professional relationship of trust and care. Mack (2000) has discussed the popularity of individuals seeking information online instead of directly from their health care providers and the effects this behavior has on patient–provider relationships. He is emphatic in his reminder that "organizations and individuals that provide health information on the Internet have obligations to be trustworthy, provide high-quality content, protect users' privacy, and adhere to standards of best practices for online commerce and online professional services in healthcare" (p. 41).

Makus (2001) suggested that both autonomy and justice are enhanced with universal access to information but that tensions may be created in patient–provider relationships as a result of this access to outside information. Health care workers need to realize that they are no longer the sole providers and gatekeepers of health-related information; ideally, they should embrace information empowerment and suggest websites to patients that contain reliable, accurate, and relevant information.

It is clear that patients' increasing use of the Internet for health care information may prompt entirely new types of ethical issues, such as who is responsible if a patient is harmed as a result of following online health advice. Derse and Miller (2008) discuss this issue extensively and conclude that a clear line separates information and practice. Practice occurs when there is direct or personal communication between the provider and the patient, when the advice is tailored to the patient's specific health issue, and when there is a reasonable expectation that the patient will act in reliance on the information.

A summit sponsored by the Internet Healthcare Coalition (http://www.ihealthcoalition.org) in 2000 developed the E-Health Code of Ethics (eHealth code, n.d.), which includes eight standards for the ethical development of health-related Internet sites: (1) candor, (2) honesty, (3) quality, (4) informed consent, (5) privacy, (6) professionalism, (7) responsible partnering, and (8) accountability. For more information about each of these standards, access the full discussion of the E-Health Code of Ethics (http://www.ihealthcoalition.org/ehealth-code).

It is important to realize that the standards for ethical development of health-related Internet sites are voluntary; there is no overseer perusing these sites and issuing safety alerts for users. Although some sites carry a specific symbol indicating that they have been reviewed and are trustworthy (HONcode and Trust-e), the health care provider cannot control which information patients access or how they perceive and act related to the health information they find online.

Theoretical Approaches to Health Care Ethics

Theoretical approaches to health care ethics have evolved in response to societal changes. In a 30-year retrospective article for the *Journal of the American Medical Association*, Pellegrino (1993) traced the evolution of health care ethics from the Hippocratic ethic to principlism to the current antiprinciplism movement.

The Hippocratic tradition emerged from relatively homogeneous societies where beliefs were similar and most societal members shared common values. The emphasis was on **duty**, virtue, and gentlemanly conduct.

Principlism arose as societies became more heterogeneous and members began experiencing a diversity of incompatible beliefs and values; it emerged as a foundation for ethical decision making. Principles were expansive enough to be shared by all rational individuals, regardless of their background and individual beliefs. This approach continued into the 1900s and was popularized by two bioethicists, Beauchamp and Childress (1977, 1994), in the last quarter of the 20th century. Principles are considered broad guidelines that provide guidance or direction but leave substantial room for case-specific judgment. From principles, one can develop more detailed rules and policies.

Beauchamp and Childress (1994) proposed four guiding principles: (1) respect for autonomy, (2) nonmaleficence, (3) beneficence, and (4) justice:

- **Autonomy** refers to the individual's freedom from controlling interferences by others and from personal limitations that prevent meaningful choices, such as adequate understanding. Two conditions are essential for autonomy: **liberty**, meaning the independence from controlling influences, and the individual's capacity for intentional action.
- **Nonmaleficence** asserts an obligation not to inflict harm intentionally and forms the framework for the standard of due care to be met by any professional. Obligations of nonmaleficence are obligations of not inflicting harm and not imposing risks of harm. **Negligence**—a departure from the standard of due care toward others—includes intentionally imposing risks that are unreasonable and unintentionally but carelessly imposing risks.
- **Beneficence** refers to actions performed that contribute to the welfare of others. Two principles underlie beneficence: Positive beneficence requires the provision of benefits, and utility requires that benefits and drawbacks be balanced. One must avoid negative beneficence, which occurs when constraints are placed on activities that, even though they might not be unjust, could in some situations cause detriment or harm to others.
- **Justice** refers to fair, equitable, and appropriate treatment in light of what is due or owed to a person. Distributive justice refers to fair, equitable, and appropriate distribution in society determined by justified norms that structure the terms of social cooperation.

Beauchamp and Childress also suggest three types of rules for guiding actions: substantive, authority, and procedural. (Rules are more restrictive in scope than principles and are more specific in content.) Substantive rules are rules of **truth** telling, confidentiality, privacy, and **fidelity** and those pertaining to the allocation and rationing of health care, omitting treatment, physician-assisted suicide, and informed consent. Authority rules indicate who may and should perform actions. Procedural rules establish procedures to be followed.

The principlism advocated by Beauchamp and Childress has since given way to the **antiprinciplism** movement, which emerged in the 21st century with the expansive technological changes and the tremendous rise in ethical dilemmas accompanying these changes. Opponents of principlism include those who claim that its principles do not represent a theoretical approach as well as those who claim that its principles are too far removed from the concrete particularities of everyday human existence; are too conceptual, intangible, or abstract; or disregard or do not take into account a person's psychological factors, personality, life history, sexual orientation, or religious, ethnic, and cultural background. Different approaches to making ethical decisions are next briefly explored, providing the reader with an understanding of the varied methods professionals may use to arrive at an ethical decision.

The **casuist approach** to ethical decision making grew out of the call for more concrete methods of examining ethical dilemmas. Casuistry is a case-based ethical reasoning method that analyzes the facts of a case in a sound, logical, and ordered or structured manner. The facts are compared to decisions arising out of consensus in previous paradigmatic or model cases. One casuist proponent, Jonsen (1991), prefers particular and concrete paradigms and analogies over the universal and abstract theories of principlism.

The Husted bioethical decision-making model centers on the health care professional's implicit agreement with the patient or client (Husted & Husted, 1995). It is based on six contemporary bioethical standards: (1) autonomy, (2) freedom, (3) veracity, (4) privacy, (5) beneficence, and (6) fidelity.

The **virtue ethics** approach emphasizes the virtuous character of individuals who make the choices. A **virtue** is any characteristic or disposition desired in others or oneself. It is derived from the Greek word *aretai*, meaning "excellence," and refers to what one expects of oneself and others. Virtue ethicists emphasize the ideal situation and attempt to identify and define ideals. Virtue ethics dates back to Plato and Socrates. When asked "whether virtue can be taught or whether virtue can be acquired in some other way, Socrates answers that if virtue is knowledge, then it can be taught. Thus, Socrates assumes that whatever can be known can be taught" (Scott, 2002, para. 9). According to this view, the cause of any moral weakness is not a matter of character flaws but rather a matter of ignorance. In other words, a person acts immorally because the individual does not know what is really good for him or her. A person can, for example, be overpowered by immediate pleasures and forget to consider the long-term **consequences.** Plato emphasized that to lead a moral life and not succumb to immediate pleasures and gratification, one must have a moral vision. He identified four cardinal virtues: (1) **wisdom,** (2) **courage,** (3) **self-control,** and (4) justice.

Aristotle's **Nicomachean** principles (Aristotle, 350 BC) also contribute to virtue ethics. According to this philosopher, virtues are connected to will and motive because the intention is what determines if one is or is not acting virtuously. Ethical considerations, according to his **eudaemonistic** principles, address the question "What is it to be an excellent person?" For Aristotle, this ultimately means acting in a temperate manner according to a rational mean between extreme possibilities.

Virtue ethics has experienced a recent resurgence in popularity (Healthcare Ethics, 2007). Two of the most influential moral and medical authors, Pellegrino and Thomasma (1993), have maintained that virtue theory should be related to other theories within a comprehensive philosophy of the health professions. They argue that moral events are composed of four elements (the agent, the act, the circumstances, and the consequences) and state that a variety of theories must be interrelated to account for different facets of moral judgment.

Care ethics is responsiveness to the needs of others that dictates providing care, preventing harm, and maintaining relationships. This viewpoint has been in existence for some time. Engster (n.d.) states that "Carol Gilligan's *In a Different Voice* (1982) established care ethics as a major new perspective in contemporary moral and political discourse" (p. 2). The relationship between care and virtue is complex, however. Benjamin and Curtis (1992) base their framework on care ethics; they propose that "critical reflection and inquiry in ethics involves the complex interplay of a variety of human faculties, ranging from empathy and moral imagination on the one hand to analytic precision and careful reasoning on the other" (p. 12). Care ethicists are less stringently guided by rules, focusing rather on the needs of others and the individual's responsibility to meet those needs. As opposed to the aforementioned theories that are centered on the individual's rights, an ethic of care emphasizes the personal part of an interdependent relationship that affects how decisions are made. In this theory, the specific situation and context in which the person is embedded become a part of the decision-making process.

The consensus-based approach to bioethics was proposed by Martin (1999), who claims that American bioethics harbors a variety of ethical methods that emphasize different ethical factors, including principles, circumstances, character, interpersonal needs, and personal meaning. Each method reflects an important aspect of ethical experience, adds to the others, and enriches the ethical imagination. Thus, working with these methods provides the challenge and the opportunity necessary for the perceptive and shrewd bioethicist to transform them into something new with value through the process of building ethical consensus. Diverse ethical insights can be integrated to support a particular bioethical decision, and that decision can be understood as a new, ethical whole.

Applying Ethics to Informatics

With the Knowledge Age has come global closeness, meaning the ability to reach around the globe instantaneously through technology. Language barriers are being broken through technologically based translators that can enhance interaction and exchange of data and information. Informatics practitioners are bridging continents, and international panels, committees, and organizations are beginning to establish standards and rules for the implementation of informatics. This international perspective must be taken into consideration when informatics dilemmas are examined from an ethical standpoint; it promises to influence the development of ethical approaches that begin to accept that health care practitioners are working within international networks and must recognize, respect, and regard the diverse political, social, and human factors within informatics ethics.

The various ethical approaches can be used to help health care professionals make ethical decisions in all areas of practice. The focus of this text is on informatics.

Informatics theory and practice have continued to grow at a rapid rate and are infiltrating every area of professional life. New applications and ways of performing skills are being developed daily. Therefore, education in informatics ethics is extremely important.

Typically, situations are analyzed using past experience and in collaboration with others. Each situation warrants its own deliberation and unique approach because each individual patient seeking or receiving care has his or her own preferences, quality of life, and health care needs in a situational milieu framed by financial, provider, setting, institutional, and social context issues. Health care professionals must take into consideration all of these factors when making ethical decisions.

The use of expert systems, **decision support** tools, evidence-based practice, and artificial intelligence in the care of patients creates challenges in terms of who should use these tools, how they are implemented, and how they are tempered with clinical judgment. All clinical situations are not the same, and even though the result of interacting with these systems and tools is enhanced information and knowledge, the health care professional must weigh this information in light of each patient's unique clinical circumstances, including that individual's beliefs and wishes. Patients are demanding access to quality care and the information necessary to control their lives. Health care professionals need to analyze and synthesize the parameters of each distinctive situation using a specific decision-making framework that helps them make the best decisions. Getting it right the first time has a tremendous impact on expected patient outcomes. The focus should remain on patient outcomes while the informatics tools available are ethically incorporated.

Facing ethical dilemmas on a daily basis and struggling with unique client situations may cause many health care professionals to question their own actions and the actions of their colleagues and patients. One must realize that colleagues and patients may reach very different decisions, but that does not mean anyone is wrong. Instead, all parties reach their ethical decision based on their own review of the situational facts and understanding of ethics. As one deals with diversity among patients, colleagues, and administrators, one must constantly strive to use ethical imagination to reach ethically competent decisions.

Balancing the needs of society, his or her employer, and patients could cause the health care professional to face ethical challenges on an everyday basis. Society expects judicious use of finite health care resources. Employers have their own policies, standards, and practices that can sometimes inhibit the practice of the health care professional. Each patient is unique and has life experiences that affect his or her health care perspective, choices, motivation, and adherence. Combine all of these factors with the challenges posed by informatics, and it is clear that the evolving health care arena calls for an informatics-competent, politically active, consumer-oriented, business-savvy, ethical professional to rule this ever-changing landscape known as health care.

The goal of any ethical system should be that a rational, justifiable decision is reached. Ethics is always there to help the practitioner decide what is right. Indeed, the measure of an adequate ethical system or theory or approach is, in part, its ability to be useful in novel contexts. A comprehensive, robust theory of ethics should be up to the task of addressing a broad variety of new applications and challenges at the intersection of informatics and health care.

The information concerning an ethical dilemma must be viewed in the context of the dilemma to be useful. **Bioinformatics** could gather, manipulate, classify, analyze, synthesize, retrieve, and maintain databases related to ethical cases, the effective reasoning applied to various ethical dilemmas, and the resulting ethical decisions. This input would certainly be potent—but the resolution of dilemmas cannot be achieved simply by examining relevant cases from a database. Instead, health care professionals must assess each situational context and the patient's specific situation and needs and make their ethical decisions based on all of the information they have at hand.

Ethics is exciting, and competent health care professionals need to know about ethical dilemmas and solutions in their professions. Ethicists have often been thought of as experts in the arbitrary, ambiguous, and ungrounded judgments of other people. They know that they make the best decisions they can based on the situation and stakeholders at hand. Just as health care professionals try to make the best health care decisions with and for their patients, ethically driven practitioners must do the same. Each health care provider must critically think through the situation to arrive at the best decision.

To make ethical decisions about informatics technologies and patients' intimate health care data and information, the health care provider must be competent in informatics. To the extent that information technology is reshaping health care practices or promises to improve patient care, health care professionals must be trained and competent in the use of these tools. This competency needs to be evaluated through instruments developed by professional groups or societies; such assessment will help with consistency and quality. For the health care professional to be an effective patient advocate, he or she must understand how information technology affects the patient and the subsequent delivery of care. Information science and its effects on health care are both interesting and important. It follows that information technology and its **ethical, social, and legal implications** should be incorporated into all levels of professional education.

The need for confidentiality was perhaps first articulated by Hippocrates; thus, if anything is different in today's environment, it is simply the ways in which confidentiality can be violated. Perhaps the use of computers for clinical decision support and data mining in research will raise new ethical issues. Ethical dilemmas associated with the integration of informatics must be examined to provide an ethical framework that considers all of the stakeholders. Patients' rights must be protected in the face of a health care provider's duty to his or her employer and society at large when initiating care and assigning finite health care resources. An ethical framework is necessary to help guide health care providers in reference to the ethical treatment of electronic data and information during all stages of collection, storage, manipulation, and dissemination. These new approaches and means come with their own ethical dilemmas. Often they are dilemmas not yet faced because of the cutting-edge nature of these technologies.

Just as processes and models are used to diagnose and treat patients in practice, so a model in the analysis and synthesis of ethical dilemmas or cases can also be applied.

An ethical model for ethical decision making (**Box 5-1**) facilitates the ability to analyze the dilemma and synthesize the information into a plan of action (McGonigle, 2000). The model presented here is based on the letters in the word *ethical*. Each letter guides and prompts the health care provider to think critically (think and rethink) through the situation presented. The model is a tool because, in the final analysis, it allows the health care professional to objectively ascertain the essence of the dilemma and develop a plan of action.

BOX 5-1   ETHICAL MODEL FOR ETHICAL DECISION MAKING

- **E**xamine the ethical dilemma (conflicting values exist).
- **T**horoughly comprehend the possible alternatives available.
- **H**ypothesize ethical arguments.
- **I**nvestigate, compare, and evaluate the arguments for each alternative.
- **C**hoose the alternative you would recommend.
- **A**ct on your chosen alternative.
- **L**ook at the ethical dilemma and examine the outcomes while reflecting on the ethical decision.

APPLYING THE ETHICAL MODEL

Examine the ethical dilemma:
- Use your problem-solving, decision-making, and critical thinking skills.
- What is the dilemma you are analyzing? Collect as much information about the dilemma as you can, making sure to gather the relevant facts that clearly identify the dilemma. You should be able to describe the dilemma you are analyzing in detail.
- Ascertain exactly what must be decided.
- Who should be involved in the decision-making process for this specific case?
- Who are the interested players or stakeholders?
- Reflect on the viewpoints of these key players and their value systems.
- What do you think each of these stakeholders would like you to decide as a plan of action for this dilemma?
- How can you generate the greatest good?

Thoroughly comprehend the possible alternatives available:
- Use your problem-solving, decision-making, and critical thinking skills.
- Create a list of the possible alternatives. Be creative when developing your alternatives. Be open-minded; there is more than one way to reach a goal. Compel yourself to discern at least three alternatives.
- Clarify the alternatives available and predict the associated consequences—good and bad—of each potential alternative or intervention.
- For each alternative, ask the following questions:
  - Do any of the principles or rules, such as legal, professional, or organizational, automatically nullify this alternative?
  - If this alternative is chosen, what do you predict as the best-case and worst-case scenarios?
  - Do the best-case outcomes outweigh the worst-case outcomes?
  - Could you live with the worst-case scenario?

(*continues*)

BOX 5-1 ETHICAL MODEL FOR ETHICAL DECISION MAKING (continued)

▢ Will anyone be harmed? If so, how will they be harmed?
▢ Does the benefit obtained from this alternative overcome the risk of potential harm that it could cause to anyone?

Hypothesize ethical arguments:
- Use your problem-solving, decision-making, and critical thinking skills.
- Determine which of the five approaches apply to this dilemma.
- Identify the moral principles that can be brought into play to support a conclusion as to what ought to be done ethically in this case or similar cases.
- Ascertain whether the approaches generate converging or diverging conclusions about what ought to be done.

Investigate, compare, and evaluate the arguments for each alternative:
- Use your problem-solving, decision-making, and critical thinking skills.
- Appraise the relevant facts and assumptions prudently.
  ▢ Is there ambiguous information that must be evaluated?
  ▢ Are there any unjustifiable factual or illogical assumptions or debatable conceptual issues that must be explored?
- Rate the ethical reasoning and arguments for each alternative in terms of their relative significance.
  ▢ 4 = extreme significance
  ▢ 3 = major significance
  ▢ 2 = significant
  ▢ 1 = minor significance
- Compare and contrast the alternatives available with the values of the key players involved.
- Reflect on these alternatives:
  ▢ Does each alternative consider all of the key players?
  ▢ Does each alternative take into account and reflect an interest in the concerns and welfare of all of the key players?
  ▢ Which alternative will produce the greatest good or the least amount of harm for the greatest number of people?
- Refer to your professional codes of ethical conduct. Do they support your reasoning?

Choose the alternative you would recommend:
- Use your problem-solving, decision-making, and critical thinking skills.
- Make a decision about the best alternative available.
  ▢ Remember the Golden Rule: Does your decision treat others as you would want to be treated?
  ▢ Does your decision take into account and reflect an interest in the concerns and welfare of all of the key players?
  ▢ Does your decision maximize the benefit and minimize the risk for everyone involved?
- Become your own critic; challenge your decision as you think others might. Use the ethical arguments you predict they would use and defend your decision.
  ▢ Would you be secure enough in your ethical decision-making process to see it aired on national television or sent out globally over the Internet?
  ▢ Are you secure enough with this ethical decision that you could have allowed your loved ones to observe your decision-making process, your decision, and its outcomes?

BOX 5-1   ETHICAL MODEL FOR ETHICAL DECISION MAKING (continued)

Act on your chosen alternative:
- Use your problem-solving, decision-making, and critical thinking skills.
- Formulate an implementation plan delineating the execution of the decision.
   - ☐ This plan should be designed to maximize the benefits and minimize the risks.
   - ☐ This plan must take into account all of the resources necessary for implementation, including personnel and money.
- Implement the plan.

Look at the ethical dilemma and examine the outcomes while reflecting on your ethical decision:
- Use your problem-solving, decision-making, and critical thinking skills.
- Monitor the implementation plan and its outcomes. It is extremely important to reflect on specific case decisions and evaluate their outcomes to develop your ethical decision-making ability.
- If new information becomes available, the plan must be reevaluated.
- Monitor and revise the plan as necessary.

Source: The ethical model for ethical decision making was developed by Dr. Dee McGonigle and is the property of Educational Advancement Associates (EAA). The permission for its use in this text has been granted by Mr. Craig R. Goshow, Vice President, EAA.

Case Analysis Demonstration

The following case study is intended to help readers think through how to apply the ethical model. Review the model and then read through the case. Try to apply the model to this case or follow along as the model is implemented. Readers are challenged to determine their decision in this case and then compare and contrast their response with the decision the authors reached.

> *Allison is a nutrition specialist for a large metropolitan hospital. She is expecting an instructor from the local university at 2:00 p.m. to review and discuss the use of the EHR to assess nutritional status and the use of the EHR resources to develop and implement nutritional therapies. They were planning to develop scenarios for the nutrition students scheduled for the following day. Just as the university professor arrives, Allison's supervisor calls her to attend a meeting that starts in 5 minutes. She must attend this meeting. To expedite the scenario planning for the following day, Allison gives her EHR access password to the instructor.*

Examine the Ethical Dilemma

Allison made a commitment to meet with the university instructor to develop nutrition scenarios at 2:00 p.m. The meeting she was required to attend prevented Allison from living up to that commitment. Allison had an obligation to her supervisor/employer and a competing obligation to the professor. She solved the dilemma of competing obligations by providing her EHR access password to the university professor.

By sharing her password, Allison most likely violated hospital policy related to the security of health care information. She may also have violated the International Code of Ethics and Code of Good Practice adopted by the International Confederation of Dietetic Associations (2014), which stated that dietitians must ensure that practice meets legislative requirements, in this case the protection of information of a confidential nature. Because the university professor was also a dietician and had a legitimate interest in the protected health care information, it could be argued that Allison did not commit a violation of the code of ethics.

Thoroughly Comprehend the Possible Alternatives Available

Some possible **alternative** actions include the following: (1) Allison could have asked the professor to wait until she returned from the meeting, (2) Allison could have delegated another staff member to assist the professor, or (3) Allison could have logged on to the system for the professor.

Hypothesize Ethical Arguments

The utilitarian approach applies to this situation. An ethical action is one that provides the greatest good for the greatest number; the underlying principles in this perspective are beneficence and nonmaleficence. The rights to be considered are as follows: right of the individual to choose for himself or herself (autonomy), right to truth (**veracity**), right of privacy (the ethical right to privacy avoids conflict and, like all rights, promotes harmony), right not to be injured, and right to what has been promised (fidelity).

Does the action respect the **moral rights** of everyone? The principles to consider are autonomy, veracity, and fidelity.

As for the fairness or justice, how fair is an action? Does it treat everyone in the same way, or does it show favoritism and discrimination? The principles to consider are justice and distributive justice.

Thinking about the common good assumes that one's own good is inextricably linked to the good of the community; community members are bound by the pursuit of common values and goals and ensure that the social policies, social systems, institutions, and environments on which one depends are beneficial to all. Examples of such outcomes are affordable health care, effective public safety, a just legal system, and an unpolluted environment. The principle of distributive justice is considered.

Virtue assumes that one should strive toward certain ideals that provide for the full development of humanity. Virtues are attitudes or character traits that enable one to be and to act in ways that develop the highest potential; examples include honesty, courage, compassion, generosity, fidelity, integrity, fairness, self-control, and prudence. Like habits, virtues become a characteristic of the person. The virtuous person is the ethical person. Ask yourself, What kind of person should I be? What will promote the development of character within myself and my community? The principles considered are fidelity, veracity, beneficence, nonmaleficence, justice, and distributive justice.

In this case, there is a clear violation of an institutional policy designed to protect the privacy and confidentiality of medical records. However, the professor had a legitimate interest in the information and a legitimate right to the information. Allison trusted that the professor would not use the system password to obtain information outside the scope of the legitimate interest. However, Allison cannot be sure that the professor would not access inappropriate information. Further, Allison is responsible for how her access to the electronic system is used. Balancing the rights of everyone—the professor's right to the information, the patients' rights to expect that their information is safeguarded, and the right of the supervisor to request her presence at a meeting—is important and is the crux of the dilemma. Does the work-related meeting obligation outweigh the obligation to the professor? Yes, probably. Allison did the right thing by attending the meeting. By giving out her system access password, Allison also compromised the rights of the other patients' information in the EHR who expect that their confidentiality and privacy would be safeguarded.

Virtue ethics suggests that individuals use power to bring about human benefit. One must consider the needs of others and the responsibility to meet those needs. Allison must simultaneously provide care, prevent harm, and maintain professional relationships.

Allison may want to effect a long-term change in hospital policy for the common good. It is reasonable to assume that this event was not an isolated incident and that the problem may recur in the future. Can the institutional policy be amended to provide professors with legitimate access to the EHR? As suggested in the HIPAA administrative guidelines, the professor could receive the same staff training regarding appropriate and inappropriate use of access and sign the agreement to safeguard the records. If the institution has tracking software, the professor's access could be monitored to watch for inappropriate use. From the analysis, it is clear that the best immediate solution is to delegate another dietitian to assist the professor with the case scenario development until Allison is able to return.

Investigate, Compare, and Evaluate the Arguments for Each Alternative

Review and think through the items listed in **Table 5-1**.

Choose the Alternative You Would Recommend

The best immediate solution is to delegate another staff member to assist the professor. The best long-term solution is to change the hospital policy to include access for professors, as described previously.

Act on Your Chosen Alternative

Allison should delegate another staff member to assist the professor in developing scenarios for student learning.

TABLE 5-1   DETAILED ANALYSIS OF ALTERNATIVE ACTIONS

Alternative	Good Consequences	Bad Consequences	Do Any Rules Nullify	Expected Outcome	Potential Benefit > Harm
1. Wait until meeting is over	No policy violation Patient rights safeguarded	Not the best use of the professor's time	No	Best: Meeting will require a short time Worst: Meeting may take a long time	Patient rights protected Collegial relationship jeopardized Patient rights may take precedence
2. Delegate to another staff member	No policy violated	Other staff may be equally busy or might not be as familiar with patients	No	Best: Assignments will be completed Worst: May not have benefit of expert advice	Confidentiality of record is assured May compromise student learning Patient rights may take precedence
3. Log on to the system for the professor	Professor can begin making assignments	May still be a violation of policy regarding system access	Rules regarding to medical record	Best: Assignments can be completed Worst: Abuse of access to information	Potential compromise of records Patient is cared for

Look at the Ethical Dilemma and Examine the Outcomes While Reflecting on the Ethical Decision

As already indicated in the alternative analyses, delegation may not be an ideal solution because the dietitian who is assigned to assist the professor may not possess the same extensive information about all of the patients as Allison. It is, however, the best immediate solution to the dilemma and is certainly safer than compromising the integrity of the hospital's computer system. As noted previously, Allison may want to pursue a long-term solution to a potentially recurring problem by helping the professor gain legitimate access to the computer system with the professor's own password. The system administrator would then have the ability to track who used the system and which types of information were accessed during use.

This sample case analysis provides the authors' perspective on this case and the ethical decision made. If your decision did not match this perspective, what was the basis for the difference of opinion? If you worked through the model, you might have reached a different decision based on your individual background and perspective. This does not make the decision right or wrong. A decision should reflect the best decision one can make given review, reflection, and critical thinking about a specific situation.

New Frontiers in Ethical Issues

The expanding use of new information technologies in health care will bring about new and challenging ethical issues. Consider that patients and health care providers no longer have to be in the same place for a quality interaction. How, then, does one deal with licensing issues if the electronic consultation takes place across a state line? Derse and Miller (2008) describe a second-opinion medical consultation on the Internet where the information was provided to the referring physician and not directly to the patient. In essence, provider-to-provider consultation does not constitute practicing in a state in which you are not licensed. As new technologies for health care delivery are developed, new ethical challenges may arise. It is important for all health care providers to be aware of the code of ethics for their specific practices and to understand the laws governing their practice and private health information.

In an ideal world, health care professionals must not be affected by conflicting loyalties; nothing should interfere with judicious, ethical decision making. As the technologically charged waters of health care are navigated, one must hone a solid foundation of ethical decision making and practice it consistently.

Legal Aspects of Health Informatics

In addition to the ethical considerations for practice, health professionals must abide by laws governing the use of health information. This text will explore two key pieces of legislation that have shaped the health informatics landscape: the Health Insurance Portability and Accountability Act (HIPAA) of 1996 and the HITECH Act of 2009.

HIPAA was signed into law by President Bill Clinton in 1996. Hellerstein (1999) summarized the intent of the act as follows: to curtail health care fraud and abuse, enforce standards for health information, guarantee the security and privacy of health information, and ensure health insurance portability for employed persons. Consequences were put into place for institutions and individuals who violate the requirements of this act. For this text, we concentrate on the health information security and privacy aspects of HIPAA, which are outlined as follows.

The privacy provisions of the federal law, HIPAA, apply to health information created or maintained by health care providers who engage in certain electronic transactions, health plans, and health care clearinghouses. The U.S. Department of Health and Human Services (HHS) issued the regulation, "Standards for Privacy of Individually Identifiable Health Information," applicable to **entities** covered by HIPAA. The **Office of Civil Rights** (OCR) is the departmental component responsible for implementing and enforcing the privacy regulation (see the Statement of Delegation of Authority to the Office for Civil Rights, as published in the *Federal Register* on December 28, 2000 [HHS, 2006, para. 1]).

The need and means to guarantee the security and privacy of health information was the focus of numerous debates. Comprehensive standards for the implementation of this portion of the act eventually were finalized, but the process to adopt final standards took years. In August 1998, HHS released a set of proposed rules addressing health information management. Proposed rules specific to health information privacy and security were released in November 1999. The purpose of the proposed rules was to balance patients' rights to privacy and providers' needs for access to information (Hellerstein, 2000).

Hellerstein (2000) summarized the proposed privacy rules. The rules do the following:

- Define protected health information as "information relating to one's physical or mental health, the provision of one's health care, or the payment for that health care, that has been maintained or transmitted electronically and that can be reasonably identified with the individual it applies to" (Hellerstein, 2000, p. 2).
- Propose that authorization by patients for release of information is not necessary when the release of information is directly related to treatment and payment for treatment. Specific patient authorization is not required for research, medical or police emergencies, legal proceedings, and collection of data for public health concerns. All other releases of health information require a specific form for each release, and only information pertinent to the issue at hand is allowed to be released. All releases of information must be formally documented and accessible to the patient on request.
- Establish patient ownership of the health care record and allow for patient-initiated corrections and amendments.
- Mandate administrative requirements for the protection of health care information. All health care organizations are required to have a privacy official and an office to receive privacy violation complaints. A specific training program for employees that includes a certification of completion and a signed statement by all employees that they will uphold privacy procedures must be developed and implemented. All employees must re-sign the agreement to uphold privacy every 3 years. Sanctions for violations of policy must be clearly defined and applied.
- Mandate that all outside entities that conduct business with health care organizations (e.g., attorneys, consultants, and auditors) must meet the same standards as the organization for information protection and security.
- Allow protected health information to be released without authorization for research studies. Patients may not access their information in blinded research studies because this access may affect the reliability of the study outcomes.

- Propose that protected health information may be deidentified before release in such a manner that the identity of the patient is protected. The health care organization may code the deidentification so that the information can be reidentified once it has been returned.
- Apply only to health information maintained or transmitted by electronic means.

As concerns mounted and deadlines loomed, the health care arena prepared to comply with the requirements of the law. The administrative simplification portion of this law was intended to decrease the financial and administrative burdens by standardizing the electronic transmission of certain administrative and financial transactions. This section also addressed the security and privacy of health care data and information for the covered entities of health care providers who transmit any health information in electronic form in connection with a covered transaction, health plans, and health care clearinghouses (HHS, 2007).

The privacy requirements, which went into effect on April 14, 2003, limited the release of protected health information without the patient's knowledge and consent. Covered entities must comply with the requirements. Notably, they must dedicate a privacy officer, adopt and implement privacy procedures, educate their personnel, and secure their electronic patient records. Most individuals are familiar with the need to notify patients of their privacy rights, having signed forms on interacting with health care providers.

According to the HHS (2002), the privacy rule provides certain rights to patients: the right to request restrictions to access of the health record, the right to request an alternative method of communication with a provider, the right to receive a paper copy of the notice of privacy practices, the right to file a complaint if the patient believes his or her privacy rights were violated, the right to inspect and copy one's health record, the right to request an amendment to the health record, and the right to see an account of disclosures of one's health record. This places the burden of maintaining privacy and accuracy on the health care system rather than the patient.

On October 16, 2003, the electronic transaction and code set standards became effective. At the time, they did not require electronic transmission but rather mandated that if transactions were conducted electronically, they must comply with the required federal standards for electronically filed health care claims. "The Secretary has made the **Centers for Medicare & Medicaid Services** (CMS) responsible for enforcing the electronic transactions and code sets provisions of the law" ("Guidance on Compliance with HIPAA Transactions and Code Sets," 2003, para. 3).

The security requirements went into effect on April 21, 2005, and required the covered entities to put safeguards in place that protect the confidentiality, integrity, and availability of protected health information when stored and transmitted electronically.

The safeguards that were addressed were administrative, physical, and technical. The administrative safeguards refer to the documented formal policies and procedures that are used to manage and execute the security measures. They govern the protection of health care data and information and the conduct of the personnel. The physical safeguards refer to the policies and procedures that must be in place to limit physical access to electronic information systems. Technical safeguards are the policies and procedures used to control access to health care data and information. Safeguards need to be in place to control access, whether the data and information are at rest, residing on a machine or storage medium, being processed, or in transmission, such as being backed up to storage or disseminated across a network.

The HITECH Act (Leyva & Leyva, 2011), enacted on February 17, 2009, is part of the **American Recovery and Reinvestment Act (ARRA)**. The ARRA, also known as the "Stimulus" law, was enacted to stimulate various sectors of the U.S. economy during the most severe recession this country had experienced since the Great Depression of the late 1920s and early 1930s. The HIT industry was one area where lawmakers saw an opportunity to stimulate the economy and improve the delivery of health care at the same time. This explains why the title of the HITECH Act contains the phrase "for Economic and Clinical Health."

The ARRA is a lengthy piece of legislation that is organized into two major sections: Division A and Division B. Each division contains several titles. Title XIII of Division A of the ARRA is the HITECH Act. It addresses the development, adoption, and implementation of HIT **policies** and **standards** and provides enhanced **privacy** and **security** protections for patient information—an area of the law that is of paramount concern in nursing informatics. Title IV of Division B of the ARRA is considered part of the HITECH Act. It addresses Medicare and Medicaid HIT and provides significant financial incentives to health care professionals and hospitals that adopt and engage in the "**meaningful use**" of EHR technology.

Overview of the HITECH Act

At the time the HITECH Act was enacted, it was estimated that less than 8% of U.S. hospitals used a basic EHR system in at least one of their clinical units and that less than 2% of U.S. hospitals had an EHR system in all of their clinical settings (Ashish, 2009). Not surprisingly, the cost of an EHR system was a major barrier to widespread adoption of this technology in most health care facilities. The HITECH Act sought to change that situation by providing incentives to health facilities so that each person in the United States would have an EHR. In addition, a nationwide HIT infrastructure would be developed so that access to a person's EHR would be readily available to every health care provider who treats the patient, no matter where the patient may be located at the time treatment is rendered. According to the **Office of the National Coordinator for Health Information Technology** (ONC, 2015), three out of four hospitals now have at least a basic EHR with clinician notes, and for larger acute care hospitals, nearly 97% have EHR technology certified by HHS.

Definitions

The HITECH Act includes some important definitions that anyone involved in health informatics should know:

- **"Certified EHR Technology"**: an EHR that meets specific governmental standards for the type of record involved, whether it is an ambulatory EHR used by office-based health care practitioners or an inpatient EHR used by hospitals. The specific standards that are to be met for any such EHRs are set forth in federal regulations.
- **"Enterprise Integration"**: "the electronic linkage of healthcare providers, health plans, the government and other interested parties, to enable the electronic exchange and use of health information among all the components in the healthcare infrastructure."
- **"Health Care Provider"**: hospitals, skilled nursing facilities, nursing homes, long-term care facilities, home health agencies, hemodialysis centers, clinics, community mental health centers, ambulatory surgery centers, group practices, pharmacies and pharmacists, laboratories, physicians, and therapists, among others.
- **"HIT"**: "hardware, software, integrated technologies or related licenses, intellectual property, upgrades, or packaged solutions sold as services that are designed for or support the use by healthcare entities or patients for the electronic creation, maintenance, access, or exchange of health information."
- **"Qualified Electronic Health Record"**: "an electronic record of health-related information on an individual." A "qualified" EHR contains a patient's demographic and clinical health information, including the medical history and a list of health problems, and is capable of providing support for clinical decisions and entry of physician orders. It must also have the capacity "to capture and query information relevant to health care quality" and "exchange electronic health information with, and integrate such information from other sources" (Readthestimulus.org, 2009, pp. 32–35).

Purposes

The HITECH Act established the ONC within HHS. The ONC is headed by the national coordinator, who is responsible for overseeing the development of a nationwide HIT infrastructure that supports the use and exchange of information to achieve the following goals:

1. Improve health care quality by enhancing coordination of services between and among the various health care providers a patient may have, fostering more appropriate health care decisions at the time and place of delivery of services, and preventing medical errors and advancing the delivery of **patient-centered care**.
2. Reduce the cost of health care by addressing inefficiencies, such as duplication of services within the health care delivery system, and by reducing the number of medical errors.
3. Improve people's health by promoting prevention, early detection, and management of chronic diseases.

4. Protect public health by fostering early detection and rapid response to infectious diseases, bioterrorism, and other situations that could have a widespread impact on the health status of many individuals.
5. Facilitate clinical research.
6. Reduce **health disparities.**
7. Better secure patient health information.

Improving health care quality has been an ongoing challenge in the United States. According to the **Agency for Healthcare Research and Quality** (AHRQ, 2009), quality health care is care that is "safe, timely, patient centered, efficient, and equitable" (p. 1).

Providers need reliable information about their performance to guide improvement activities. Realistically, HIT infrastructure is needed to ensure that relevant data are collected regularly, systematically, and unobtrusively while protecting patient privacy and confidentiality . . . . Systems need to generate information that can be understood by end users and that are interoperable across different institutions' data platforms …
Quality improvement typically requires examining patterns of care across panels of patients rather than one patient at a time . . . . Ideally, performance measures should be calculated automatically from health records in a format that can be easily shared and compared across all providers involved with a patient's care. (AHRQ, 2009, p. 13)

EHR technology also will make it easier for all providers involved in a patient's care to readily access that patient's complete and current health care record, thereby allowing providers to make well-informed, efficient, and effective decisions about a patient's care at the time those decisions need to be made. This is of tremendous benefit to the patient and promotes a higher level of patient-centered care. It also allows effective coordination of care between and among all providers involved in the patient's care, including doctors, nurses, therapists, nutritionists, hospitals, nursing homes, rehabilitation facilities, home health agencies, laboratories, and other diagnostic centers, thereby ensuring the continuum of patient care.

Perhaps the most important task facing the national coordinator during the development and implementation of a nationwide HIT infrastructure is ensuring the security of the patient health information within that system. The ability to secure and protect confidential patient information has always been of paramount importance to clinicians, who view this consideration as an ethical and legal obligation of practice. Patients value their privacy, and they have a right to expect that their confidential health information will be properly safeguarded.

The HITECH Act also provides significant monetary incentives for providers who engage in meaningful use of health information technology. "Meaningful use" is defined as "using electronic health records (EHRs) in a meaningful manner, which includes, but is not limited to electronically capturing health information in a coded format, using that information to track key clinical conditions, communicating that information to help coordinate care, and initiating the reporting of clinical quality measures and public health information" (Centers for Medicare and Medicaid Services, 2010, para. 3).

Monetary incentives are available to clinicians and facilities that implement EHR systems that meet the specific standards. Providers that fail to adopt such systems within a specified time frame may be subject to significant governmental penalties.

How the HITECH Act Changed HIPAA

HIPAA Privacy and Security Rules

Health care professionals have been complying with HIPAA for years. Recall that HIPAA was enacted by the federal government for several purposes, including better portability of health insurance as a worker moved from one job to another; deterrence of fraud, abuse, and waste within the health care delivery system; and simplification of the administrative functions associated with the delivery of health care, such as reimbursement claims sent to Medicare and Medicaid. Simplification of administrative functions entailed the adoption of electronic transactions that included sensitive health care information. To protect the privacy and security of health information, two sets of federal regulations were implemented. The Privacy Rule became effective in 2003, and the Security Rule became effective in 2005. Many practitioners that refer to HIPAA are not referring to the comprehensive federal statute enacted in 1996 but rather to the Privacy Rule and the Security Rule—that is, the federal regulations that were adopted years after HIPAA became law.

Under the Privacy Rule, patients have a right to expect privacy protections that limit the use and disclosure of their health information. Under the Security Rule, providers are obligated to safeguard their patients' health information from improper use or disclosure, maintain the integrity of the information, and ensure its availability. Both rules apply to **protected health information** (PHI), defined as any physical or mental health information created, received, or stored by a "covered entity" that can be used to identify an individual patient, regardless of the form of the health information (i.e., it can be electronic, handwritten, or verbal) (V|lex, 2011). Covered entities include hospitals and other health care providers that transmit any health information electronically as well as health insurance companies and health care clearinghouses (V|lex, 2011).

Clinicians have become very knowledgeable about the requirements of the Privacy and Security Rules. They are familiar with their obligations to protect patient information and the rights afforded to their patients under these regulations. Patients are entitled to a notice of privacy practices from their health care provider. Inpatients are entitled to opt out of the facility's directory, thereby protecting disclosure of information that they are even a patient in the facility. Under certain circumstances, patients must authorize disclosure of their PHI before it can be released by the provider. Patients can request and obtain access to their own health care records and may request that corrections and additions be made to their records. Providers must consider a patient's request to amend a health care record, but they are not required to make such an amendment if the request is unwarranted. Unauthorized access or use or any loss of health care information must be disclosed to any patient affected by the breach. Patients may request an accounting of anyone who accessed their health care information, and the provider is required to provide that information in a timely manner. Finally, patients have a right to complain if they perceive that the privacy or security of their health care information has been compromised in some way. Such complaints can be made directly to the provider or to the OCR.

The OCR, which is part of HHS, is responsible for enforcing HIPAA. It provides significant information and guidance to clinicians who must comply with the Privacy and Security Rules. It has been tracking complaints and investigating violations since 2003. Guidance and information about the complaint process and the violations that the OCR has handled are available on its website at http://www.hhs.gov/ocr/privacy/hipaa /modelnotices.html. As an example, one such violation involved a practitioner who had privileges within a health care system. She accessed her ex-husband's medical records without his authorization by using the systemwide EHRs. A complaint was filed, and the OCR investigated the matter. The OCR resolved the complaint with the health care system. As part of this resolution, the health care system curtailed the practitioner's access to its EHRs, and it required her to undergo remedial training. In addition, it reported the practitioner to her professional board (HHS, Office of Civil Rights, n.d.)

Many businesses are moving to enact a "bring your own device" (BYOD) policy for employees. This policy, which helps to streamline the lives of employees by maintaining personal and business information on one device, can also result in cost savings for the organization overall. BYOD is an issue, however, when dealing with PHI. Health care organizations typically do not encourage use of personal devices for professional matters, and in many instances they actually have policies in place forbidding employees from using personal devices in the workplace. According to HIT Consultant (2013), approximately 50% of health care organizations report that personal mobile devices can be used to access the Internet within their facilities, but these devices are not given access to the organization's network. Typically, only devices that are issued by the organization, secured, and routinely audited are able to access to the network. Health care professionals must exercise caution when bringing their personal devices into the health care organization to ensure that they are not violating any specifics of the BYOD policy.

Compliance with the Privacy and Security Rules is mandatory for all covered entities, and the HITECH Act extends compliance with these requirements directly to other entities that are business associates of a covered entity. Requirements include designation of privacy and information security officials to protect health information and appropriate handling of any complaints. Sanctions must be imposed if a violation of HIPAA occurs. The Privacy and Security Rules also mandate that certain physical and technical safeguards be implemented for PHI, and they require entities to conduct periodic training of all staff to ensure compliance with these safeguards. Most entities adhere to industry standards and provide their personnel with yearly training. In addition, entities are to conduct regular audits to ensure compliance, and any breaches in the privacy or security of PHI must be remedied immediately. It is important to avoid a security incident, defined as "the attempted or successful unauthorized access, use, disclosure, modification, or destruction of information or interference with system operations in an information system" (CMS, 2008, p. 1). Such incidents trigger certain notification requirements.

The HITECH Act–Enhanced HIPAA Protections

The HITECH Act has had a significant impact on HIPAA's Privacy and Security Rules in the following ways:

- HHS is to provide annual guidance about how to secure health information.
- Notification requirements in the event of a breach in the security of health information have been enhanced.
- HIPAA requirements now apply directly to any business associates of a covered entity.
- The rules that pertain to providing an accounting to patients who want to know who accessed their health information have changed.
- Enforcement of HIPAA has been strengthened.

These measures are being implemented to provide further assurance that health information will be protected as the country transitions to a nationwide HIT infrastructure. Several other organizations are also involved in the privacy and security aspects of the HIT infrastructure development (see **Box 5-2**).

Avoiding security incidents has become a paramount concern for health care organizations and providers. Providers must protect their information and prevent unauthorized persons from accessing, using, disclosing, changing, or destroying a patient's health information or otherwise interfering with the operations of a health information system, such as an EHR. To facilitate a provider's ability to do this, the HITECH Act requires HHS to provide annual guidance to secure health information. PHI can be secured or unsecured. PHI is considered unsecured if the provider does not follow the guidance provided by HHS for implementing technologies and methodologies that make PHI "unusable, unreadable, or indecipherable to unauthorized individuals" (HHS, 2009). PHI can be secured through encryption, shredding and other forms of complete destruction, or electronic media sanitation.

The distinction between secured and unsecured PHI is important because providers that experience a breach in the privacy or security of their PHI must adhere to certain notification requirements depending on the type of PHI affected by the breach. The HITECH Act enhanced the breach notification requirements of HIPAA. If the PHI is unsecured, the provider must take certain steps to notify those individuals who have been affected. Providers can avoid these onerous breach notification requirements if the PHI is secured in accordance with the specifications of HHS.

A breach is considered discovered as soon as an employee other than the individual who committed the breach knows or should have known of the breach, such as unauthorized access or even an unsuccessful attempt to access information. For example, if a respiratory therapist knows that a colleague has accessed or attempted to access the

BOX 5-2 OTHER ORGANIZATIONS ASSISTING HIPAA

Dee McGonigle, Kathleen Mastrian, and Nedra Farcus

Several other organizations have been involved in HIPAA implementation. The **American National Standards Institute** (ANSI) X12N and **Health Level 7** (HL7) standards organizations worked together to develop an electronic standard for claims attachments to recommend to HHS (Spencer & Bushman, 2006, para. 2). ANSI was founded in 1918 and has served as the coordinator of the U.S. voluntary standards and conformity assessment system (ANSI, n.d., para. 1). ANSI provides a forum where the private and public sectors can cooperatively work together toward the development of voluntary national consensus standards and the related compliance programs (para. 2). HL7 (n.d.) is one of several American National Standards Institute–accredited **standards–developing organizations** (SDOs) operating in the health care arena (para. 1). It states that its mission is to provide standards for interoperability that improve care delivery, optimize work flow, reduce ambiguity, and enhance knowledge transfer among all stakeholders, including health care providers, government agencies, the vendor community, fellow SDOs, and patients (para. 5).

HL7 was initially associated with HIPAA in 1996 through the creation of a claims attachments special interest group charged with standardizing the supplemental information needed to support health care insurance and other e-commerce transactions. The initial deliverable of this group was six claim attachments. This special interest group is currently known as the Attachment Special Interest Group. As the attachment projects continue, they are slated to include skilled nursing facilities, home health care, preauthorization, and referrals.

The "Level Seven" in HL7's name refers to the highest level of the **International Organization for Standardization** (ISO) communications model for the **Open Systems Interconnection** (OSI) application level. The application level addresses the definition of the data to be exchanged, the timing of the interchange, and the communication of certain errors to the application. The seventh level supports such functions as security checks, participant identification, availability checks, exchange mechanism negotiations, and, most importantly, data exchange structuring (HL7, n.d., para. 5).

The OSI was an attempt to standardize networking by the ISO. HL7 addresses the distinct requirements of the systems in use in hospitals and other facilities, is concerned more with application than with the other levels, and considers user authentication and privacy (Webopedia, 2008). The lower levels of OSI address hardware, software, and data reformatting.

HL7's mission is supported through two separate groups: the Extensible Markup Language (XML) special interest group and the structured documents technical committee. The XML special interest group makes recommendations on use of XML standards for all of HL7's platform- and vendor-independent health care specifications (HL7, n.d., para. 21). XML began as a simplified subset of the standard generalized markup language; its major purpose is to facilitate the exchange of structured data across different information systems, especially via the Internet. It is considered an extensible language because it permits users to define their own elements, thereby supporting customization to enable purpose-specific development. The structured documents technical committee supports the HL7 mission through development of structured document standards for health care (para. 21). HL7 also organizes, maintains, and sustains a repository for the vocabulary terms used in its messages to provide a shared, well-defined, and unambiguous knowledge base of the meaning of the data transferred.

ISO (2008a) is a network of the national standards institutes of 157 countries. It includes one member per country, and a central secretariat in Geneva, Switzerland, coordinates the system (para. 1). ISO is a nongovernmental organization; its members are not delegations of national governments (unlike the case in the United Nations system). Nevertheless, ISO occupies a special position between the public and private sectors. On the one hand,

BOX 5-2   OTHER ORGANIZATIONS ASSISTING HIPAA (continued)

many of its member institutes are part of the governmental structure of their countries or are mandated by their government. On the other hand, other members have their roots uniquely in the private sector, having been set up by national partnerships of industry associations (ISO, 2008a, para. 2).

This placement enables ISO to become a bridging organization where members can reach agreement on solutions that meet both the requirements of business and the broader needs of society, consumers, and users. These international agreements become standards that use the prefix "ISO" followed by the number of the standard. An example is the health informatics, health cards, numbering system, and registration procedure for issuer identifiers, ISO 20302:2006; it is designed to confirm, via a numbering system and registration procedure, the identities of both the health care application provider and the health cardholder so that information may be exchanged by using cards issued for health care service (ISO, 2008b, para. 12). ISO provides standards for interoperability that improve care delivery, optimize work flow, reduce ambiguity, and enhance knowledge transfer among all of its stakeholders, including health care providers, government agencies, the vendor community, fellow SDOs, and patients. The standards are used on a voluntary basis because ISO has no power to force their enactment.

All of the organizations described here have guidelines, standards, and rules to help health care entities collect, store, manipulate, dispose of, and exchange secure PHI. Many SDOs work to help develop standards. HIPAA guarantees the security and privacy of health information and curtails health care fraud and abuse while enforcing standards for health information.

UNITED STATES AND BEYOND

Health care was not the only focus of U.S. legislative acts. One often sees "GLBA" and "SOX" when searching for information on HIPAA. The **Gramm-Leach-Bliley Act** (GLBA) is federal legislation in the United States to control how financial institutions handle the private information they collect from individuals. The **Sarbanes-Oxley (SOX) Act** is legislation put in place to protect shareholders and the public from deceptive accounting practices in organizations.

Privacy and data regulations are also being established around the world, such as the Data Protection Act 1998 in the United Kingdom (Ministry of Justice, 2008); the Dutch Data Protection Authority (2007), which released privacy legislation guidelines on publishing personal data on the Internet; and Finland's Personal Data File Act 1988 and Personal Data Act 1999 (Data Protection Board, n.d.). New Zealand's Health Information Privacy Code 1994 had amendment number 6 come into effect in November 2007; this amendment defined entities such as the ethics committee; hospital, health, or disability services; health professional body; registered health professional; and health practitioner (Privacy Commissioner, 2007). Argentina's Privacy and Data Protection (2007) states that it is the first Latin American country to be awarded the status of "adequate country" from the point of view of European Data Protection authorities—a breakthrough that is expected to encourage other countries in the region to work toward improving data protection rights for individuals (Privacy and Data Protection, 2007, para. 7). In Canada, the Personal Information Protection and Electronic Documents Act received royal assent in 2000 (Office of the Privacy Commissioner of Canada, 2004). Safe Harbor deals with the transfer of personal data from the European Union to the United States; the regulations in Article 25 and 26 of the European Data Protection Directive serve as the basis for governing this transfer. According to these regulations, transferring data to third countries is in principle possible only if these countries guarantee an adequate level of protection as required by the directive (Federal Commissioner for Data Protection and Freedom of Information, n.d., para. 1). It is quite evident that privacy and security have become global concerns.

record of a patient for whom the colleague is not providing care (e.g., the practitioner who accessed her ex-husband's EHR, as discussed previously), the employer is deemed to have discovered the breach as soon as the colleague learned of it. The discovery of a breach triggers the beginning of the time frame during which the provider must fulfill the notification requirements. A provider must fulfill these requirements within a reasonable period of time; under no circumstances may a provider take more than 60 days from discovery of the breach. It is easy to understand why providers require their employees to report knowledge of such breaches immediately to the privacy or information security officer. A provider's failure to adhere to the breach notification requirements could result in OCR sanctions, including monetary penalties.

Whenever a breach involves unsecured PHI, covered entities are responsible for alerting each individual affected by mail (or by e-mail if preferred by the individual). If there is insufficient contact information for 10 or more patients, the provider is required to place conspicuous postings on the home page of its website or in major print or broadcast media (without identifying patients). A toll-free telephone number must be provided so that affected individuals can call for information about the breach. For breaches involving unsecured PHI of more than 500 individuals, a prominent media outlet must also be notified. Notice must be given to HHS as well, and HHS will post the information on its public website (HHS, 2009). It is easy to see why providers would want to avoid these requirements by making sure their PHI is secured. Having to post such notices undermines the trust that exists between health care providers and the patients and communities they serve.

The HITECH Act has improved the privacy and security of patient health information by applying the requirements of HIPAA directly to the business associates of covered entities. In the past, it was up to the covered entity to enter into contracts with its business associates to ensure compliance with HIPAA. Now business associates are responsible for their own compliance. An example of such a business associate is a HIT company hired by a hospital to implement or upgrade an EHR system. The technology company has access to the hospital's EHR system and must comply with the HIPAA Privacy and Security Rules, just as covered entities must comply with these rules. This includes being subject to enforcement by the OCR for any violations.

Existing accounting rules are enhanced under the HITECH Act, giving patients the right to **access** their EHR and receive an accounting of all disclosures. Before the HITECH Act, HIPAA regulations provided an exception to the accounting requirements. Providers and other covered entities were not required to include in the accounting any disclosures that were made to facilitate the **treatment** of patients, the **payment** for services, or the **operations** of the entity—a provision commonly known as the "TPO exception." This exception ended in January 2011 for providers that recently implemented new EHR systems. For those providers with EHR systems that were implemented before the HITECH Act, the TPO exception ended in January 2014. It is easy to understand why this exception has ended. As all providers implement comprehensive EHR systems, it will be very easy to generate an electronic record with an accounting of anyone who accessed a patient's record.

Finally, the HITECH Act strengthened the enforcement of HIPAA. HHS can conduct audits, which will be even easier to accomplish once a nationwide HIT infrastructure is in place. In addition, stiffer **civil monetary penalties** (CMPs) for violations of HIPAA became effective as soon as the HITECH Act became law in February 2009. CMPs are divided into three tiers. A Tier 1 CMP, in which the covered entity had no reason to know of a violation, is $100 per incident, up to a cap of $25,000 per year. A Tier 2 CMP, in which the covered entity had reasonable cause to know of a violation, is $1,000 per incident, up to a cap of $100,000 per year. A Tier 3 CMP, in which the covered entity engaged in willful neglect that resulted in a breach, is $10,000 per incident, up to a cap of $250,000 per year. In addition, the HITECH Act gives authority to impose an additional CMP of $50,000 to $1.5 million if the covered entity does not properly correct a violation. Criminal penalties also can be imposed when warranted. It is imperative that providers avoid these penalties.

Before enactment of the HITECH Act, the federal government alone enforced HIPAA. Now, state attorneys general can play a significant role in the enforcement and prosecution of HIPAA violations. Once the HITECH Act became law, state attorneys general were authorized to pursue civil claims for HIPAA violations and collect up to $25,000 plus attorneys' fees. As of 2012, individuals who are damaged by such violations became eligible to share in any monetary awards obtained by these state officials.

Implications for Practice

Being Involved and Staying Informed

The development and implementation of a nationwide EHR system holds great promise for professional practice and health informatics. All health care professions will benefit from the many enhancements such an infrastructure has to offer, including the ability to improve the delivery of care and the quality of that care, the ability to make more efficient and timely care decisions for patients, the ability to avoid errors that may harm patients, and the ability to promote health and wellness for the patients whom professionals serve. On a broader scale, researchers will have the ability to more readily access data that can be used to continue to foster evidence-based practice. The possibilities seem endless. For those who devote their professional careers to health informatics or plan to do so, the opportunities abound. Much work remains to be done as this country transitions to a nationwide HIT infrastructure, however, and there are monetary incentives available from the government for adopting systems that comply with the meaningful use requirement.

All health care professionals need to be engaged in this process, whether they treat patients, are managers within health care organizations, teach, develop computer programs, or help create institutional or governmental policies. Practitioners, as the end users of developing technologies, cannot afford to be left behind in these exciting times. Their voices must be heard, whether it is within the facility where they work as changes to the EHR system are contemplated or whether it is in the public policy arena. How often are the end users the last to know that a new EHR system has been adopted by their hospital? How many times have health care professionals been trained to use a system that would have benefited from their input before it was implemented or even purchased? Health care professionals often are not invited to the table when entities make decisions about informatics, so they should not be afraid to ask to be included, whether it is to be heard within the workplace or within the governmental agencies that are overseeing the changes that are taking place.

Even professionals who do not get involved in this process need to stay current with the rapid changes that are taking place. Information about federal initiatives is available from the ONC and the OCR. Both offices are housed within HHS and are excellent resources for additional information about the HITECH Act and HIPAA. Regulations to implement the HITECH Act and enhance the HIPAA protections required by it are being proposed and adopted at a rapid pace. The ONC can be accessed at http://www.healthit.gov/newsroom/about-onc. The OCR can be accessed at http://www.hhs.gov/ocr/privacy/hipaa/modelnotices.html. State resources also are available.

Protecting Yourself

Health care professionals who strive to protect the privacy and security of patient information are protecting themselves from ethical lapses and violations of law. Check your professional code of ethics for how to protect a patient's rights to privacy and confidentiality.

Associated with the right to privacy, the professional has a duty to maintain confidentiality of all patient information. Health professionals who engage with social media need to be especially cognizant of the potential for breaching the confidentiality of patient information. The patient's well-being could be jeopardized and the fundamental trust between patient and provider destroyed by unnecessary access to data or by the inappropriate disclosure of identifiable patient information. The rights, well-being, and safety of the individual patient should be the primary factors in arriving at any professional judgment concerning the disposition of confidential information received from or about the patient, whether oral, written, or electronic. Data and information may be shared only with those members of the health care team who have a need to know that information. Only information pertinent to a patient's treatment and welfare should be disclosed and only to those directly involved with the patient's care.

Ethical and Legal Issues and Social Media

As connectivity has improved owing to emerging technologies, a rapid explosion in the phenomenon known as **social media** has occurred. Social media are defined as "a group of Internet-based applications that build on the ideological and technological foundations of Web 2.0 and that allow the creation and exchange of user-generated content" (Spector & Kappel, 2012, p. 1). Just as the electronic health record serves as a real-time event in recording patient–provider contact, so the use of social media represents an instantaneous form of communication. Health care providers can enhance the patient care delivery system, promote professional collegiality, and provide timely communication and education regarding health-related matters by using this forum ("White Paper," 2011, p. 1). In all cases, however, providers must exercise judicious use of social media to protect patients' rights. Health professionals must understand their obligation to their chosen profession, particularly as it relates to personal behavior and the perceptions of their image as portrayed through social media. Above all, we must be mindful that once communication is written and posted on the Internet, there is no way to retract what was written; it is a permanent record that can be tracked, even if the post is deleted (Englund, Chappy, Jambunathan, & Gohdes, 2012, p. 242).

Social media platforms include such electronic communication outlets as Facebook, Twitter, LinkedIn, and YouTube. Other widely used means of instantaneous communications include wikis, blogs, tweeting, Skype, and the "hangout" on Google+. We can safely predict that these types of social networking programs will continue to evolve, posing even more potential threats to information privacy while at the same time providing great opportunities for professional networking and exchange of ideas.

Use of social networking has increased dramatically among all age-groups, including a 78% increase in use among the 50- to 64-year-old age-group and a 42% increase in use among persons older than 65 years over a time frame of a little more than 3 years. Facebook reported in June 2012 that it had 955 million active monthly users, a figure that is much higher now. Twitter's influence on health care is suggested by the fact that more than 100 million pieces of health care information have been tweeted, with as many as 140 million tweets being recorded in a day's time (Prasad, 2013, p. 492). Moreover, people spend more than 700 billion minutes per month actively engaged with the Facebook site (Miller, 2011, p. 307). The Pew Research Internet Project (2014) reports social media use among adults who are online at 74%, providing a great opportunity for health professionals to engage with patients and other providers in an ethical and professional manner.

The rapid growth of social media has found many health care professionals unprepared to face the new challenges or to exploit the opportunities that exist with these forums. The need to maintain confidentiality presents a major obstacle to the health care industry's widespread adoption of such technology; thus, social networking has not yet been fully embraced by many health professionals (Anderson, 2012, p. 1). Englund et al. (2012) note that undergraduate nursing students may face ambiguous and understudied professional and ethical implications when using social networking venues, a fact that is likely to be true for all health professions.

The popularity of social and mobile networking applications is one indication of how new Web-based technologies are changing communication preferences. The Web is no longer a destination place but instead has become a vehicle of communication where individuals use apps, which are installed or downloaded, to connect with others. Individuals act as their own portal and can connect from anywhere with their various communities. This makes it difficult to separate out various communities and social networks. Where once it was relatively easy to separate work relationships from friends and family, networked communities tend to overlap, blurring the boundaries between them. The phenomenon of overlapping networks means that the unintended audience is almost always greater than the intended one. A status update that may be construed as harmless and funny to one's friends could be taken an entirely different way by family or colleagues. This is not to say that networked communities are harmful or bad. Indeed, the benefits of such communities far exceed their negatives. However, the immediacy and the permanence of the updates shared mean that the user must think about the impact beyond the intended audience in ways never before required (Johnson & Swain, 2011).

Another confounding factor is the increased use of mobile devices by health professionals as well as the public (Swartz, 2011, p. 345). The mobile device known as the **smartphone** has the capability to take still pictures as well as make live recordings; it has found its way into treatment rooms around the globe.

As a consequence of more stringent confidentiality laws and more widespread availability and use of social and mobile media, numerous ethical and legal dilemmas have been posed to health professionals. What are not well defined are the expectations of health care providers regarding this technology. In some cases, providers employed in the emergency department setting have been subjected to video and audio recordings by patients and families when they perform procedures and give care during the emergency department visit. Providers would be wise to inquire—before an incident occurs—about the hospital policy regarding audio/video recording by patients and families as well as the state laws governing two-party consent laws. Such laws require consent of all parties to any recording or eavesdropping activity (Lyons & Reinisch, 2013, p. 54).

Sometimes the enthusiasm for patient care and learning can lead to ethics and legal violations. In one case, an inadvertent violation of privacy laws occurred when a nurse in a small town blogged about a child in her care whom she referred to as her "little handicapper." The post also noted the child's age and the fact that the child used a wheelchair. A complaint about this breach of confidentiality was reported to the Board of Nursing. A warning was issued to the nurse blogging this information, although a more stringent disciplinary action could have been taken (Spector & Kappel, 2012, p. 2). Even a seemingly innocent comment on social media about how hard one's day was could be misconstrued as a direct complaint about a specific patient.

In another case cited by Spector and Kappel (2012), a student nurse cared for a 3-year-old leukemia patient whom she wanted to remember after finishing her pediatric clinical experience. She took the child's picture, and in the background of the photo the patient's room number was clearly displayed. The child's picture was posted on the student nurse's Facebook page along with her statement of how much she cared about this child and how proud she was to be a student nurse. Someone forwarded the picture to the nurse supervisor of the children's hospital. Not only was the student expelled from the program, but the clinical site offer made by the children's hospital to the nursing school was rescinded. In addition, the hospital faced citations for violations of HIPAA because of the student nurse's transgression (p. 3).

A white paper published by the National Council of State Boards of Nursing (2011) provides a thorough discussion of the issues associated with nurses' use of social media and provides a series of case studies for discussion that could easily be applied to other health professions. In addition, you should visit your professional website to see specific information on appropriate and inappropriate use of social media. **Table 5-2** provides some quick links to social media information for several health professions.

The similarities between professional ethical obligations and the legal requirements of HIPAA and other federal and state privacy and confidentiality laws are readily apparent to health care professionals. By complying with their ethical code, many professionals were complying with the Privacy and Security Rules before they were required to do so. Since the adoption of the HIPAA Privacy and Security Rules and the HITECH Act, it has been more important than ever for health care professionals to understand their obligations in this area and avoid the pitfalls of violations.

In addition to the sanctions imposed by the OCR, violations can lead to disciplinary actions by employers and professional licensing boards as well as litigation. Such actions can have a serious negative impact on the professional's reputation and financial well-being. If a health care professional is terminated for invading a patient's privacy or breaching the confidentiality of a patient's information, some state laws require reporting the information to all prospective employers of the professional; other laws require reporting to the state licensing board. These boards may have the authority to publicly discipline a health care professional who has engaged in professional misconduct by invading a patient's privacy, which includes inappropriately accessing a patient's EHR, and breaching confidentiality of patient information, such as allowing or tolerating unauthorized access to a patient's EHR. These types of situations can also cause patients to file complaints with the OCR and lawsuits against the offenders. All professionals must be ever mindful of their obligations to report a breach in the privacy or security of PHI to their employers, even if it entails reporting a colleague.

TABLE 5-2 SOCIAL MEDIA POLICIES BY PROFESSIONAL ORGANIZATIONS	
Organization	**Social Media Information**
American Association of Respiratory Care	https://www.aarc.org/careers/career-advice/using-social-media-in-your-job-search/talking-politics-social-media
American Occupational Therapy Association	http://www.aota.org/Practice/Manage/Social-Media.aspx
American Physical Therapy Association	http://www.apta.org/SocialMedia/Tips
American Dental Hygienists Association	https://www.adha.org/resources-docs/7614_Policy_Manual.pdf
Academy of Nutrition and Dietetics	http://www.eatrightpro.org/resource/leadership/board-of-directors/academy-policies/social-media-policy
	Case Studies: http://www.eatrightpro.org/~/media/eatrightpro%20files/career/code%20of%20ethics/social_media_ethics_case_study.ashx

Finally, some view the EHR as a convenient method for employers to monitor the performance of its employees. Clearly, an EHR system provides a wealth of information that can be and often is required to be monitored. Audits are required to make sure that no breaches in the system's security occur. Audits are not necessarily required to determine, for example, who is failing to complete the hospital's documentation requirements in a timely fashion, who is improperly altering (attempting to correct) the record, or who is dispensing more pain medication than the average. Professionals have been challenged by employers who allege failure to document, improper or false documentation, and suspected diversion of narcotics. These types of situations are unsettling and may be on the rise as more providers adopt or augment EHR systems. Thus, it behooves every professional who works with such a system to obtain proper training and to know the policies and procedures that pertain to its use.

Social media can and should be used in an appropriate manner by professionals to educate and promote health behaviors in the clients they serve, communicate with clients if they choose this method of communication, and network with other professionals by sharing information (deidentified) and knowledge. As Gagnon and Sabus (2015) suggest, "The reach of social media for health and wellness presents exciting opportunities for the health care professional with a well-executed social media presence. Social media give health care providers a far-reaching platform on which to contribute high-quality online content and amplify positive and accurate health care information and messages. It also provides a forum for correcting misinformation and addressing misconceptions" (p. 410). They advocate for health care professionals to practice digital professionalism and for social media use to be one of the professional competencies for health professional education. Bazan (2015) suggested that social media can be used to consult with other health care providers, such as in a professional Facebook group using direct private messaging between the two providers, but cautions that posting to the main social site cannot contain any hint of PHI. He also shares information about a progressive practice that communicates with patients via private messaging on Facebook. Remember that everything you do electronically leaves a digital footprint! Proceed with caution and be certain that your digital interactions comply completely with professional ethics, laws, and organizational policies.

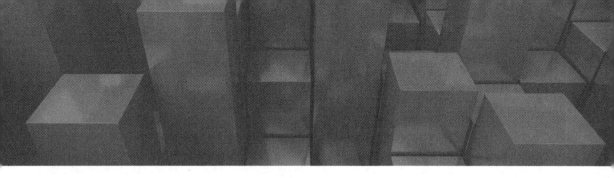

Summary

As science and technology advance and policymakers and health care providers continue to shape health care practices including information management, it is paramount that health care professionals embrace ethical decision making. Health care professionals are typically honest, trustworthy, and ethical, and they understand that they are duty bound to focus on the needs and rights of their patients. At the same time, their day-to-day work is conducted in a world of changing health care landscapes populated by new technologies, diverse patients, varied health care settings, and changing policies set by their employers, insurance companies, providers, and legislation. Health care professionals need to juggle all of these balls simultaneously, a task that often results in far too many gray areas or ethical decision-making dilemmas with no clear correct course of action.

Patients rely on the ethical and legal competence of their health care providers, believing that their situation is unique and will be respected and evaluated based on their own needs, abilities, and limitations. The health care professional cannot allow conflicting loyalties to interfere with judicious, ethical, and legal decision making. Just as in the opening example of the *Apollo* mission, it is uncertain where this technologically heightened information era will lead, but if a solid foundation of ethical decision making is relied on, duties and rights will be judiciously and ethically fulfilled.

The HITECH Act and the HIPAA Privacy and Security Rules are intended to enhance the rights of individuals. These laws provide patients with greater access and control over their PHI. They can control its uses, dissemination, and disclosures. Covered entities must establish not only a required level of security for PHI but also sanctions for employees who violate the organization's privacy policies and administrative processes for responding to patient requests regarding their information. Therefore, they must be able to track the PHI, note access from the perspective of which information was accessed and by whom, and identify any disclosures. Finally, readers should recognize that there is global awareness of the need for privacy protections for personal information or PHI. Over the next few years, international efforts will accelerate, enhancing international data exchange.

Thought-Provoking Questions

1. Identify moral dilemmas in health informatics that would best be approached with the use of an ethical decision-making framework, such as the use of smartphones to interact with patients as well as other technologies that monitor and assess patient health and exchange patient data/information.
2. Discuss the evolving health care ethics traditions within their social and historical contexts.

3. Differentiate among the theoretical approaches to health care ethics as they relate to the theorists' perspectives of individuals and their relationships.
4. Select one of the health care ethics theories and support its use in examining ethical issues in health informatics. Then select one of the health care ethics theories and argue against its use in examining ethical issues in health informatics.
5. One of the largest problems with health care information security has always been inappropriate use by authorized users. How do HIPAA and the HITECH Act help to curb this problem?
6. How do you envision HL7, HIPAA, and the HITECH Act evolving in the next decade?
7. If you were the privacy officer in your organization, how would you address the following?
   a. Tracking each point of access of the patient's database, including who entered the data.
   b. Encouraging employees to report privacy and security breaches.
   c. The health care professionals are using smartphones, iPads, and other mobile devices. How do you address privacy when data can literally walk out of your setting?
   d. You observe one of the health care professionals using his smartphone to take pictures of a patient. He sees you and says, in front of the patient, "I am not capturing her face!" How do you respond to this situation?

Apply Your Knowledge

Anna owns a document scanning business and has hired 12 16-year-old students from the local high school to help with document scanning. The majority of the scan jobs that they do typically consist of business documents. They take the documents, scan them in by hand, page by page, and then import them to CD. When there is a paper problem, they copy the original and then discard it, using the copy.

Anna has just been contracted by Low Mountain Health Center to scan old patient records onto CDs. She is excited. The 100 boxes of medical records arrive within 1 week of signing the contract, and Anna immediately puts them in the scanning storage to be done ASAP. The students begin to work with these records without any further training.

Consider the following as you use the ETHICAL model to analyze the case:

1. What is the problem? (Clearly state the problem)
2. What are the ethical issues involved?
3. Assess the ethical principles, which ones would guide you in this case?
4. Determine three alternatives for Anna that would bring her into HIPAA compliance.
5. What are the consequences for each alternative you generated?

Additional Resources

E-Health Code of Ethics http://www.ihealthcoalition.org/ehealth-code
Internet Healthcare Coalition http://www.ihealthcoalition.org
Office of Civil Rights http://www.hhs.gov/ocr/privacy/hipaa/modelnotices.html
Office of the National Coordinator for Health Information Technology http://www.healthit.gov/newsroom/about-onc

References

Agency for Healthcare Research and Quality. (2009). *National healthcare quality report (NHQR) 2009: Crossing the quality chasm: A new healthcare system for the 21st century*. Washington, DC: National Academies Press.

Anderson, K. (2012, September). Patient care and social media. *Australian Nursing Journal, 22*. http://go.galegroup.com.silk.library.umass.edu/ps/i.do?id=GALE%CA301964363&v=2.1&u =mlin_w_umassamh&it=r&p+AONE&sw=w

Ashish, J. (2009). Use of electronic health records in U.S. hospitals. *New England Journal of Medicine, 360*(16), 1628–1638.

Bazan, J. (2015). HIPAA in the age of social media. *Optometry Times, 7*(2), 16–18.

Beauchamp, T. L., & Childress, J. F. (1977). *Principles of biomedical ethics*. New York: Oxford University Press.

Beauchamp, T. L., & Childress, J. F. (1994). *Principles of biomedical ethics* (4th ed.). New York: Oxford University Press.

Benjamin, M., & Curtis, J. (1992). *Ethics in nursing* (3rd ed.). New York: Oxford University Press.

Centers for Medicare and Medicaid Services. (2010). Meaningful use. https://www .cms.gov /EHRIncentivePrograms/30_Meaningful_Use.asp

Data Protection Board. (n.d.). Legislation for the protection of privacy. http://www.tietosuoja .fi/27305.htm

Derse, A., & Miller, T. (2008). Net effect: Professional and ethical challenges of medicine online. *Cambridge Quarterly of Healthcare Ethics, 17*(4), 453–464. Retrieved from Health Module (Document ID: 1540615461).

Dutch Data Protection Authority. (2007, December). Dutch DPA publication of personal data on the Internet. http://www.dutchdpa.nl/downloads_overig/en_20071108 _richtsnoeren_internet.pdf?refer=true&theme=purple

eHealth code. (n.d.). http://www.ihealthcoalition.org/ehealth-code

Englund, H., Chappy, S., Jambunathan, J., & Gohdes, E. (2012, November/December). Ethical reasoning and online social media. *Nurse Educator, 37*, 242–247. http://dx.doi.org/10.1097 /NNE.0b013e31826f2c04

Engster, D. (n.d.). Can care ethics be institutionalized? Toward a caring natural law theory. https://lmstest.manhattan.edu/pluginfile.php/39833/mod_resource/content/1 /Engster%20Care%20and%20Political%20Theory.pdf

Federal Commissioner for Data Protection and Freedom of Information. (n.d.). Safe harbor. http://www.bfdi.bund.de/cln_007/nn_671558/EN/EuropeanInternationalAffaires /Artikel/SafeHarbor.html

Gagnon, K., & Sabus, C. (2015). Professionalism in a digital age: Opportunities and considerations for using social media in health care. *Physical Therapy, 95*(3), 406–414. doi: 10.2522/ ptj.20130227

Guidance on compliance with HIPAA transactions and code sets. (2003). http://www.cms .gov/Regulations-and-Guidance/HIPAA-Administrative-Simplification/Transaction CodeSetsStands/index.html?redirect=/transactioncodesetsstands/02_transactionsand codesetsregulations.asp

Healthcare Ethics. (2007). Virtue ethics. http://www.ascensionhealth.org/ethics/public/issues /virtue.asp

Health Level Seven (HL7). (n.d.). What is HL7? http://www.hl7.org

Hellerstein, D. (1999). HIPAA's impact on healthcare. *Health Management Technology*. http:// findarticles.com/p/articles/mi_m0DUD/is_3_20/ai_54396227

Hellerstein, D. (2000). HIPAA and health information privacy rules: Almost there. *Health Management Technology*. http://findarticles.com/p/articles/mi_m0DUD/is_4_21/ai_61523494

HIT Consultant. (2013). 3 do's and don'ts of effective HIPAA compliance for BYOD & mHealth. http://www.hitconsultant.net/2013/06/11/3-dos-and-donts-of-effective -hipaacompliance-for-byod-mhealth

Howard, R. (Director). (1995). *Apollo 13* [Motion picture]. Universal City, CA: MCA Universal Studios.

Husted, G. L., & Husted, J. H. (1995). *Ethical decision-making in nursing* (2nd ed.). New York: Mosby.

International Confederation of Dietetic Associations. (2014). International code of ethics and code of good practice. http://www.internationaldietetics.org/International-Standards /International-Code-of-Ethics-and-Code-of-Good-Prac.aspx

International Organization for Standardization. (2008a). About ISO. http://www.iso.org/iso /about.htm

International Organization for Standardization. (2008b). Health informatics. http://www .iso.org/iso/iso_catalogue/catalogue_tc/catalogue_detail.htm?csnumber=35376

Johnson, G., & Swain, J. (2011). Professional development and collaboration tools. In D. McGonigle & K. Mastrian (Eds.), *Nursing informatics and the foundation of knowledge* (2nd ed). Burlington, MA: Jones and Bartlett Learning. pp. 185–195.

Jonsen, A. R. (1991). Casuistry as methodology in clinical ethics. *Theoretical Medicine, 12,* 295–307.

Leyva, C., & Leyva, D. (2011). HITECH Act. http://www.hipaasurvivalguide.com/hitech-act-text .php

Lyons, R., & Reinisch, C. (2013). The legal and ethical implications of social media in the emergency department. *Advanced Emergency Nursing Journal, 35*(1), 53–56. http://dx.doi .org/10.1097/TME.0b013e31827a4926

Mack, J. (2000). Patient empowerment, not economics, is driving e-health: Privacy and ethics issues need attention too! *Frontiers of Health Services Management, 17*(1), 39–43; discussion 49–51. Retrieved from ABI/INFORM Global (Document ID: 59722384).

Makus, R. (2001). Ethics and Internet healthcare: An ontological reflection. *Cambridge Quarterly of Healthcare Ethics, 10*(2), 127–136. Retrieved from Health Module (Document ID: 1409693941).

Martin, P. A. (1999). Bioethics and the whole: Pluralism, consensus, and the transmutation of bioethical methods into gold. *Journal of Law, Medicine & Ethics, 27*(4), 316–327.

McGonigle, D. (2000). The ethical model for ethical decision making. *Inside Case Management, 7*(8), 1–5.

Miller, L. A. (2011). Social media: Friend and foe. *Journal of Perinatal and Neonatal Nursing,* 307–309. http://dx.doi.org/10.1097/JPN.0b013e31823506e9

Ministry of Justice. (2008). Data sharing and protection. http://www.justice.gov.uk /information-access-rights/data-protection

National Council of State Boards of Nursing. (2011). White paper: A nurse's guide to the use of social media. http://www.ncsbn.org

Office of the National Coordinator for Health Information Technology. (2015, June). Non-federal acute care hospital electronic health record adoption. Health IT Quick-Stat #47. http:// dashboard.healthit.gov/quickstats/pages/FIG-Hospital-EHR-Adoption.php

Office of the Privacy Commissioner of Canada. (2004). Privacy legislation. http://www .privcom.gc.ca/legislation/02_06_07_e.asp

Pellegrino, E. D. (1993). The metamorphosis of medical ethics: A thirty-year retrospective. *Journal of the American Medical Association, 269,* 1158–1162.

Pellegrino, E., & Thomasma, D. (1993). *The virtues in medical practice.* New York: Oxford University Press.

Pew Research Internet Project. (2014). Social networking fact sheet. Retrieved from http://www .pewinternet.org/fact-sheets/social-networking-fact-sheet

Prasad, B. (2013). Social media, health care, and social networking. *Gastrointestinal Endoscopy, 77*, 492–495.

Privacy Commissioner. (2007). Health information privacy code. http://www.privacy.org.nz/health-information-privacy-code

Privacy and Data Protection. (2007). Data protection in Argentina. http://www.protecciondedatos.com.ar

Readthestimulus.org. (2009, January 16). Committee print. http://govinfo.sla.org/2009/02/08/readthestimulusorg/

Scott, A. (2002). Plato's Meno. http://www.angelfire.com/md2/timewarp/plato.html

Spector, N., & Kappel, D. M. (2012). Guidelines for using electronic and social media. *Online Journal of Nursing, 17*. http://www.medscape.com/viewarticle/780050

Spencer, J., & Bushman, M. (2006). HIPAAdvisory: The next HIPAA frontier: Claims attachments. http://www.hipaadvisory.com/action/tcs/nextfrontier.htm

Stern, J. (2013). Google Glass: What you can and can't do with Google's wearable computer. http://abcnews.go.com/Technology/google-glass-googles-wearable-gadget/story?id=19091948

Swartz, M. K. (2011, November/December). The potential for social media. *Journal of Pediatric Health Care, 25*, 345.

U.S. Department of Health and Human Services, Office of Civil Rights. (n.d.). Health information privacy: All case examples. http://www.hhs.gov/ocr/privacy/hipaa/enforcement/examples/allcases.html#case1

U.S. Department of Health and Human Services. (2002). Federal Register, Part V, Department of Health and Human Services: Standards for privacy of individually identifiable health information; Final rule. http://www.hhs.gov/ocr/privacy/hipaa/administrative/privacyrule/privrulepd.pdf

U.S. Department of Health and Human Services. (2006). Medical privacy: National standards to protect the privacy of personal health information. http://www.ihs.gov/hipaa

U.S. Department of Health and Human Services. (2007). Administrative simplification in the health care industry. http://aspe.os.dhhs.gov/admnsimp

US Department of Health and Human Services, CMS. (2008). CMS information security incident handling and breach analysis/notification process. https://www.cms.gov/informationsecurity/downloads/incident_handling_procedure.pdf

U.S. Department of Health and Human Services. (2009). Federal Register: 45 CFR Parts 160 and 164: Breach notification for unsecured protected health information; Interim. http://www.hhs.gov/ocr/privacy/hipaa/administrative/breachnotificationrule/index.html

Velasquez, M., Andre, C., Shanks, T., & Myer, M. (for the Markkula Center for Applied Ethics). (1987). What is ethics? http://www.scu.edu/SCU/Centers/Ethics/practicing/decision/whatisethics.shtml

V|lex. (2011). 45 CFR 160.103—Definitions. http://cfr.vlex.com/vid/160-103-definitions-19933565

Webopedia. (2008). The 7 layers of the OSI model. http://www.webopedia.com/quick_ref/OSI_Layers.asp

Section II

Choosing and Using Information Systems

Informatics and information technology (IT) have invaded health care, and some professionals are happy with the practice enhancements afforded by these transformational changes. Others, however, remain convinced that the changes wrought by IT are nothing more than a nuisance. In the past, health care administrators have found the implementation of technology tools to be an expensive venture with minimal rewards. This disappointment is likely related to their lack of knowledge about health informatics (HI), which caused administrators to listen to vendors or other colleagues; in essence, it was decision making based on limited and biased information. There were at least two reasons for the experience of limited rewards. First, health care professionals were rarely included in the testing and implementation of products designed for use in practice. Second, the new products they purchased had to interface with old, legacy systems that were not at all compatible or seemed compatible until the glitches arose. These glitches caused frustration for health care professionals and administrators alike. They purchased tools that should have made the professionals happy, but instead all they did was grumble.

The good news is that approaches have changed as a result of the difficult lessons learned from the early forays into technology tools. Health care professionals are now regularly involved both at the agency level and at the vendor level in the decision-making process and development of new systems and products. Older legacy systems are being replaced with newer systems that have more capacity to interface with other systems. Health care professionals and administrators have become more astute in the realm of HI, but there is still a long way to go. The *Systems Development Life Cycle* chapter introduces the system development life cycle, which is used to make important and appropriate organizational decisions for technology adoption.

Administrators need information systems that facilitate their administrative role, and they particularly need systems that provide financial, risk management, quality assurance, human resources, payroll, patient registration, acuity, communication, and scheduling functions. The administrator must be open to learning about all of the tools available. One of the most important tasks that an administrator can oversee and engage in is data mining, or the extraction of data and information from sizable data sets that have been collected and warehoused. Data mining helps to identify patterns in aggregate data, gain insights, and ultimately discover and generate knowledge applicable practice. To take advantage of these benefits, administrators must become astute informaticists—knowledge workers who harness the information and knowledge at their fingertips to facilitate the practice of their clinicians, improve patient care, and advance disciplinary science.

Clinical information systems (CIS) have traditionally been designed for use by one unit or department within an institution. However, because clinicians working in other areas of the organization need access to this information, these data and information are generally used by more than one area. The new initiatives arising with the development of the electronic health record place institutions in the position of striving to manage their CIS through the electronic health record. Currently, there are many CISs, including nursing, laboratory, pharmacy, monitoring, and order entry, plus additional ancillary systems to meet the individual institutions' needs. The *Administrative Information Systems* chapter provides an overview of administrative information systems and helps the reader understand the powerful data aggregation and data mining tools afforded by these systems.

The *Human–Technology Interface* chapter discusses the need to improve quality and safety outcomes significantly in the United States. Through the use of IT, the designs for human–technology interfaces can be radically improved so that the technology better fits both human and task requirements. A number of useful tools are currently available for the analysis, design, and evaluation phases of development life cycles and should be used routinely by informatics professionals to ensure that technology better fits both task and user requirements. In this chapter, the authors stress that the focus on interface improvement using these tools has dramatically improved patient safety. With increased attention from informatics professionals and engineers, the same kinds of improvements should be possible in other areas. This human–technology interface is a crucial area if the theories, architectures, and tools provided by the building block sciences are to be implemented.

Each organization must determine who can access and use its information systems and provide robust tools for securing information in a networked environment. The *Electronic Security* chapter addresses the important safeguards for protecting information. As new technologies designed to enhance patient care are adopted, barriers to implementation and resistance by practitioners to change are frequently encountered. The *Work Flow and Meaningful Use* chapter provides insights into clinical work flow analysis and provides advice on improving efficiency and effectiveness to achieve meaningful use of caring technologies.

Pause to reflect on the Foundation of Knowledge model (**Figure II-1**) and its relationship to both personal and organizational knowledge management. Consider that organizational decision making must be driven by appropriate information and knowledge developed in the organization and applied with wisdom. Equally important to adopting technology within an organization is the consideration of the knowledge base and knowledge capabilities of the individuals within that organization. Administrators must use the system development life cycle wisely and carefully consider organizational work flow as they adopt HI technology for meaningful use.

The reader of this section is challenged to ask the following questions: (1) How can I apply the knowledge gained from my practice setting to benefit my patients and enhance my practice. (2) How can I help my colleagues and patients understand and use the current technology that is available. (3) How can I use my wisdom to create the theories, tools, and knowledge of the future?

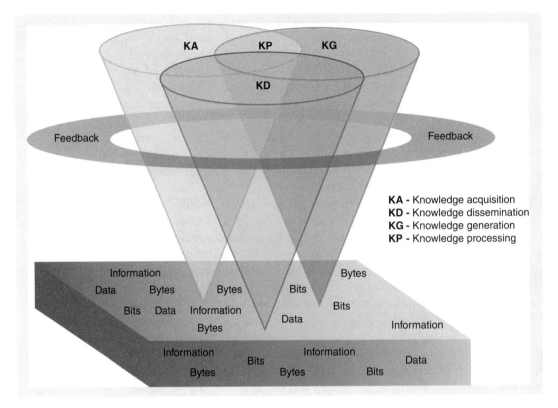

Figure II-1 Foundation of Knowledge Model
Source: Designed by Alicia Mastrian.

6

Systems Development Life Cycle

Dee McGonigle and Kathleen Mastrian

OBJECTIVES

1. Describe the systems development life cycle (SDLC).
2. Explore selected approaches to the SDLC.
3. Assess interoperability and its importance in addressing and meeting the challenges of implementing the HITECH Act in health care.
4. Reflect on the past to move forward into the future to determine how new systems will be developed, integrated, and made interoperable in health care.

Introduction

The following case scenario demonstrates the need to have all of the stakeholders involved from the beginning to the end of the **systems development life cycle** (SDLC). Creating the right team to manage the development is a key. Various methodologies have been developed to guide this process. This chapter reviews the following approaches to SDLC: waterfall, rapid prototyping or rapid application development (RAD), object-oriented system development (OOSD), and the dynamic system development method (DSDM). When reading about each approach, think about the case scenario and how important it is to understand the specific situational needs and the various methodologies for bringing a system to life. As in this case, it is generally necessary or beneficial to use a hybrid approach that blends two or more models for a robust development process.

As the case demonstrates, the process of developing systems or SDLC is an ongoing development with a life cycle. The first step in developing a system is to understand the problem or business needs. It is followed by understanding the solution or how to address those needs, developing a plan, implementing

Key Terms
Chief information officer
Computer-aided software engineering
Dynamic system development method
End users
Health management information system
Hospital information system
Information technology
Integration
Interoperability
Iteration
Milestones
MoSCoW
Object-oriented systems development
Open-source software
Prototype
Rapid application development
Rapid prototyping
Repository
(continues)

the plan, evaluating the implementation, and, finally, maintenance, review, and destruction. If the system needs major upgrading outside of the scope of the maintenance phase, if it needs to be replaced because of technological advances, or if the business needs change, a new project is launched, the old system is destroyed, and the life cycle begins anew.

SDLC is a way to deliver efficient and effective information systems that fit with the strategic business plan of an organization. The business plan stems from the mission of the organization. In the world of health care, its development includes a needs assessment for the entire organization, which should include outreach linkages (as seen in the case scenario) and partnerships and merged or shared functions. The organization's participating physicians and other ancillary professionals and their offices are included in thorough needs assessments. When developing a strategic plan, the design must take into account the existence of the organization within the larger health care delivery system and assess the various factors outside of the organization itself, including technological, legislative, and environmental issues that impact the organization. The plan must identify the needs of the organization as a whole and propose solutions to meet those needs or a way to address the issues.

SDLC can occur within an organization, be outsourced, or be a blend of the two approaches. With outsourcing, the team hires an outside organization to carry out all or some of the development. Developing systems that truly meet business needs is not an easy task and is quite complex. Therefore, it is common to run over budget and miss milestones. When reading this chapter, reflect on the case scenario and in general the challenges teams face when developing systems.

CASE SCENARIO

Envision two large health care facilities that merge resources to better serve their community. This merger is called the Wellness Alliance, and its mission is to establish and manage community health programming that addresses the health needs of the rural, underserved populations in the area. The Wellness Alliance would like to establish pilot clinical sites in five rural areas to promote access and provide health care to these underserved consumers. Each clinical site will have a full-time program manager and eight part-time employees (secretary, nurse, physical therapist, speech pathologist, occupational therapist, dietitian, respiratory therapist, and doctor). Each program manager will report to the wellness program coordinator, a newly created position within the Wellness Alliance.

Because you are the health care professional with extensive experience, you have been appointed as the wellness program coordinator. Your directive is to establish these clinical sites within 3 months and report back in 6 months as to the following: (1) community health programs offered, (2) level of community involvement in outreach health programs and clinical site–based programming, (3) consumer visits made to the clinical site, and (4) personnel performance.

You are excited and challenged, but soon reality sets in: You know that you have five different sites with five different program managers. You need some way to gather the vital information from each of them in a similar manner so that the data are meaningful and useful to you as you develop your reports and evaluate the strengths and weaknesses of the pilot project. You know that you need a system that will handle all of the pilot project's information needs.

Your first stop is the **chief information officer** of the health system, an informaticist. You know her from the **health management information system** miniseminar that she led. After explaining your needs, you share with her the constraint that this system must be in place in 3 months when the sites are up and running before you make your report. When she begins to ask questions, you realize that you do not know the answers. All you know is that you must be able to report on which community health programs were offered, track the level of community involvement in outreach health programs and clinical site-based programming, monitor consumer visits made to the clinical site, and monitor the performance of site personnel. You know that you want accessible, real-time tracking, but as far as programming and clinical site-related activities are concerned, you do not have a precise description of either the process or the procedures that will be involved in implementing the pilot or the means by which they will gather and enter data.

The chief information officer requires that you and each program manager remain involved in the development process. She assigns an **information technology** (IT) analyst to work with you and your team in the development of a system that will meet your current needs. After the first meeting, your head is spinning: The IT analyst has challenged your team not only to work out the process for your immediate needs but also to envision what your needs will be in the future. At the next meeting, you tell the analyst that your team does not feel comfortable trying to map everything out at this point. He states that there are several ways to go about building the system and software by using the systems development life cycle (SDLC). Noticing the blank look on everyone's faces, he explains that the SDLC is a series of actions used to develop an information system. The SDLC is similar to the process we use to care for patients, in which we must assess, diagnose, plan, implement, evaluate, and revise. If the plan developed in this way does not meet the patient's need or if a new problem arises, the health care professional either revises and updates the plan or starts anew. Likewise, you will plan, analyze, design, implement, operate, support, and secure the proposed community health system.

The SDLC is an iterative process—a conceptual model that is used in project management describing the phases involved in building or developing an information system. It moves from assessing feasibility or project initiation, to design analysis, to system specification, to programming, to testing, to implementation, to maintenance, and to destruction—literally from beginning to end. As the IT analyst describes this process, once again he sees puzzled looks. He quickly states that even the destruction of the system is planned—that is, how it will be retired, broken down, and replaced with a new system. Even during upgrades, destruction tactics can be invoked to secure the data and even decide if servers are to be disposed of or repurposed. The security people will tell you that this is their phase, where they make sure that any sensitive information is properly handled and decide whether the data are to be securely and safely archived or destroyed.

After reviewing all of the possible methods and helping you to conduct your feasibility and business study, the analyst chooses the dynamic system development method (DSDM). This SDLC model was chosen because it works well when the time span is short and the requirements are fluctuating and mainly unknown at the outset. The IT analyst explains that this model works well on tight schedules and is a highly iterative and incremental approach stressing continuous user input and involvement. As part of this highly iterative process, the team will revisit and loop through the same development activities numerous times; this repetitive examination provides ever-increasing levels of detail, thereby improving accuracy. The analyst explains that you will use a mock-up of the **hospital information system** (HIS) and design for what is known; you will then create your own mini-system that will interface with the HIS. Because time is short, the analysis, design, and development phases will occur

(continues)

CASE SCENARIO (continued)

simultaneously while you are formulating and revising your specific requirements through the iterative process so that they can be integrated into the system.

The functional model iteration phase will be completed in 2 weeks based on the information that you have given to the analyst. At that time, the prototype will be reviewed by the team. The IT analyst tells you to expect at least two or more iterations of the prototype based on your input. You should end with software that provides some key capabilities. Design and testing will occur in the design and build iteration phase and continue until the system is ready for implementation, the final phase. This DSDM should work well because any previous phase can be revisited and reworked through its iterative process.

One month into the SDLC process, the IT analyst tells the team that he will be leaving his position at Wellness Alliance. He introduces his replacement. She is new to Wellness Alliance and is eager to work with the team. The initial IT analyst will be there 1 more week to help the new analyst with the transition. When he explains that you are working through DSDM, she looks a bit panicky and states that she has never used this approach. She has used the waterfall, prototyping, iterative enhancement, spiral, and object-oriented methodologies—but never the DSDM. From what she heard, DSDM is new and often runs amok because of the lack of understanding as to how to implement it appropriately. After 1 week on the project, the new IT analyst believes that this approach was not the best choice. As the leader of this SDLC, she is growing concerned about having a product ready at the point when the clinical sites open. She might combine another method to create a hybrid approach with which she would be more comfortable; she is thinking out loud and has everyone very nervous.

The IT analyst reviews the equipment that has arrived for the sites and is excited to learn that the Mac computers were ordered from Apple. They will be powerful and versatile enough for your needs.

Two months after the opening of the clinical sites, you as the wellness program coordinator are still tweaking the system with the help of the IT analyst. It is hard to believe how quickly the team was able to get a robust system in place. As you think back on the process, it seems so long ago that you reviewed the HIS for deficiencies and screenshots. You reexamined your requirements and watched them come to life through five prototype iterations and constant security updates. You trained your personnel on its use, tested its performance, and made final adjustments before implementation. Your own stand-alone system that met your needs was installed and fully operational on the Friday before you opened the clinic doors on Monday, 1 day ahead of schedule. You are continuing to evaluate and modify the system, but that is how the SDLC works: It is never finished but rather is constantly evolving.

Waterfall Model

The **waterfall model** is one of the oldest methods and literally depicts a waterfall effect—that is, the output from each previous phase flows into or becomes the initial input for the next phase. This model is a sequential development process in that there is one pass through each component activity from conception or feasibility through implementation in a linear order. The deliverables for each phase result from the inputs and any additional information that is gathered. There is minimal or no iterative development where one takes advantage of what was learned during the development of earlier deliverables. Many projects are broken down into six phases (**Figure 6-1**), especially small to medium-size projects.

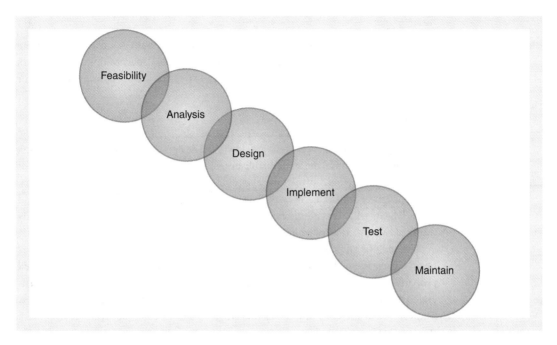

Figure 6-1 Waterfall Phases

Feasibility

As the term implies, the feasibility study is used to determine whether the project should be initiated and supported. This study should generate a project plan and estimated budget for the SDLC phases. Often, the **TELOS strategy**—technological and systems, economic, legal, operational, and schedule feasibility—is followed. Technological and systems feasibility addresses the issues of technological capabilities, including the expertise and infrastructure to complete the project. Economic feasibility is the cost–benefit analysis, weighing the benefits versus the costs to determine whether the project is fiscally possible to do and worth undertaking. Formal assessments should include return on investment. Legal feasibility assesses the legal ramifications of the project, including current contractual obligations, legislation, regulatory bodies, and liabilities that could affect the project. Operational feasibility determines how effective the project will be in meeting the needs and expectations of the organization and actually achieving the goals of the project or addressing and solving the business problem. Schedule feasibility assesses the viability of the time frame, making sure it is a reasonable estimation of the time and resources necessary for the project to be developed in time to attain the benefits and meet constraints. TELOS helps to provide a clear picture of the feasibility of the project.

Analysis

During the analysis phase, the requirements for the system are teased out from a detailed study of the business needs of the organization. As part of this analysis, work flows and business practices are examined. It may be necessary to consider options for changing the business process.

Design

The design phase focuses on high- and low-level design and interface and data design. At the high-level phase, the team establishes which programs are needed and ascertains how they will interact. At the low-level phase, team members explore how the individual programs will actually work. The interface design determines what the look and feel will be or what the interfaces will look like. During data design, the team critically thinks about and verifies which data are required or essential.

The analysis and design phases are vital in the development cycle, and great care is taken during these phases to ensure that the software's overall configuration is defined properly. Mock-ups or prototypes of screenshots, reports, and processes may be generated to clarify the requirements and get the team or stakeholders on the same page, limiting the occurrence of glitches that might result in costly software development revisions later in the project.

Implement

During this phase, the designs are brought to life through programming code. The right programming language, such as C++, Pascal, Java, and so forth, is chosen based on the application requirements.

Test

The testing is generally broken down into five layers: (1) the individual programming modules, (2) **integration**, (3) volume, (4) the system as a whole, and (5) beta testing. Typically, the programs are developed in a modular fashion, and these individual modules are then subjected to detailed testing. The separate modules are subsequently synthesized, and the interfaces between the modules are tested. The system is evaluated with respect to its platform and the expected amount or volume of data. It is then tested as a complete system by the team. Finally, to determine if the system performs appropriately for the user, it is beta tested. During beta testing, users put the new system through its paces to make sure that it does what they need it to do to perform their jobs.

Maintain

Once the system has been finalized from the testing phase, it must be maintained. This could include user support through actual software changes necessitated through use or time.

The waterfall approach is linear and progresses sequentially. The main lack of iterative development is seen as a major weakness, according to Purcell (2015). No projects are static, and typically changes occur during the SDLC. As requirements change, there is no way to address them formally using the waterfall method after project requirements are developed. The waterfall model should be used for simple projects when the requirements are well known and stable from the outset.

Rapid Prototyping or Rapid Application Development

As technology advances and faster development is expected, **rapid prototyping**, also known as **rapid application development** (RAD), provides a fast way to add functionality through prototyping and user testing. It is easier for users to examine actual **prototypes** rather than documentation. A rapid requirements-gathering phase relies on workshops and focus groups to build a prototype application using real data. This prototype is then beta tested with users, and their feedback is used to perfect or add functionality and capabilities to the system. According to Alexandrou (2010), "RAD (rapid application development) proposes that products can be developed faster and of higher quality" (para. 1). The RAD approach uses informal communication, repurposes components, and typically follows a fast-paced schedule. Object-oriented programming using such languages as C++ and Java promotes software repurposing and reuse.

The major advantage is the speed with which the system can be deployed; a working, usable system can be built within 3 months. The use of prototyping allows the developers to skip steps in the SDLC process in favor of getting a mock-up in front of the user. At times, the system may be deemed acceptable if it meets a predefined minimum set of requirements rather than all of the identified requirements. This rapid deployment also limits the project's exposure to change elements. Unfortunately, the fast pace can be its biggest disadvantage in some cases. Once one is locked into a tight development schedule, the process may be too fast for adequate testing to be put in place and completed. The most dangerous lack of testing is in the realm of security.

The RAD approach is chosen because it builds systems quickly through user-driven prototyping and adherence to quick, strict delivery **milestones**. This approach continues to be refined and honed, and other contemporary manifestations of RAD continue to emerge in the agile software development realm.

Object-Oriented Systems Development

The **object-oriented systems development** (OOSD) model blends SDLC logic with object-oriented modeling and programming power (Stair & Reynolds, 2016). Object-oriented modeling makes an effort to represent real-world objects by modeling the real-world entities or things (e.g., clinic, patient, account, health care professional) into abstract computer software objects. Once the system is object oriented, all of the interactions or exchanges take place between or among the objects. The objects are derived from classes, and each object is comprised of data and the actions that can be enacted on those data.

Class hierarchy allows objects to inherit characteristics or attributes from parent classes, which fosters object reuse resulting in less coding. The object-oriented programming languages, such as C++ and Java, promote software repurposing and reuse. Therefore, the class hierarchy must be clearly and appropriately designed to reap the benefits of this SDLC approach, which uses object-oriented programming to support the interactions of objects.

For example, in the case scenario, a system could be developed for the Wellness Alliance to manage the community health programming for the clinic system being set up for outreach. There could be a class of programs, and *well-baby care* could be an object in the class of programs; *programs* is a relationship between Wellness Alliance and well-baby care. The program class has attributes, such as *clinic site*, *location address*, or *attendees* or *patients*. The relationship itself may be considered an object having attributes, such as *pediatric programs*. The class hierarchy from which all of the system objects are created with resultant object interactions must be clearly defined.

The OOSD model is a highly iterative approach. The process begins by investigating where object-oriented solutions can address business problems or needs, determining user requirements, designing the system, programming or modifying object modeling (class hierarchy and objects), implementing, user testing, modifying, and implementing the system and ends with the new system being reviewed regularly at established intervals and modifications being made as needed throughout its life.

Dynamic System Development Method

The **dynamic system development method** (DSDM) is a highly iterative and incremental approach with a high level of user input and involvement. The iterative process requires repetitive examination that enhances detail and improves accuracy. The DSDM has three phases: (1) preproject, (2) project life cycle (feasibility and business studies, functional model iteration, design and build iteration, and implementation), and (3) postproject.

In the preproject phase, buy-in or commitment is established and funding secured. This helps to identify the stakeholders (administration and **end users**) and gain support for the project.

In the second phase, the project's life cycle begins. This phase includes five steps: (1) feasibility, (2) business studies, (3) functional model iteration, (4) design and build iteration, and (5) implementation. In steps 1 and 2, the feasibility and business studies are completed. The team ascertains if this project meets the required business needs while identifying the potential risks during the feasibility study. In step 1, the deliverables are a feasibility report, project plan, and a risk log. Once the project is deemed feasible, step 2, the business study, is begun. The business study extends the feasibility report by examining the processes, stakeholders, and their needs. It is important to align the stakeholders with the project and secure their buy-in because it is necessary to have user input and involvement throughout the entire DSDM process. Therefore, bringing them in at the beginning of the project is imperative.

Using the **MoSCoW** approach, the team works with the stakeholders to develop a prioritized requirements list and a development plan. MoSCoW stands for "Must have, Should have, Could have, and Would have." The "must have" requirements are needed to meet the business needs and are critical to the success of the project. "Should have" requirements are those that would be great to have if possible, but the success of the project does not depend on their being addressed. The "could have" requirements are those that would be nice to have met, and the "would have" requirements can be put off until later; these may be undertaken during future developmental iterations. Timeboxing is generally used to develop the project plan. In timeboxing, the project is divided into sections, each having its own fixed budget and dates or milestones for deliverables. The MoSCoW approach is then used to prioritize the requirements within each section; the requirements are the only variables because the schedule and budget are set. If a project is running out of time or money, the team can easily omit the requirements that have been identified as the lowest priority to meet their schedule and budget obligations. This does not mean that the final deliverable, the actual system, would be flawed or incomplete. Instead, it meets the business needs. According to Haughey (2010), the 80/20 rule, or Pareto principle, can be applied to nearly everything. The Pareto principle states that 80% of the project comes from 20% of the system requirements; therefore, the 20% of requirements must be the crucial requirements or those with the highest priority. One also must consider the pancake principle: The first pancake is not as good as the rest, and one should know that the first development will not be perfect. This is why it is extremely important to clearly identify the "must have" and "should have" requirements.

In the third step of the project life cycle phase, known as functional model iteration, the deliverables are a functional model and prototype ready for user testing. Once the requirements are identified, the next step is to translate them into a functional model with a functioning prototype that can be evaluated by users. This could take several iterations to develop the desired functionality and incorporate the users' input. At this stage, the team should examine the quality of the product and revise the list requirements and risk log. The requirements are adjusted, the ones that have been realized are deleted, and the remaining requirements are prioritized. The risk log is revised based on the risk analysis completed during and after prototype development.

The design and build iteration step focuses on integrating functional components and identifying the nonfunctional requirements that need to be in the tested system. Testing is crucial; the team will develop a system that the end users can safely use on a daily basis. The team will garner user feedback and generate user documentation. These efforts provide this step's deliverable: a tested system with documentation for the next and final phase of the development process.

In the final step of the project life cycle phase, known as implementation, deliverables are the system (ready to use), documentation, and trained users. The requirements list should be satisfied, along with the users' needs. Training users and implementing the approved system is the first part of this phase, and the final part consists of a full review. It is important to review the impact of the system on the business processes and to determine if it addressed the goals or requirements established at the beginning of the project. This final review determines if the project is completed or if further development is necessary. If further development is needed, preceding phases are revisited. If the project is complete and satisfies the users, then it moves into maintenance and ongoing development.

The final phase is labeled "postproject." In this phase, the team verifies that the system is functioning properly. Once verified, the maintenance schedule is begun. Because the DSDM is iterative, this postproject phase is seen as ongoing development, and any of the deliverables can be refined. This is what makes the DSDM such an iterative development process.

DSDM is one of an increasing number of agile methodologies being introduced, such as Scrum and Extreme Programming. These new approaches address the organizational, managerial, and interpersonal communication issues that often bog down SDLC projects. Empowerment of teams and user involvement enhance the iterative and programming strengths provided in these SDLC models.

Computer-Aided Software Engineering Tools

When reviewing SDLC, the **computer-aided software engineering** (CASE) tools that will be used must be described. CASE tools promote adherence to the SDLC process since they automate several required tasks; this provides standardization and thoroughness in the total systems development method (Stair & Reynolds, 2016). These tools help to reduce cost and development time while enriching the quality of the product. CASE tools contain a **repository** with information about the system: models, data definitions, and references linking models together. They are valuable in their ability to make sure the models follow diagramming rules and are consistent and complete.

The various types of tools can be referred to as upper CASE tools or lower CASE tools. The upper CASE tools support the analysis and design phases, whereas the lower CASE tools support implementation. The tools can also be general or specific in nature, with the specific tools being designed for a particular methodology.

Two examples of CASE tools are Visible Analyst and Rational Rose. According to Andoh-Baidoo, Kunene, and Walker (n.d.), Visible Analyst "supports structured and object-oriented design (UML)," whereas Rational Rose "supports solely object-oriented design (UML)" (p. 372). Both tools can "build and reverse database schemas for SQL and Oracle" and "support code generation for pre.NET versions of Visual Basic" (p. 372). Visible Analyst can also support shell code generation for pre.NET versions of C and COBOL, whereas Rational Rose can support complete code for C++ and Java. In addition, Andoh-Baidoo et al. found that Rational Rose "provides good integration with Java, and incorporates common packages into class diagrams and decompositions through classes" (p. 372).

CASE tools have many advantages, including decreasing development time and producing more flexible systems. On the downside, they can be difficult to tailor or customize and use with existing systems.

Open-Source Software and Free/Open-Source Software

Another area that must be discussed with SDLC is **open-source software** (OSS). An examination of job descriptions or advertisements for candidates shows that many IS and IT professionals need a thorough understanding of SDLC and OSS development tools (e.g., PHP, MySQL, and HTML). With OSS, any programmer can implement, modify, apply, reconstruct, and restructure the rich libraries of source codes available from proven, well-tested products. As Karopka, Schmuhl, and Demski (2014) noted,

> *Free/Libre Open Source Software (FLOSS) has been successfully adopted across a wide range of different areas and has opened new ways of value creation. Today there are hundreds of examples of successful FLOSS projects and products ranging from Linux to Android, from Open/Libre Office to MySQL, from the Apache Web Server to hundreds of embedded GNU/Linux kernels in different types of systems. Especially in times of financial crisis and austerity the adoption of FLOSS principles opens interesting alternatives and options to tremendously lower total cost of ownership (TCO) and open the way for a continuous user-driven improvement process. (para. 6)*

To transform health care, it is necessary for clinicians to use information systems that can share patient data (Goulde & Brown, 2006; NORC, 2014). This all sounds terrific, and many people wonder why it has not happened yet, but the challenges are many. How does one establish the networks necessary to share data between and among all health care facilities easily and securely? "Health care IT is beginning to adopt OSS to address these challenges" (Goulde & Brown, p. 4). Early attempts at OSS ventures in the health care realm failed because of a lack of support or buy-in for sustained effort, technological lags, authority and credibility, and other such issues. "Spurred by a greater sense of urgency to adopt IT, health industry leaders are showing renewed interest in open source solutions" (Goulde & Brown, p. 5). Karopka et al. (2014) concluded that

> *North America has the longest tradition in applying FLOSS-HC delivery. It is home of many mature, stable and widely disseminated FLOSS applications. Some of them are even used on a global scale. The deployment of FLOSS systems in healthcare delivery is comparatively low in Europe. (para. 48)*

Health care is realizing the benefits of FLOSS. According to Goulde and Brown (2006), "other benefits of open source software—low cost, flexibility, opportunities to innovate—are important but independence from vendors is the most relevant for health care" (p. 10).

Interoperability

Interoperability, the ability to share information across organizations, will remain paramount under the HITECH Act (see Chapter 5). The ability to share patient data is extremely important, both within an organization and across organizational boundaries. According to the Health Information and Management Systems Society (HIMSS, 2015), "An acceptable 2015 [interoperability standards] Advisory and more complete 2016 Advisory will not be achievable without the inclusion of health IT security standards" (para. 4). Few health care systems take advantage of the full potential of the current state of the art in computer science and health informatics (HIMSS, 2010). The consequences of this situation include a drain on financial resources from the economy, the inability to truly mitigate the occurrence of medical errors, and a lack of national preparedness to respond to natural and man-made epidemics and disasters. HIMSS has created the Integration and Interoperability Steering Committee to guide the industry on allocating resources to develop and implement standards and technology needed to achieve interoperability (para. 2).

As we enter into SDLCs, we must be aware of how this type of development will affect both our own health care organization and the health care delivery system as a whole. In an ideal world, we would all work together to create systems that are integrated within our own organization while having the interoperability to cross organizational boundaries and unite the health care delivery system to realize the common goal of improving the quality of care provided to consumers.

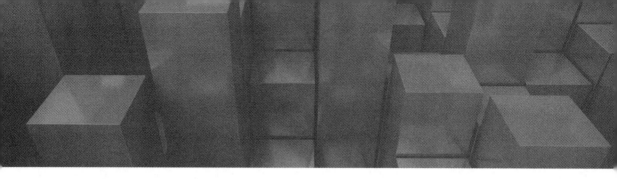

Summary

At times during the SDLC, new information affects the outputs from earlier phases; the development effort may be reexamined or halted until these modifications can be reconciled with the current design and scope of the project. At other times, teams are overwhelmed with new ideas from the iterative SDLC process that result in new capabilities or features that exceed the initial scope of the project. Astute team leaders will preserve these ideas or initiatives so they can be considered at a later time. The team should develop a list of recommendations to improve the current software when the project is complete. This iterative and dynamic exchange makes the SDLC robust.

As technology and research continue to advance, new SDLC models are being pioneered and revised to enhance development techniques. The interpretation and implementation of any model selected reflect the knowledge and skill of the team applying the model. The success of the project is often directly related to the quality of the organizational decision making throughout the project—that is, how well the plan was followed and documented. United efforts to create systems that are integrated and interoperable will define the future of health care.

Thought-Provoking Questions

1. How would you describe cognitive informatics? Reflect on a plan of care that you have developed or implemented for a patient. How could cognitive informatics be used to create tools to help with this important work?
2. Think of a clinical setting you are familiar with and envision artificial intelligence tools. Are there any current tools in use? Which tools would enhance practice in this setting and why?
3. Reflect on the SDLC in relation to the quality of the organizational decision making throughout the project. What are some of the major stumbling blocks faced by health care organizations?
4. Why is it important for all health care professionals to understand the basics of how information systems are selected and implemented?

Apply Your Knowledge

The SDLC is similar to the process we use to care for patients, in which we must assess, diagnose, plan, implement, evaluate, and revise. If the plan developed in this way does not meet the patient's need or if a new problem arises, the health care professional either revises and updates the plan or starts anew. When a health care organization is looking to implement a new system, careful consideration must be given to how the system will be implemented.

1. Complete the following table to help you compare and contrast the approaches to system development.

Approach	Description	Advantages	Disadvantages
Waterfall			
Rapid prototyping or rapid application development (RAD)			
Object-oriented system development (OOSD)			
Dynamic system development method (DSDM)			

2. When new technologies are implemented in health care systems, health care professionals may resist the technology. Consider a situation where you were forced to make a change. How did you feel? What are some strategies that might have made the change more palatable to you?

References

Alexandrou, M. (2010). Rapid application development (RAD) methodology. http://www.mariosalexandrou.com/methodologies/rapid-application-development.asp

Andoh-Baidoo, F., Kunene, K., & Walker, R. (n.d.). An evaluation of CASE tools as pedagogical aids in software development courses. http://www.swdsi.org/swdsi2009/Papers/9K10.pdf

Goulde, M., & Brown, E. (2006). Open source software: A primer for health care leaders. http://www.protecode.com/an-open-source-world-a-primer-on-licenses-obligations-and-your-company

Haughey, D. (2010). Pareto analysis step by step. http://www.projectsmart.co.uk/pareto-analysis-step-by-step.html

Health Information and Management Systems Society. (2015). HIMSS has ideas for 2015 interoperability standards advisory. http://healthitinteroperability.com/news/himss-has-ideas-for-2015-interoperability-standards-advisory

Health Information and Management Systems Society. (2010). Integration and interoperability. http://www.himss.org/library/interoperability-standards?navItemNumber=13323

Karopka, T., Schmuhl, H., & Demski, H. (2014). Free/Libre open source software in health care: A review. *Healthcare Informatics Research*, 20(1), 11–22. PMCID: PMC3950260. http://www.ncbi.nlm.nih.gov/pmc/articles/PMC3950260

NORC. (2014). Data sharing to enable clinical transformation at the community level: IT takes a village. http://www.healthit.gov/sites/default/files/beacondatasharingbrief062014.pdf

Purcell, J. (2015). Comparison of software development lifecycle methodologies. https://software-security.sans.org/resources/paper/cissp/comparison-software-development-lifecycle-methodologies

Stair, R., & Reynolds, G. (2016). *Principles of information systems* (12th ed.). Boston: Cengage Learning.

Administrative Information Systems

Marianela Zytkowski, Susan Paschke, Dee McGonigle,
and Kathleen Mastrian

OBJECTIVES

1. Explore agency-based health information systems.
2. Evaluate how administrators use core business systems in their practice.
3. Assess the function and information output from selected information systems used in health care organizations.

Introduction

To compete in the ever-changing health care arena, organizations require quick and immediate access to a variety of types of information, data, and bodies of knowledge for daily clinical, operational, financial, and human resource activities. Information is continuously shared between units and departments within health care organizations and is also required or requested from other health care organizations, regulatory and government agencies, educational and philanthropic institutions, and consumers.

The health care context is distinct from other organizations that use information systems. Fichman, Kohli, and Krishnan (2011) identify six important elements of health care that influence the development and implementation of information systems:

- The stakes are life and death
- Health care information is highly personal
- Health care is highly influenced by regulation and competition
- Health care is professionally driven and hierarchical

- Health care is multidisciplinary
- Health care information systems implementation is complex with important implications for learning and adaptation (pp. 420–423)

Health care organizations integrate a variety of clinical and administrative types of **information systems**. These systems collect, process, and distribute patient-centered data to aid in managing and providing care. Together, they create a comprehensive record of the patient's medical history and support organizational processes. Each of these systems is unique in the way it functions and provides information to clinicians, therapists, and administrators. An understanding of how each of these types of systems works within health care organizations is fundamental in the study of informatics.

Types of Health Care Organization Information Systems

Case Management Information Systems

Case management information systems identify resources, patterns, and variances in care to prevent costly complications related to chronic conditions and to enhance the overall outcomes for patients with chronic illness. These systems span past episodes of treatment and search for trends among the records. Once a trend is identified, case management systems provide **decision support** promoting preventive care. Care plans are a common tool found in case management systems. A **care plan** is a set of care guidelines that outline the course of treatment and the recommended interventions that should be implemented to achieve optimal results. By using a **standardized plan of care**, these systems present clinicians with treatment protocols to maximize patient outcomes and support best practices. Information technology in health care is positioned to support the development of interdisciplinary care plans. In the health informatics pathway, Standard 5 deals with documentation: "Health informatics professionals will understand the content and diverse uses of health information. They will accurately document and communicate appropriate information using legal and regulatory processes" (National Consortium for Health Science Education, 2012, para. 11).

Case management information systems are especially beneficial for patient populations with a high cost of care and complex health needs, such as the elderly or patients with chronic disease conditions. Avoiding complications requires identifying the right resources for care and implementing preventive treatments across all health care visits. Ultimately, this preventive care decreases the costs of care for patients with chronic illnesses and supports a better quality of life. Such systems increase the value of individual care while controlling the costs and risks associated with long-term health care.

Case management systems are increasingly being integrated with electronic health records. Information collected by these systems is processed in a way that helps to reduce risks, ensure quality, and decrease costs. A presentation of results of the 2012 Health Information Technology Survey conducted by the Case Management Society of America (2014) revealed several key trends in information technology, including the increased use of social media and wireless communications, the use of information technology to support care transitions and prevent readmissions, expanded use of patient engagement technologies (text messaging, e-mail, portals, and smartphone apps), and work toward the integration of case management software into the electronic health record.

Key Terms (continued)
Relational database management system
Repository
Rows
Scheduling systems
Stakeholders
Standardized plan of care
Structured Query Language
Tables
Tiering
Triage
Tuple

Communication Systems

Communication systems promote interaction among health care providers and between providers and patients. Such systems have historically been kept separate from other types of health information systems and from one another. Health care professionals overwhelmingly recognize the value of these systems, however, so they are now more commonly integrated into the design of other types of systems as a newly developing standard within the industry. Examples of communication systems include call light systems, wireless telephones, pagers, e-mail, and instant messaging, which have traditionally been forms of communication targeted at clinicians. Other communication systems target patients and their families. Some patients are now able to access their electronic chart from home via an Internet connection. They can update their own medical record to inform their physician of changes to their health or personal practices that impact their physical condition. Inpatients in hospital settings also receive communication directly to their room. Patients and their families may, for example, review individualized messages with scheduled tests and procedures for the day and confirm menu choices for their meals. These types of systems may also communicate educational messages, such as smoking cessation advice.

As health care begins to introduce more of this technology into practice, the value of having communication tools integrated with other types of systems is being widely recognized. Integrating communication systems with clinical applications provides a real-time approach that facilitates interactions among the entire health care team, patients, and their families to enhance care. These systems enhance the flow of communication within an organization and promote an exchange of information to care better for patients. The next generation of communication systems will be integrated with other types of health care systems and guaranteed to work together smoothly. The Research Brief discusses the economic impact of communication inefficiencies in U.S. hospitals.

As hospitals and practices strive to become more patient centered, communication technologies will be an integral part of this goal. Many of us have experienced the anxiety of waiting for news about a loved one during a surgical procedure. Newer communication techniques, such as surgical tracking boards that communicate about the process, help to ease these anxieties. Gordon et al. (2015) report high patient and family satisfaction with a HIPAA compliant surgical instant messaging system to communicate real-time surgical progress with patient designated recipients. They stated that

> while this study focused on the discipline of surgery, we can easily imagine the benefits of this type of communications application outside of the surgical model that we have studied. The results of any laboratory, pathology, or radiography studies can be instantaneously shared with concerned family members all over the globe. In the critical care setting, doctors can communicate with a patient's extended support group more efficiently and in a less stress-inducing environment than the typical crowded consultation room outside of the intensive care unit. News of the arrival of a newborn baby boy or girl can be sent to eager aunts, uncles, and grandparents back home. The opportunities for enhancing communication pertaining to medical issues are seemingly limitless. (p. 6)

What are some ways that new communication technologies could be used to increase patient and family satisfaction with health care in your discipline?

Core Business Systems

Core business systems enhance administrative tasks within health care organizations. Unlike clinical information systems (CISs), whose aim is to provide direct patient care, these systems support the management of health care within an organization. Core business systems provide the framework for reimbursement, support of best practices, quality control, and resource allocation. There are four common core business systems: (1) admission, discharge, and transfer (ADT) systems; (2) financial systems; (3) acuity systems; and (4) scheduling systems.

ADT systems provide the backbone structure for the other types of clinical and business systems (Hassett & Thede, 2003). These systems were among the first to be automated in health care. Admitting, billing, and bed management departments most commonly use ADT systems. These systems hold key information on which all other systems rely. For example, ADT systems maintain the patient's name; medical record number; visit or account number; and demographic information, such as age, gender, home address, and contact information. Such systems are considered the central source for collecting this type of patient information and communicating it to other types of health care information systems.

Financial systems manage the expenses and revenue for providing health care. The finance, auditing, and accounting departments within an organization most commonly use financial systems. These systems determine the direction for maintenance and growth for a given facility. They often interface to share information with materials management, staffing, and billing systems to balance the financial impact of these resources within an organization. Financial systems report fiscal outcomes, which can then be tracked and related to the organizational goals of an institution. These systems are key components in the decision-making process as health care institutions prepare

---

RESEARCH BRIEF

Researchers attempted to quantify the costs of poor communication, termed "communication inefficiencies," in hospitals. This qualitative study was conducted in seven acute care hospitals of varying sizes via structured interviews with key informants at each facility. The interview questions focused on four broad categories: (1) communication bottlenecks, (2) negative outcomes as a result of those bottlenecks, (3) subjective perceptions of the potential effectiveness of communication improvements on the negative outcomes, and (4) ideas for specific communication improvements. The researchers independently coded the interview data and then compared results to extract themes.

All of the interviewees indicated that communication was an issue. Inefficiencies revolved around time spent tracking people down to communicate with them, with various estimates provided: 3 hours per nursing shift wasted tracking people down, 20% of productive time wasted on communication bottlenecks, and a reported average of five to six telephone calls to locate a physician. Several respondents pointed to costly medical errors that were the direct result of communication issues. Communication lapses also resulted in inefficient use of clinician resources and increased length of stay for patients.

The researchers developed a conceptual model of communication quality with four primary dimensions: (1) efficiency of resource use, (2) effectiveness of resource use, (3) quality of work life, and (4) service quality. They concluded that the total cost of communication inefficiencies in U.S. hospitals is more than $12 billion annually and estimated that a 500-bed hospital could lose as much as $4 million annually because of such problems. They urge the adoption of information technologies to redesign work flow processes and promote better communication.

Source: The full article appears in Agarwal, Sands, Schneider, and Smaltz (2010).

---

their fiscal budgets. They often play a pivotal role in determining the strategic direction for an organization.

Acuity systems monitor the range of patient types within a health care organization using specific indicators. They track these indicators based on the current patient population within a facility. By monitoring the patient acuity, these systems provide feedback about how intensive the care requirement is for an individual patient or group of patients. Identifying and classifying a patient's acuity can promote better organizational management of the expenses and resources necessary to provide care. Acuity systems help predict the ability and capacity of an organization to care for its current population. They also forecast future trends to allow an organization to successfully strategize on how to meet upcoming market demands.

Scheduling systems coordinate staff, services, equipment, and allocation of patient beds. They are frequently integrated with the other types of core business systems. By closely monitoring staff and physical resources, these systems provide data to the financial systems. For example, resource-scheduling systems may provide information about operating room use or availability of intensive care unit beds and regular nursing unit beds. These systems also provide great assistance to financial systems when they are used to track medical equipment within a facility. Procedures and care are planned when the tools and resources are available. Scheduling systems help to track resources within a facility while managing the frequency and distribution of those resources.

Order Entry Systems

Order entry systems are one of the most important systems in use today. They automate the way that orders have traditionally been initiated for patients—that is, clinicians place orders using these systems instead of creating traditional handwritten transcriptions onto paper. Order entry systems provide major safeguards by ensuring that physician orders are legible and complete, thereby providing a level of patient safety that was historically missing with paper-based orders. **Computerized physician (provider) order entry systems** provide decision support and automated alert functionality that was unavailable with paper-based orders.

The seminal report by the Institute of Medicine estimated that medical errors cost the United States approximately $37.6 billion each year; nearly $17 billion of those costs are associated with preventable errors. Consequently, the federal Agency for Healthcare Research and Quality Patient Safety Network (2015), continued to recommend eliminating reliance on handwriting for ordering medications.

Because of the global concern for patient safety as a result of incorrect and misinterpreted orders, health care organizations are incorporating order entry systems into their operations as a standard tool for practice. Such systems allow for clear and legible orders, thereby both promoting patient safety and streamlining care. Although much of the health information technology literature suggests that physicians are resistant to adopting health information technology, a recent study by Elder, Wiltshire, Rooks, BeLue, and Gary (2010) found that physicians who use **information technology** were more satisfied overall with their careers. Chapter 12 provides more information about the use of computerized physician order entry systems in clinical care.

Patient Care Support Systems

Most specialty disciplines within health care have an associated **patient care information system**. These patient-centered systems focus on collecting data and disseminating information related to direct care. Several of these systems have become mainstream types of systems used in health care. The four systems most commonly encountered in health care include (1) clinical documentation systems, (2) pharmacy information systems, (3) laboratory information systems, and (4) radiology information systems.

Clinical documentation systems, also known as "clinical information systems," are the most commonly used type of **patient care support system** within health care organizations. CISs are designed to collect patient data in realtime. They enhance care by putting data at the clinician's fingertips and enabling decision making where it needs to occur—that is, at the bedside. For that reason, these systems often are easily accessible at the point of care for caregivers interacting with the patient. CISs are **patient centered**, meaning they contain the observations, interventions, and outcomes noted by the care team. Team members enter information, such as the plan of care, hemodynamic data, laboratory results, clinical notes, allergies, and medications. All members of the treatment team use clinical documentation systems; for example, pharmacists, allied health workers, nurses, physicians, support staff, and many others access the clinical record for the patient using these systems. Frequently these types of systems are also referred to as the electronic patient record or **electronic health record**. Chapter 11 provides a comprehensive overview of CISs and the electronic health record.

Pharmacy information systems also have become mainstream patient care support systems. They typically allow pharmacists to order, manage, and dispense medications for a facility. They also commonly incorporate information regarding allergies and height and weight to ensure effective medication management. Pharmacy information systems streamline the order entry, dispensing, verification, and authorization process for medication administration. They often interface with clinical documentation and order entry systems so that clinicians can order and document the administration of medications and prescriptions to patients while having the benefits of decision support alerting and interaction checking.

Laboratory information systems were perhaps some of the first clinical information systems (after the financial systems) ever used in health care. Because of their long history of use within health care, laboratory systems have been models for the design and implementation of other types of patient care support systems. Laboratory information systems report on blood, body fluid, and tissue samples, along with biological specimens collected at the bedside and received in a central laboratory. They provide clinicians with reference ranges for tests indicating high, low, or normal values to make care decisions. Often, the laboratory system provides result information directing clinicians toward the next course of action within a treatment regimen.

The final type of patient care support system commonly found within health care is the **radiology information system** (RIS) found in radiology departments. These systems schedule, result, and store information related to diagnostic radiology procedures. One feature found in most radiology systems is a **picture archiving and communication system** (PACS). The PACS may be a stand-alone system, kept separate from the main radiology system, or it can be integrated with the RIS and CIS. These systems collect, store, and distribute medical images, such as computed tomography scans, magnetic resonance images, and X-rays. PACS replace traditional hard-copy films with digital media that are easy to store, retrieve, and present to clinicians. The benefit of RIS and PACS is their ability to assist in diagnosing and storing vital patient care support data. Imaging studies can be available in minutes as opposed to 2 to 6 hours for images in a film-based system. The digital workstations provide enhanced imaging capabilities and onscreen measurement tools to improve diagnostic accuracy. Finally, the archive system stores images in a database that is readily accessible so that images can be easily retrieved and compared to subsequent testing or shared instantly with consultants.

The mobility of patients both geographically and within a single health care delivery system challenges information systems because data must be captured wherever and whenever the patient receives care. In the past, **managed care information systems** were implemented to address these issues. According to Ciotti and Zodda (1996), a managed care information system "can nimbly cross organizational boundaries, includes an enterprise-wide **master patient index** (MPI), and offers access across provider, geographic, and departmental lines" (para. 10). Consequently, data can be obtained at any and all of the areas where a patient interacts with the health care system. Patient tracking mechanisms continue to be honed, but the financial impact of health care also has changed these systems to some extent. The information systems currently in use enable nurses and physicians to make clinical decisions while being mindful of their financial ramifications. In the future, vast improvements in information systems and systems that support health information exchange are likely to continue to emerge.

Many health care organizations now aggregate data in a **data warehouse** (DW) for the purpose of mining the data to discover new relationships and to build organizational knowledge. Rojas (2015) stated that

> *hospitals and medical centers have more to gain from big data analytics than perhaps any other industry. But as data sets continue to grow, healthcare facilities are discovering that success in data analytics has more to do with storage methods than with analysis software or techniques. Traditional data silos are hindering the progress of big data in the healthcare industry, and as terabytes turn into petabytes, the most successful hospitals are the ones that are coming up with new solutions for storage and access challenges. (para. 1)*

None of the disparate information systems was able to communicate with any of the others, resulting in poor communication, billing errors, and issues with continuity of care. By developing a single comprehensive database, health care systems are able to facilitate interprofessional communication and maintain compliance with privacy regulations. Based on their size, **triage** and **tiering** might be necessary:

> *Consider the case of Intermountain, a chain of 22 hospitals in Salt Lake City. With 4.7 petabytes of data under its management, cloud storage becomes cost prohibitive. The network estimates the hospital chain's data will grow by 25–30 percent each year until it reaches 15 petabytes five years from now. With such massive data needs, Intermountain found ways to cut costs and streamline efficiency. One way was through data tiering, which is the creation of data storage tiers that can be accessed at the appropriate speeds. Tiering is currently done manually through triaging, but several different organizations are exploring auto-tiering, which automatically stores data according to availability needs. (Rojas, 2015, paras. 9–10)*

The most basic element of a database system is the data. The term *data* refers to raw facts that can consist of unorganized text, graphics, sound, or video. Information is data that has been processed—it has meaning; information is organized in a way that people find meaningful and useful. Even useful information can be lost if one is mired in unorganized information. Computers can come to the rescue by helping to create order out of chaos. Computer science and information science are designed to help cut down the amount of information to a more manageable size and organize it so that users can cope with it more efficiently through the use of databases and database programs technology.

Learning about basic databases and database management programs is paramount so that users can apply data and information management principles in health care.

Databases are structured or organized collections of data that are typically the main component of an information system. Databases and database management software allow the user to input, sort, arrange structure, organize, and store data and turn those data into useful information. An individual can set up a personal database to organize recipes, music, names and addresses, notes, bills, and other data. In health care, databases and information systems make key information available to health care providers and ancillary personnel to promote the provision of quality patient care. **Box 7-1** provides a detailed description of a database.

BOX 7-1   OVERVIEW OF DATABASE CONSTRUCTION

Databases consist of **fields** (**columns**) and **records** (**rows**). Within each record, one of the fields is identified as the **primary key** or **key field** This primary key contains a code, name, number, or other information that acts as a unique identifier for that record. In the health care system, for example, a patient is assigned a patient number or ID that is unique for that patient. As you compile related records, you create **data files** or **tables** A data file is a collection of related records. Therefore, databases consist of one or more related data files or tables.

An **entity** represents a table, and each field within the table becomes an **attribute** of that entity. The database developer must critically think about the attributes for each specific entity. For example, the entity "disease" might have the attributes of "chronic disease," "acute disease," or "communicable disease." The name of the entity, "disease," implies that the entity is about diseases. The fields or attributes are "chronic," "acute," or "communicable."

The **entity–relationship diagram** specifies the relationship among the entities in the database. Sometimes the implied relationships are readily apparent based on the entities' definitions; however, all relationships should be specified as to how they relate to one another. Typically, three relationships are possible: (1) one to one, (2) one to many, and (3) many to many. A one-to-one relationship exists between the entities of the table about a patient and the table about the patient's birth. A one-to-many relationship could exist when one entity is repeatedly used by another entity. Such a one-to-many relationship could then be a table query for age that could be used numerous times for one patient entity. The many-to-many relationship reflects entities that are all used repeatedly by other entities. This is easily explained by the entities of patient and nurse. The patient could have several nurses caring for him or her, and the nurse could have many patients assigned to him or her (see **Figure 7-1**).

The relational model is a database model that describes data in which all data elements are placed in relation in two-dimensional tables; the relations or tables are analogous to files. A **relational database management system (RDMS)** is a system that manages data using this kind of relational model. A relational database could link a patient's table to a treatment table (e.g., by a common field, such as the patient ID number). To keep track of the tables that constitute a database, the **database management system** uses software called a **data dictionary**. The data dictionary contains a listing of the tables and their details, including field names, validation settings, and data types. The data type refers to the type of information, such as a name, a date, or a time.

The database management system is an important program because before it was available, many health systems and businesses had dozens of database files with incompatible formats. Because patient data come from a variety of sources, these separated, isolated data files required duplicate entry of the same information, thereby increasing the risk of data entry error. The design of the relational databases eliminates data duplication. Some examples of popular database management system software include Microsoft's Access or Visual FoxPro, Corel's Paradox, Oracle's Oracle Database 10g, and IBM's DB2.

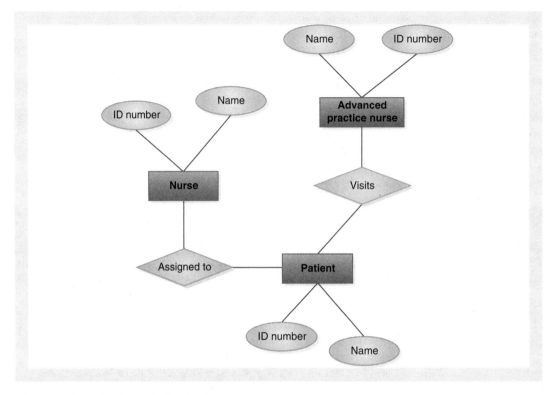

Figure 7-1 Example of an Entity Relationship Diagram (ERD)

On a large scale, a data warehouse is an extremely large database or **repository** that stores all of an organization's or institution's data and makes these data available for **data mining**. The DW can combine an institution's many different databases to provide management personnel with flexible access to the data. On the smaller scale, a **data mart** represents a large database where the data used by one of the units or a division of a health care system are stored and maintained. For example, a university hospital system might store clinical information from its many affiliate hospitals in a DW, and each separate hospital might have a data mart housing its data.

There are many ways to access and retrieve information in databases. Searching information in databases can be done through the use of a **query**, as is used in Microsoft's Access database. A query asks questions of the database to retrieve specific data and information. **Box 7-2** provides a detailed description of the **Structured Query Language** (SQL).

Data mining software sorts thorough data to discover patterns and ascertain or establish relationships. This software discovers or uncovers previously unidentified

BOX 7-2   SQL

SQL was originally called SEQUEL, or Structured English Query Language. SQL, still pronounced "sequel," now stands for Structured Query Language; it is a database querying language rather than a programming language. It is a standard language for accessing and manipulating databases. SQL is "used with relational databases; it allows users to define the structure and organization of stored data, verify and maintain data integrity, control access to the data, and define relationships among the stored data items" (University of California at San Diego, 2010, para. 8). In this way, it simplifies the process of retrieving information from a database in a functional or usable form while facilitating the reorganization of data within the databases.

The relational database management system is the foundation or basis for SQL. An RDMS stores data in "database objects called tables" (W3Schools.com, 2010, para. 6). A table is a collection of related data that consists of columns and rows; as noted earlier, columns are also referred to as fields, and rows are also referred to as records or **tuples**. Databases can have many tables, and each table is identified by a name (see the Database Example: School of Nursing Faculty).

SQL statements handle most of the actions users need to perform on a database. SQL is an **International Organization for Standardization** (ISO) standard and **American National Standards Institute** (ANSI) standard, but many different versions of the SQL language exist (Indiana University, 2010). To remain compliant with the ISO and ANSI standards, SQL must handle or support the major commands of SELECT, UPDATE, DELETE, INSERT and WHERE in a similar manner (W3Schools.com, 2010). The SELECT command allows you to extract data from a database. UPDATE updates the data, DELETE deletes the data, and INSERT inserts new data. WHERE is used to specify selection criteria, thereby restricting the results of the SQL query. Thus, SQL allows you to create databases and manipulate them by storing, retrieving, updating, and deleting data.

The database example provided here reflects the faculty listing for a school of nursing. The table that contains the data is identified by the name "Faculty." The faculty members are each categorized by the following fields (columns): Last Name, First Name, Department Affiliation, Office Phone Number, Office Location, and UserID. Each individual faculty member's information is a record (tuple or row).

DATABASE EXAMPLE: SCHOOL OF NURSING FACULTY

Using the SQL command SELECT, all of the records in the "Faculty" table can be selected:
SELECT * FROM Faculty
This command would SELECT all (*) of the records FROM the table known as FACULTY. The asterisk (*) is used to select all of the columns.

relationships among the data in a database by conducting an exploratory analysis looking for hidden patterns in data. Using such software, the user searches for previously undiscovered or undiagnosed patterns by analyzing the data stored in a DW. **Drill-down** is a term that means the user can view DW information by drilling down to lower levels of the database to focus on information that is pertinent to his or her needs at the moment.

As users move through databases within the health care system, they can access anything from enterprise-wide DWs to data marts. For example, an infection control professional might notice a pattern of methicillin-resistant *Staphylococcus aureus* infections in the local data mart (a single hospital within a larger system). The professional might want to find out if the outbreak is local (data mart) or more widespread in the system (DW). He or she might also query the database to determine if certain patient attributes (e.g., age or medical diagnosis) are associated with the incidence of infection.

These kinds of data mining capabilities are also quite useful for health care practitioners who wish to conduct clinical research studies. For example, one might query a database to tease out attributes (patient characteristics) associated with asthma-related hospitalizations. For a more detailed description and review of data mining, see Chapter 16.

According to Mishra, Sharma, and Pandey (2013), there is a new set of challenges and opportunities for managing data, data mining, and establishing algorithms in the clouds. Data mining in the clouds is emerging and evolving. This frontier is becoming a potent way to take advantage of the power of cloud computing and combine it with SQL. The world as we know it is changing: "Clouds" are leading us to develop revolutionary data mining technologies. There are five typical clinical applications for databases: (1) hospitals, (2) clinical research, (3) clinical trials, (4) ambulatory care, and (5) public health. Some health care systems are connecting their hospitals together by choosing a single CIS to capture data on a systemwide basis. In such health care organizations, multiple application programs share a pool of related data. Think about how potent such databases might potentially be in managing organizations and providing insights into new relationships that may ultimately transform the way work is done.

Department Collaboration and Exchange of Knowledge and Information

The implementation of systems within health care is the responsibility of many people and departments. All systems require a partnership of collaboration and knowledge sharing to implement and maintain successful standards of care. **Collaboration** is the sharing of ideas and experiences for the purposes of mutual understanding and learning. **Knowledge exchange** is the product of collaboration when sharing an understanding of information promotes learning from past experiences to make better future decisions.

Depending on the type of project, collaboration may occur at many different levels within an organization. At an administrative level, collaboration among key stakeholders is critical to the success of any project. **Stakeholders** have the most responsibility for completing the project. They have the greatest influence in the overall design of the system, and ultimately they are the people who are most impacted by a system implementation. Together with the organizational executive team, stakeholders collaborate on the overall budget and time frame for a system implementation.

Collaboration may also occur among the various departments impacted by the system. These groups frequently include representatives from information technology, clinical specialty areas, support services, and software vendors. Once a team is assembled, it defines the objectives and goals of the system. The team members work strategically to align their goals with the goals of the organization where the system is to be used. The focus for these groups is on planning, resource management, transitioning, and ongoing support of the system. Their collaboration determines the way in which the project is managed, the deliverables for the project, the individuals held accountable for the project, the time frame for the project, opportunities for process improvement using the system, and the means by which resources are allocated to support the system.

From collaboration comes the exchange of information and ideas through knowledge sharing. Specialists exchange knowledge within their respective areas of expertise to ensure that the system works for an entire organization. From one another, they learn requirements that make the system successful. This exchange of ideas is what makes health care information systems so valuable. A multidisciplinary approach ensures that systems work in the complex environment of health care organizations that have diverse and complex patient populations.

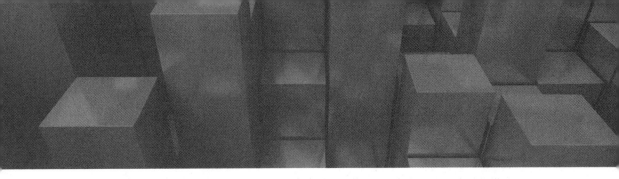

Summary

The integration of technology within health care organizations offers limitless possibilities. As new types of systems emerge, health care professionals will become smarter and more adept at incorporating these tools into their daily practice. Success will be achieved when health care incorporates technology systems in a way that they are viewed not as separate tools to support health care practices but rather as necessary instruments to provide health care. Patients, too, will become savvier at using health care information systems as a means of communication and managing their personal and preventive care. In the future, these two mind-sets will become expectations for health care and not simply a high-tech benefit, as they are often viewed today.

Ultimately, it is not the type of systems that are adopted that is important but rather the method in which they are put into practice. In an ideal world, robust and transparent information technologies will support clinical and administrative functions and promote safe, quality, and cost-effective care.

Thought-Provoking Questions

1. Which type of technology exists today in your discipline that could be converted into new types of information systems to be used in health care?
2. How could collaboration and knowledge sharing at a single organization be used to help individuals preparing for information technology at a different facility?
3. Discuss the administrative information systems and their applications.

Apply Your Knowledge

All members of the health care team must be willing to work together and collaborate to deliver quality patient care. Consider the various administrative information systems discussed in this chapter. Think about each of the systems in relation to your discipline.

1. Make a list of each of the systems discussed in this chapter and reflect on the system and how the system may impact your practice.
2. What is interoperability?
3. Why is it important to embrace interoperability?

References

Agarwal, R., Sands, D., Schneider, J., & Smaltz, D. (2010). Quantifying the economic impact of communication inefficiencies in U.S. hospitals. *Journal of Healthcare Management*, *55*(4), 265–281.

Agency for Healthcare Research and Quality Patient Safety Network. (2015). Patient safety primers: Medication errors. http://psnet.ahrq.gov/primer.aspx?primerID=23

Case Management Society of America. (2014, September 12). *The IT Factor: Years of Study Reveal Healthcare Trends*. http://www.cmsa.org/Individual/NewsEvents/2010HealthITSurvey/tabid/539/Default.aspx

Ciotti, V., & Zodda, F. (1996). Selecting managed care information systems. *Journal of the Healthcare Financial Management Association*, *50*(6), 35–36. http://findarticles.com/p/articles/mi_m3257/is_n6_v50/ai_18515376

Elder, K., Wiltshire, J., Rooks, R., BeLue, R., & Gary, L. (2010, Summer). Health information technology and physician career satisfaction. *Perspectives in Health Information Management*, 1–18. (Document ID: 2118694921)

Fichman, R. G., Kohli, R., & Krishnan, R. (2011). Editorial overview: The role of information systems in healthcare: Current research and future trends. *Information Systems Research*, *22*(3), 419–428. doi: 10.1287/isre.1110.0382

Gordon, C. R., Rezzadeh, K. S., Li, A., Vardanian, A., Zelken, J., Shores, J. T., & Jarrahy, R. (2015). Digital mobile technology facilitates HIPAA-sensitive perioperative messaging, improves physician-patient communication, and streamlines patient care. *Patient Safety in Surgery*, *9*(1), 1–7. doi: 10.1186/s13037-015-0070-9

Hassett, M., & Thede, L. (2003). Information in practice: Clinical information systems. In B. Cunningham (Ed.), *Informatics and nursing opportunities and challenges* (2nd ed., rev., pp. 222–239). Philadelphia: Lippincott Williams & Wilkins.

Indiana University. (2010). University information technology services knowledge base: What is SQL? http://kb.iu.edu/data/ahux.html

Mishra, N., Sharma, S., & Pandey, A. (2013). High performance cloud data mining algorithm and data mining in clouds. http://www.iosrjournals.org/iosr-jce/papers/Vol8-Issue4/I0845461.pdf

National Consortium for Health Science Education. (2012). National health science career cluster model: Health informatics pathway standards & accountability criteria. http://www.healthscienceconsortium.org/wp-content/uploads/2015/07/Health-Informatics-Standards.pdf

Rojas, N. (2015). Data Science Central: Healthcare industry finds new solutions to big data storage challenges. http://www.datasciencecentral.com/profiles/blogs/healthcare-industry-finds-new-solutions-to-big-data-storage

University of California at San Diego. (2010). Data warehouse terms. http://blink.ucsd.edu/technology/help-desk/queries/warehouse/terms.html#s

W3Schools.com. (2010). Introduction to SQL. http://www.w3schools.com/SQL/sql_intro.asp

The Human–Technology Interface

Judith A. Effken, Dee McGonigle,
and Kathleen Mastrian

OBJECTIVES

1. Describe the human–technology interface.
2. Explore human–technology interface problems.
3. Reflect on the future of the human–technology interface.

Introduction

Several years ago, one of this chapter's authors stayed in a new hotel on the outskirts of London. When she entered her room, she encountered three wall-mounted light switches in a row but with no indication of which lights they operated. In fact, the mapping of switches to lights was so peculiar that she was more often than not surprised by the light that came on when she pressed a particular switch. One might conclude that the author had a serious problem, but she prefers to attribute her difficulty to poor design.

When these kinds of technology design issues surface in health care, they are more than just an annoyance. Poorly designed technology can lead to errors, lower productivity, or even the removal of the system (Alexander & Staggers, 2009). Unfortunately, as more and more kinds of increasingly complex health information technology applications are integrated, the problem becomes even worse (Johnson, 2006). However, health care professionals are very creative and, if at all possible, will design work-arounds that allow them to circumvent troublesome technology. However, work-arounds are only a Band-Aid; they are not a long-term solution.

Key Terms
Cognitive task analysis
Cognitive walkthrough
Cognitive work analysis
Earcons
Ergonomics
Field study
Gulf of evaluation
Gulf of execution
Heuristic evaluation
Human–computer interaction
Human factors
Human–technology interaction
Human–technology interface
Mapping
Situational awareness
Task analysis
Usability
Workaround

In his classic book *The Psychology of Everyday Things*, Norman (1988) argued that life would be a lot simpler if people who built the things that others encounter (such as light switches) paid more attention to how they would be used. At least one everyday thing meets Norman's criteria for good design: the scythe. Even people who have never encountered one will pick up a scythe in the manner needed to use it because the design makes only one way feasible. The scythe's design fits perfectly with its intended use and a human user. Would it not be great if all technology were so well fit to human use? In fact, this is not such a far-fetched idea. Scientists and engineers are making excellent strides in understanding human–technology interface problems and proposing solutions to them.

By the end of this chapter, the reader will be able to (1) define what is meant by the "human–technology interface." (2) describe problems with human–technology interfaces currently available in health care. and (3) describe models, strategies, and exemplars for improving interfaces during the analysis, design, and evaluation phases of the development life cycle.

The Human–Technology Interface

What is the **human–technology interface**? Broadly speaking, anytime a human uses technology, some type of hardware or software enables and supports the interaction. It is this hardware and software that defines the interface. The array of light switches described previously was actually an interface (although not a great one) between the lighting technology in the room and the human user.

In today's health care settings, one encounters a wide variety of human–technology interfaces. Those who work in hospitals may use bar-coded identification cards to log their arrival time into a human resources management system. Using the same cards, they might log into their patients' electronic health record (EHR), access their drugs from a drug administration system, and even administer their drugs using bar-coding technology. Other examples of human–technology interfaces one might encounter include a defibrillator, a patient-controlled analgesia (PCA) pump, any number of physiologic monitoring systems, electronic thermometers, and telephones and pagers.

The human interfaces for each of these technologies are different and can even differ among different brands or versions of the same device. For example, to enter data into an EHR, one might use a keyboard, a light pen, a touchscreen, or voice. Health care technologies may present information via computer screen, printer, or a personal digital assistant (PDA). Patient data might be displayed in the form of text, pictures (e.g., the results of a brain scan), or even sound (an echocardiogram), and the information may be arrayed or presented differently, based on roles and preferences. Some human–technology interfaces mimic face-to-face human encounters. For example, faculty members are increasingly using videoconferencing technology to communicate with their students. Similarly, telehealth allows health care professionals to use telecommunication and videoconferencing software to communicate more effectively and more frequently with patients at home by using the technology to monitor patients' vital signs, supervise their wound care, or demonstrate a procedure. According to Gephart and Effken (2013), "The National eHealth Collaborative Technical Expert Panel recommends fully integrating patient-generated data (e.g., home monitoring of daily weights, blood glucose, or blood pressure readings) into the clinical workflow of healthcare providers" (para. 3). Telehealth technology has fostered other virtual interfaces, such as systemwide intensive care units in which intensivists and specially trained nurses monitor critically ill patients in intensive care units, some of whom may be in rural locations. Sometimes telehealth interfaces allow patients to interact with a virtual clinician (actually a computer program) that asks questions, provides social support, and tailors education to identify patient needs based on the answers to screening questions. These human–technology interfaces have been remarkably successful; sometimes patients even prefer them to live clinicians.

Human–technology interfaces may present information using text, numbers, pictures, icons, or sound. Auditory, visual, or even tactile alarms may alert users to important information. Users may interact with (or control) the technology via keyboards, digital pens, voice activation, or even touch.

A small but growing number of clinical and educational interfaces rely heavily on tactile input. For example, many students learn to access an intravenous site using virtual technology. Other, more sophisticated virtual reality applications help physicians learn to do endoscopies or practice complex surgical procedures in a safe environment. Still others allow drug researchers to design new medications by combining virtual molecules (here, the tactile response is quite different for molecules that can be joined from those that cannot). In each of these training environments, accurately depicting tactile sensations is critical. For example, feeling the kind and amount of pressure required to penetrate the desired tissues but not others is essential to a realistic and effective learning experience.

The growing use of large databases for research has led to the design of novel human–technology interfaces that help researchers visualize and understand patterns in the data that generate new knowledge or lead to new questions. Many of these interfaces now incorporate multidimensional visualizations in addition to scatter plots, histograms, or cluster representations (Vincent, Hastings-Tolsma, & Effken, 2010). Some designers, such as Quinn and Meeker (2000) (Quinn being the founder of the Design Rhythmics Sonification Research Laboratory at the University of New Hampshire), use variations in sound to help researchers hear the patterns in large data sets. In Quinn's (2000) "climate symphony," different musical instruments, tones, pitches, and phrases are mapped onto variables, such as the amounts and relative concentrations of minerals to help researchers detect patterns in ice core data covering more than 110,000 years. Climate patterns take centuries to emerge and can be difficult to detect. The music allows the entire 110,000 years to be condensed into just a few minutes, making detection of patterns and changes much easier.

The human–technology interface is ubiquitous in health care and takes many forms. A look at the quality of these interfaces follows. Be warned: It is not always a pretty picture.

The Human–Technology Interface Problem

In *The Human Factor*, Vicente (2004) cited the many safety problems in health care identified by the Institute of Medicine's (1999) report and noted how the technology (defined broadly) used often does not fit well with human characteristics. As a case in point, Vicente described his own studies of nurses' PCA pump errors. Nurses made the errors, in large part, because of the complexity of the user interface, which required as many as 27 steps to program the device. Vicente and his colleagues developed a PCA in which programming required no more than 12 steps. Nurses who used it in laboratory experiments made fewer errors, programmed drug delivery faster, and reported lower cognitive workloads compared to the commercial device. Further evidence that human–technology interfaces do not work as well as they might is evident in the following events.

Doyle (2005) reported that when a bar-coding medication system interfered with their work flow, nurses devised **work-arounds**, such as removing the armband from the patient and attaching it to the bed, because the bar-code reader failed to interpret bar codes when the bracelet curved tightly around a small arm. Koppel et al. (2005) reported that a widely used computer-based provider order entry (CPOE) system meant to decrease medication errors actually facilitated 22 types of errors because the information needed to order medications was fragmented across as many as 20 screens, available medication dosages differed from those the physicians expected, and allergy alerts were triggered only after an order was written.

Han et al. (2005) reported increased mortality among children admitted to Children's Hospital in Pittsburgh after CPOE implementation. Three reasons were cited for this unexpected outcome. First, CPOE changed the work flow in the emergency room. Before CPOE, orders were written for critical time-sensitive treatment based on radio communication with the incoming transport team before the child arrived. After CPOE implementation, orders could not be written until the patient arrived and was registered in the system (a policy that was later changed). Second, entering an order required as many as 10 clicks and took as long as 2 minutes; moreover, computer screens sometimes froze, or response time was slow. Third, when the team changed its work flow to accommodate CPOE, face-to-face contact among team members diminished. Despite the problems with study methods identified by some of the informatics community, there certainly were serious human–technology interface problems.

In 2005, a *Washington Post* article reported that Cedars-Sinai Medical Center in Los Angeles had shut down a $34 million system after 3 months because of the medical staff's rebellion. Reasons for the rebellion included the additional time it took to complete the structured information forms, failure of the system to recognize misspellings (as nurses had previously done), and intrusive and interruptive automated alerts (Connolly, 2005). Even though physicians actually responded appropriately to the alerts, modifying or canceling 35% of the orders that triggered them, designers had not found the right balance of helpful-to-interruptive alerts. The system simply did not fit the clinicians' work flow.

Such unintended consequences (Ash, Berg, & Coiera, 2004) or unpredictable outcomes (Aarts, Doorewaard, & Berg, 2004) of health care information systems may be attributed, in part, to a flawed implementation process, but there were clearly also **human–technology interaction** issues. That is, the technology was not well matched to the users and the context of care. In the pediatric case, a system developed for medical–surgical units was implemented in a critical care unit.

Human–technology interface problems are the major cause of as many as 87% of all patient monitoring incidents (Walsh & Beatty, 2002). It is not always that the technology itself is faulty. In fact, the technology may perform flawlessly, but the interface design may lead the human user to make errors (Vicente, 2004).

Improving the Human–Technology Interface

Much can be learned from the related fields of cognitive engineering, **human factors**, and **ergonomics** about how to make interfaces more compatible with their human users and the context of care. Each of these areas of study is multidisciplinary and integrates knowledge from multiple disciplines (e.g., computer science, engineering, cognitive engineering, psychology, and sociology). Over the years, three axioms have evolved for developing effective **human–computer interactions** (Staggers, 2003): (1) Users must be an early and continuous focus during interface design; (2) the design process should be iterative, allowing for evaluation and correction of identified problems; and (3) formal evaluation should take place using rigorous experimental or qualitative methods.

Axiom 1: Users Must Be an Early and Continuous Focus During Interface Design

Rubin (1994) uses the term *user-centered design* to describe the process of designing products (e.g., human–technology interfaces) so that users can carry out the tasks needed to achieve their goals with "minimal effort and maximal efficiency" (p. 10). Thus, in user-centered design, the end user is emphasized.

According to Maynard (2014), "Humans have to interact with technology in various ways, from the industrial equipment we use to the ever-present smart devices. And industrial engineers have to consider the ergonomic implications of these interactions in their designs of workplace equipment" (para. 1). Vicente (2004) argued that technology should fit human requirements at five levels of analysis (physical, psychological, team, organizational, and political). Physical characteristics of the technology (e.g., size, shape, or location) should conform to the user's size, grasp, and available space. Information should be presented in ways that are consistent with known human psychological capabilities (e.g., the number of items that can be remembered is seven plus or minus two). In addition, systems should conform to the communication, work flow, and authority structures of work teams; to organizational factors, such as culture and staffing levels; and even to political factors, such as budget constraints, laws, or regulations.

A number of analysis tools and techniques have been developed to help designers better understand the task and user environment for which they are designing. Discussed next are task analysis, cognitive task analysis, and cognitive work analysis (CWA).

Task analysis examines how a task must be accomplished. Generally, analysts describe the task in terms of inputs needed for the task, outputs (what is achieved by the task), and any constraints on actors' choices on carrying out the task. Analysts then lay out the sequence of temporally ordered actions that must be carried out to complete the task in flowcharts (Vicente, 1999). A worker's tasks must be analyzed. Task analysis is very useful in defining what users must do and which functions might be distributed between the user and technology (U.S. Department of Health and Human Services, 2013). **Cognitive task analysis** usually starts by identifying, through interviews or questionnaires, the particular task and its typicality and frequency. Analysts then may review the written materials that describe the job or are used for training and determine, through structured interviews or by observing experts perform the task, which knowledge is involved and how that knowledge might be represented.

Cognitive work analysis was developed specifically for the analysis of complex, high-technology work domains, such as nuclear power plants, intensive care units, and emergency departments where workers need considerable flexibility in responding to external demands (Burns & Hajdukiewicz, 2004; Vicente, 1999). A complete CWA includes five types of analysis: (1) work domain, (2) control tasks, (3) strategies, (4) social–organizational, and (5) worker competencies. The work domain analysis describes the functions of the system and identifies the information that users need to accomplish their task goals. The control task analysis investigates the control structures through which the user interacts with or controls the system. It also identifies which variables and relations among variables discovered in the work domain analysis are relevant for particular situations so that context-sensitive interfaces can present the right information (e.g., prompts or alerts) at the right time. The strategies analysis looks at how work is actually done by users to facilitate the design of appropriate human–computer dialogues. The social–organizational analysis identifies the responsibilities of various users (e.g., doctors, nurses, clerks, or therapists) so that the system can support collaboration, communication, and a viable organizational structure. Finally, the worker competencies analysis identifies design constraints related to the users themselves (Effken, 2002).

Specialized tools are available for the first three types of CWA (Vicente, 1999). Analysts typically borrow tools (e.g., ethnography) from the social sciences for the two remaining types. Hajdukiewicz, Vicente, Doyle, Milgram, and Burns (2001) used CWA to model an operating room environment. Effken (2002) and Effken, Loeb, Johnson, Johnson, and Reyna (2001) used CWA to analyze the information needs for an oxygenation management display for an intensive care unit. Other examples of the application of CWA in health care are described by Burns and Hajdukiewicz (2004) in their chapter on medical systems (pp. 201–238).

Axiom 2: The Design Process Should Be Iterative, Allowing for Evaluation and Correction of Identified Problems

Today, both principles and techniques for developing human–technology interfaces that people can use with minimal stress and maximal efficiency are available. An excellent place to start is with Norman's (1988, pp. 188–189) principles:

1. Use both knowledge in the world and knowledge in the head. In other words, pay attention not only to the environment or to the user but also to both and to how they relate. By using both, the problem actually may be simplified.
2. Simplify the structure of tasks. For example, reduce the number of steps or even computer screens needed to accomplish the goal.
3. Make things visible: Bridge the **gulf of execution** and **gulf of evaluation**. Users need to be able to see how to use the technology to accomplish a goal (e.g., which buttons does one press and in which order to program this PCA?); if they do, then designers have bridged the gulf of execution. They also need to be able to see the effects of their actions on the technology (e.g., if a health care professional prescribes an intervention to treat a certain condition, the actual patient response may not be perfectly clear). This bridges the gulf of evaluation.
4. Get the mappings right. Here, the term **mapping** is used to describe how environmental facts (e.g., the order of light switches or variables in a physiologic monitoring display) are accurately depicted by the information presentation.
5. Exploit the power of constraints, both natural and artificial. Because of where the eyes are located in the head, humans have to turn their heads to see what is happening behind them; however, that is not true of all animals. As the location of one's eyes constrains what one can see, so also do physical elements, social factors, and even organizational policy constrain the way tasks are accomplished. By taking these constraints into account when designing technology, it can be made easier for humans use.
6. Design for error. Mistakes happen. Technology should eliminate predictable errors and be sufficiently flexible to allow humans to identify and recover from unpredictable errors.
7. When all else fails, standardize. To get a feel for this principle, think how difficult it is to change from a Macintosh to a Windows environment or from the Windows operating system to Vista.

Kirlik and Maruyama (2004) described a real-world human–technology interface that follows Norman's principles. The authors observed how a busy expert short-order cook strategically managed to grill many hamburgers at the same time but each to the customer's desired level of doneness. The cook put those burgers that were to be well-done on the back and far right portion of the grill, those to be medium well-done in the center of the grill, and those to be rare at the front of the grill but farther to the left. The cook moved all burgers to the left as grilling proceeded and turned them over during their travel across the grill. Everything the cook needed to know was available in this simple interface. As a human–technology interface, the grill layout was elegant. The interface used knowledge housed both in the environment and in the expert cook's head; also, things were clearly visible both in the position of the burgers and in the way they were moved. The process was clearly and effectively standardized, with built-in constraints. What might it take to create such an intuitive human–technology interface in health care?

Several useful books have been written about effective interface design (e.g., Burns & Hajdukiewicz, 2004; Cooper, 1995; Mandel, 1997). In addition, a growing body of research is exploring new ways to present clinical data that might facilitate clinicians' problem identification and accurate treatment (Agency for Healthcare Research and Quality, 2010). Just as in other industries, health care is learning that big data can provide big insights if it can be visualized, accessed, and meaningful (Intel IT Center, 2013). Often designers use graphical objects to show how variables relate. The first to do so were likely Cole and Stewart (1993), who used changes in the lengths of the sides and area of a four-sided object to show the relationship of respiratory rate to tidal volume. Other researchers have demonstrated that histograms and polygon displays are better than numeric displays for detecting changes in patients' physiologic variables (Gurushanthaiah, Weinger, & Englund, 1995). When Horn, Popow, and Unterasinger (2001) presented physiologic data via a single circular object with 12 sectors (where each sector represented a different variable), nurses reported that it was easy to recognize abnormal conditions but difficult to comprehend the patient's overall status. This kind of graphical object approach has been most widely used in anesthesiology, where a number of researchers have shown improved clinician **situational awareness** or problem detection time by mapping physiologic variables onto display objects that have meaningful shapes, such as using a bellows-like object to represent ventilation (Agutter et al., 2003; Blike, Surgenor, Whallen, & Jensen, 2000; Michels, Gravenstein, & Westenskow, 1997; Zhang et al. 2002).

Effken (2006) compared a prototype display that represented physiologic data in a structured pictorial format with two bar graph displays. Both the first bar graph display and the prototype presented data in the order that experts were observed to use them. The second bar graph display presented the data in the way that nurses collected them. In an experiment in which resident physicians and novice nurses used simulated drugs to treat observed oxygenation management problems using each display, residents' performance was improved with the displays ordered as experts used them, but nurses' performance was not improved. Instead, nurses performed better when the variables were ordered as they were used to collecting them, demonstrating the importance of understanding user roles and the tasks they need to accomplish.

Data also need to be represented in ways other than visually. Gaver (1993) proposed that because ordinary sounds map onto familiar events, they could be used as icons to facilitate easier technology navigation and use and to provide continuous background information about how a system is functioning. In health care, auditory displays have been used to provide clinicians with information about patients' vital signs (e.g., in pulse oximetry), such as by altering volume or tone when a significant change occurs (Sanderson, 2006).

Admittedly, auditory displays are probably more useful for quieter areas of the hospital, such as the operating room. Perhaps that is why researchers have most frequently applied the approach in anesthesiology. For example, Loeb and Fitch (2002) reported that anesthesiologists detected critical events more quickly when auditory information about heart rate, blood pressure, and respiratory parameters was added to a visual display. Auditory tones also have been combined as **earcons** to represent relationships among data elements, such as the relationship of systolic to diastolic blood pressure (Watson & Gill, 2004).

Axiom 3: Formal Evaluation Should Take Place Using Rigorous Experimental or Qualitative Methods

Perhaps one of the highest accolades that any interface can achieve is to say that it is transparent. An interface becomes transparent when it is so easy to use that users no longer think about it but only about the task at hand. For example, a transparent clinical interface would enable clinicians to focus on patient decisions rather than on how to access or combine patient data from multiple sources. In **Figure 8-1**, instead of the nurse interacting with the computer, the nurse and the patient interact through the technology interface. The more transparent the interface, the easier the interaction should be.

Usability is a term that denotes the ease with which people can use an interface to achieve a particular goal. Usability of a new human–technology interface needs to be evaluated early and often throughout its development. Typical usability indicators include ease of use, ease of learning, satisfaction with using, efficiency of use, error tolerance, and fit of the system to the task (Staggers, 2003). Some of the more commonly used approaches to usability evaluation are discussed next.

Surveys of Potential or Actual Users

Chernecky, Macklin, and Waller (2006) assessed cancer patients' preferences for website design. Participants were asked their preferences for a number of design

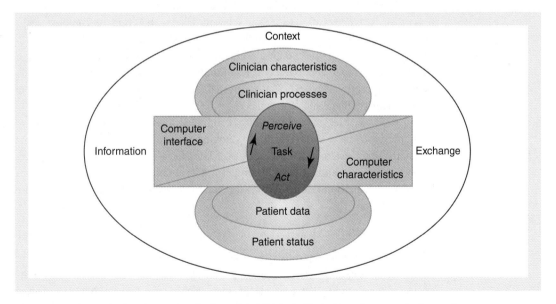

Figure 8-1   Nurse–Patient Interaction Framework in Which the Technology Supports the Interaction

Source: Adapted from Staggers and Parks (1993). Reprinted by permission of AMIA.

characteristics, such as display color, menu buttons, text, photo size, icon metaphor, and layout, by selecting on a computer screen their preferences for each item from two or three options.

Focus Group

Typically used at the very start of the design process, focus groups can help the designer better understand users' responses to potential interface designs and to content that might be included in the interface.

Cognitive Walkthrough

In a **cognitive walkthrough**, evaluators assess a paper mock-up, working prototype, or completed interface by observing the steps users are likely to take to use the interface to accomplish typical tasks. This analysis helps designers determine how understandable and easy to learn the interface is likely to be for these users and the typical tasks (Wharton, Rieman, Lewis, & Polson, 1994).

Heuristic Evaluation

A **heuristic evaluation** has become the most popular of what are called "discount usability evaluation" methods. The objective of a heuristic evaluation is to detect problems early in the design process, when they can be most easily and economically corrected. The methods are termed "discount" because they typically are easy to do, involve fewer than 10 experts (often experts in relevant fields such as human–computer technology or cognitive engineering), and are much less expensive than other methods. They are called "heuristic" because evaluators assess the degree to which the design complies with recognized usability rules of thumb or principles (the heuristics), such as those proposed by Nielsen (1994) and available on his website (http://www.useit.com/papers/heuristic/heuristic_list.html).

For example, McDaniel et al. (2002) conducted a usability test of an interactive computer-based program to encourage smoking cessation by low-income women. As part of the initial evaluation, health care professionals familiar with the intended users reviewed the design and layout of the program. The usability test revealed several problems with the decision rules used to tailor content to users that were corrected before implementation.

Formal Usability Test

Formal usability tests typically use either experimental or observational studies of actual users using the interface to accomplish real-world tasks. A number of researchers use these methods. For example, Staggers, Kobus, and Brown (2007) conducted a usability study of a prototype electronic medication administration record. Participants were asked to add, modify, or discontinue medications using the system. The time they needed to complete the task, their accuracy in the task, and their satisfaction with the prototype were assessed (the last criterion through a questionnaire). Although satisfaction was high, the evaluation also revealed design flaws that could be corrected before implementation.

Field Study

In a **field study**, end users evaluate a prototype in the actual work setting just before its general release. For example, Thompson, Lozano, and Christakis (2007) evaluated the use of touchscreen computer kiosks containing child health–promoting information in several low-income, urban community settings through an online questionnaire that could be completed after the kiosk was used. Most users found the kiosk easy to use and the information it provided easy to understand. Researchers also gained a better understanding of the characteristics of the likely users (e.g., 26% had never used the Internet, and 48% had less than a high school education) and the information most often accessed (television and media use and smoke exposure).

Dykes et al. (2006) used a field test to investigate the feasibility of using digital pen and paper technology to record vital signs as a way to bridge an organization from a paper to an electronic health record. In general, satisfaction with the tool increased with use, and the devices conformed well to nurses' work flow. However, 8% of the vital sign entries were recorded inaccurately because of inaccurate handwriting recognition, entries outside the recording box, or inaccurate data entry (the data entered were not valid values). The number of modifications needed in the tool and the time that would be required to make those changes ruled out using the digital pen and paper as a bridging technology.

Ideally, every health care setting would have a usability laboratory of its own to test new software and technology in its own setting before actual implementation. However, this can be expensive, especially for small organizations. Kushniruk and Borycki (2006) developed a low-cost rapid usability engineering method for creating a portable usability laboratory consisting of video cameras and other technology that one can take out of the laboratory into hospitals and other locations to test the technology on-site using as close to a real-world environment as possible. This is a much more cost-effective and efficient solution and makes it possible to test all technologies before their implementation.

A Framework for Evaluation

Ammenwerth, Iller, and Mahler (2006) proposed a fit between individuals, tasks, and technology (FITT) model that suggests that each of these factors be considered in designing and evaluating human–technology interfaces. It is not enough to consider only the user and technology characteristics; the tasks that the technology supports must be considered as well. The FITT model builds on DeLone and McLean's (1992) information success model, Davis's (1993) technology acceptance model, and Goodhue and Thompson's (1995) task technology fit model. A notable strength of the FITT model is that it encourages the evaluator to examine the fit between the various pairs of components: user and technology, task and technology, and user and task.

Johnson and Turley (2006) compared how doctors and nurses describe patient information and found that doctors emphasized diagnosis, treatment, and management, whereas the nurses emphasized functional issues. Although both physicians and nurses share some patient information, how they thought about patients differed. For that reason, an EHR needs to present information (even the same information) to the two groups in different ways.

Hyun, Johnson, Stetson, and Bakken (2009) used a combination of two models (technology acceptance model and task–technology fit model) to design and evaluate an electronic documentation system for nurses. To facilitate the design, they employed multiple methods, including brainstorming of experts, to identify design requirements. To evaluate how well the prototype design fit both task and user, nurses were asked to carry out specific tasks using the prototype in a laboratory setting and then complete a questionnaire on ease of use, usefulness, and fit of the technology with their documentation tasks. Because the researchers engaged nurses at each step of the design process, the result was a more useful and usable system.

Future of the Human–Technology Interface

Future technological enhancements will impact how we handle the activities of daily living in our personal lives as well as how we perform as professionals. There are new capabilities emerging daily, and it is difficult to keep up at times. Touchless sensing and gesture recognition is one trend to watch. According to Uerkwitz (2014),

> *The next one we do think is gesture control and gesture recognition, but we only think it's going to do well if it complements what the other technologies already do. And so here you could take the Samsung (005930.KS) phones; they have what is called hover technology, meaning you can turn it on and off without touching the screen. I think most people probably have that turned off, most people may not even know about it. (p. 3)*

This demonstrates not only that we must anticipate the future but also that we must explore and appreciate the capabilities of the technology we are currently using. Increased attention to improving the human–technology interface through human factors approaches has already led to significant improvements in one area of health care: anesthesiology. Anesthesia machines that once had hoses that would fit into any delivery port now have hoses that can be plugged into only the proper port. Anesthesiologists have also been actively working with engineers to improve the computer interface through which they monitor their patients' status and are among the leaders in investigating the use of audio techniques as an alternative way to help anesthesiologists maintain their situational awareness. As a result of these efforts, anesthesia-related deaths dropped from 2 in 20,000 to 1 in 200,000 in less than 10 years (Vicente, 2004). It is hoped that continued emphasis on human factors (Vicente, 2004) and user-centered design (Rubin, 1994) by informatics professionals and human–computer interactions experts will have equally successful effects on other parts of the health care system. The increased amount of informatics research in this area is encouraging, but there is a long way to go.

A systematic review of clinical technology design evaluation studies (Alexander & Staggers, 2009) found 50 nursing studies. Of those, nearly half (24) evaluated effectiveness, fewer (16) evaluated satisfaction, and still fewer (10) evaluated efficiency. The evaluations were not systematic. That is, there was no attempt to evaluate the same system in different environments or with different users. Most evaluations were done in a laboratory rather than in the setting where the system would be used. The authors argued for a broader range of studies that use an expanded set of outcome measures. For example, instead of looking at user satisfaction, evaluators should dig deeper into the design factors that led to the satisfaction or dissatisfaction. In addition, performance measures, such as diagnostic accuracy, errors, and correct treatment, should be used.

Rackspace, Brauer, and Barth (2013) reported on a social study of the human cloud formed in part by data collected from wearable technologies; they focused on assessing attitudes and "exploring how cloud computing is enabling this new generation of smart devices" (p. 2). Today, smartphones, glasses, clothing, watches, cameras, and monitors for health or patient tracking, to name but a few devices, are available to this purpose.

As our technologies continue to evolve, we are creating more design issues. The proliferation of smart devices and wearable technology brings new concerns related to human–technology interfaces. According to Madden (2013), wearable technologies are adding another wrinkle into the design process—namely, human behavior. How will someone use this technology? How will individuals behave with it on their person? How will they wear it? How and when will they enable and use it? Will others be able to detect the technologies? That is, will someone be able to wear Google Glass and take pictures or videos of other people's actions easily and seamlessly move among all of the capabilities of his or her wearable technologies? The human–technology interface must address these issues. There is a long way to go.

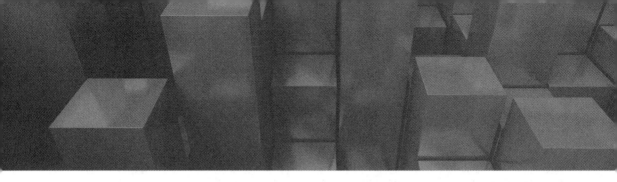

Summary

There are at least three messages the reader should take away from the discussion in this chapter. First, if there is to be significant improvement in quality and safety outcomes in the United States through the use of information technology, the designs for human–technology interfaces must be radically improved so that the technology better fits human and task requirements. However, that improvement will be possible only if clinicians identify and report problems rather than simply creating work-arounds. That means that each clinician has a responsibility to participate in the design process and to report designs that do not work.

Second, a number of useful tools are currently available for the analysis, design, and evaluation phases of development life cycles. They should be used routinely by informatics professionals to ensure that technology better fits both task and user requirements.

Third, focusing on interface improvement using these tools has had a huge impact on patient safety in the area of anesthesiology and medication administration. With increased attention from informatics professionals and engineers, the same kind of improvement should be possible in other areas regardless of the technologies actually employed there. In the ideal world, one can envision that every human–technology interface will be designed to enhance users' work flow, will be as easy to use as banking ATMs and will be fully tested before its implementation in a setting that mirrors the setting where it will be used.

Thought-Provoking Questions

1. You are a member of a team that has been asked to evaluate a prototype mobile application (app) for patients. Based on what you know about usability testing, which kind of test (or tests) might you do and why?
2. Is there a human–technology interface that you have encountered that you think needs improvement? If you were to design a replacement, which analysis techniques would you choose? Why?
3. Which type of functionality and interoperability would you want from your smartphone, watch, clothing, glasses, camera, and monitor? Provide a detailed response.

Apply Your Knowledge

The introduction to this chapter features an example of a poorly designed interface. Review this example and then do the following:

1. Think of a poorly designed interface and a well-designed technology interface from your personal life. What are the characteristics of each?

2. Consider the influence of age on the conclusion that a piece of technology is or is not user friendly.

Think of specific examples of a health care technology where the age of the user might be a factor in the perception that technology is user-friendly.

Additional Resources

Nielsen Norman Group
http://www.useit.com/papers/heuristic/heuristic_list.html

References

Aarts, J., Doorewaard, H., & Berg, M. (2004). Understanding implementation: The case of a computerized physician order entry system in a large Dutch university medical center. *Journal of the American Medical Association, 11,* 207–216.

Agency for Healthcare Research and Quality. (2010). Improving data collection across the health care system. http://www.ahrq.gov/research/findings/final-reports/iomracereport/reldata5.html

Agutter, J., Drews, F., Syroid, N., Westneskow, D., Albert, R., Strayer, et al. (2003). Evaluation of graphic cardiovascular display in a high-fidelity simulator. *Anesthesia and Analgesia, 97,* 1403–1413.

Alexander, G., & Staggers, N. (2009). A systematic review of the designs of clinical technology findings and recommendations for future research. *Advances in Nursing Science, 32*(3), 252–279.

Ammenwerth, E., Iller, C., & Mahler, C. (2006). IT-adoption and the interaction of task, technology and individuals: A fit framework and a case study. *BMC Medical Informatics and Decision Making, 6,* 3.

Ash, J. S., Berg, M., & Coiera, E. (2004). Some unintended consequences of information technology in health care: The nature of patient care information system-related errors. *Journal of the American Medical Informatics Association, 11,* 104–112.

Blike, G. T., Surgenor, S. D., Whallen, K., & Jensen, J. (2000). Specific elements of a new hemodynamics display improves the performance of anesthesiologists. *Journal of Clinical Monitoring & Computing, 16,* 485–491.

Burns, C. M., & Hajdukiewicz, J. R. (2004). *Ecological interface design.* Boca Raton, FL: CRC Press.

Chernecky, C., Macklin, D., & Waller, J. (2006). Internet design preferences of patients with cancer. *Oncology Nursing Forum, 33,* 787–792.

Cole, W. G., & Stewart, J. G. (1993). Metaphor graphics to support integrated decision making with respiratory data. *International Journal of Clinical Monitoring and Computing, 10,* 91–100.

Connolly, C. (2005, March 21). Cedars-Sinai doctors cling to pen and paper. *Washington Post,* p. A01.

Cooper, A. (1995). *About face: Essentials of window interface design.* New York: Hungry Minds, Inc.

Davis, F. D. (1993). User acceptance of information technology: System characteristics, user perceptions and behavioral impacts. *International Journal of Man–Machine Studies, 38,* 475–487.

DeLone, W. H., & McLean, E. (1992). Information systems success: The question for the dependent variable. *Information Systems Research, 3*(1), 60–95.

Doyle, M. (2005). *Impact of the Bar Code Medication Administration (BCMA) system on medication administration errors.* Unpublished doctoral dissertation, University of Arizona, Tucson.

Dykes, P. C., Benoit, A., Chang, F., Gallagher, J., Li, Q., Spurr, C., et al. (2006). The feasibility of digital pen and paper technology for vital sign data capture in acute care settings. In *AMIA*

2006 symposium proceedings (pp. 229–233). Washington, DC: American Medical Informatics Association.

Effken, J. A. (2002). Different lenses, improved outcomes: A new approach to the analysis and design of healthcare information systems. *International Journal of Medical Informatics, 65,* 59–74.

Effken, J. A. (2006). Improving clinical decision making through ecological interfaces. *Ecological Psychology, 18*(4), 283–318.

Effken, J., Loeb, R., Johnson, K., Johnson, S., & Reyna, V. (2001). Using cognitive work analysis to design clinical displays. In V. L. Patel, R. Rogers, & R. Haux (Eds.), *Proceedings of MedInfo-2001* (pp. 27–31). London: IOS Press.

Gaver, W. W. (1993). What in the world do we hear? An ecological approach to auditory event perception. *Ecological Psychology, 5,* 1–30.

Gephart, S., & Effken, J. (2013). Using health information technology to engage patients in their care. *Online Journal of Nursing Informatics (OJNI), 17* (3). http://ojni.org/issues/?p=2848

Goodhue, D. L., & Thompson, R. L. (1995). Task–technology fit and individual performance. *MIS Quarterly, 19*(2), 213–236.

Gurushanthaiah, K. I., Weinger, M. B., & Englund, C. E. (1995). Visual display format affects the ability of anesthesiologists to detect acute physiologic changes: A laboratory study employing a clinical display simulator. *Anesthesiology, 83,* 1184–1193.

Hajdukiewicz, J. R., Vicente, K. J., Doyle, D. J., Milgram, P., & Burns, C. M. (2001). Modeling a medical environment: An ontology for integrated medical informatics design. *International Journal of Medical Informatics, 62,* 79–99.

Han, Y. Y., Carcillo, J. A., Venkataraman, S. T., Clark, R. S. B., Watson, R. S., Nguyen, T., et al. (2005). Unexpected increased mortality after implementation of a commercially sold computerized physician order entry system. *Pediatrics, 116,* 1506–1512.

Horn, W., Popow, C., & Unterasinger, L. (2001). Support for fast comprehension of ICU data: Visualization using metaphor graphics. *Methods in Informatics Medicine, 40,* 421–424.

Hyun, S., Johnson, S. B., Stetson, P. D., & Bakken, S. (2009). Development and evaluation of nursing user interface screens using multiple methods. *Journal of Biomedical Informatics, 42*(6), 1004–1012.

Institute of Medicine. (1999). *To err is human: Building a safer health system.* Washington, DC: Author.

Intel IT Center. (2013). Big data visualization: Turning big data into big insights. http://www.intel.com/content/dam/www/public/us/en/documents/white-papers/big-data-visualizationturning-big-data-into-big-insights.pdf

Johnson, C. M., & Turley, J. P. (2006). The significance of cognitive modeling in building healthcare interfaces. *International Journal of Medical Informatics, 75*(2), 163–172.

Johnson, C. W. (2006). Why did that happen? Exploring the proliferation of barely usable software in healthcare systems. *Quality & Safety in Healthcare, 15*(Suppl. 1), 176–181.

Kirlik, A., & Maruyama, S. (2004). Human–technology interaction and music perception and performance: Toward the robust design of sociotechnical systems. *Proceedings of the IEEE, 92*(4), 616–631.

Koppel, R., Metlay, J. P., Cohen, A., Abaluck, B., Localio, A. R., Kimmel, S. E., et al. (2005). Role of computerized physician order entry systems in facilitating medication errors. *Journal of the American Medical Association, 293*(10), 1197–1203.

Kushniruk, A. W., & Borycki, E. M. (2006). Low-cost rapid usability engineering: Designing and customizing usable healthcare information systems. *Healthcare Quarterly (Toronto, Ont.), 9*(40), 98–100, 102.

Loeb, R. G., & Fitch, W. T. (2002). A laboratory evaluation of an auditory display designed to enhance intraoperative monitoring. *Anesthesia and Analgesia, 94*, 362–368.

Madden, S. (2013). With wearable tech like Google Glass, human behavior is now a design problem. http://gigaom.com/2013/06/15/with-wearable-tech-like-google-glass -humanbehavior-is-now-a-design-problem/

Mandel, T. (1997). *The elements of user interface design.* New York: Wiley.

Maynard, D. (2014). Molding human interaction with technology. *Industrial Engineer, 46*(3), 54–55.

McDaniel, A., Hutchinson, S., Casper, G. R., Ford, R. T., Stratton, R., & Rembush, M. (2002). Usability testing and outcomes of an interactive computer program to promote smoking cessation in low income women. In *Proceedings AMIA 2002* (pp. 509–513). Washington, DC: American Medical Informatics Association.

Michels, P., Gravenstein, D., & Westenskow, D. R. (1997). An integrated graphic data display improves detection and identification of critical events during anesthesia. *Journal of Clinical Monitoring & Computing, 13*, 249–259.

Nielsen, J. (1994). Heuristic evaluation. In J. Nielsen & R. L. Mack (Eds.), *Usability inspection methods* (pp. 25–62). New York: Wiley.

Norman, D. A. (1988). *The psychology of everyday things.* New York: Basic Books.

Quinn, M. (2000). The climate symphony: Rhythmic techniques applied to the sonification of ice core data. http://www.bcca.org/ief/dquin00c.htm

Quinn, M., & Meeker, L. (2000). Research set to music: The climate symphony and other sonifications of ice core, radar, DNA, seismic and solar wind data. http://www.drsrl.com/climate _paper.html

Rackspace, Brauer, C., & Barth, J. (2013). The human cloud: Wearable technology from novelty to productivity. A social study into the impact of wearable technology. http://sloanreview.mit .edu/article/managing-the-human-cloud

Rubin, J. (1994). *Handbook of usability testing: How to plan, design, and conduct effective tests.* New York: Wiley.

Sanderson, P. (2006). The multimodal world of medical monitoring displays. *Applied Ergonomics, 37*, 501–512.

Staggers, N. (2003). Human factors: Imperative concepts for information systems in critical care. *AACN Clinical Issues, 14*(3), 310–319.

Staggers, N., Kobus, D., & Brown, C. (2007). Nurses' evaluations of a novel design for an electronic medication administration record. *CIN: Computers, Informatics, Nursing, 25*(2), 67–75.

Staggers, N., & Parks, P. L. (1993). Description and initial applications of the Staggers & Parks nurse–computer interaction framework. *Computers in Nursing, 11*, 282–290.

Thompson, D. A., Lozano, P., & Christakis, D. A. (2007). Parent use of touchscreen computer kiosks for child health promotion in community settings. *Pediatrics, 119*(3), 427–434.

Uerkwitz, A. (2014). Opportunities in next generation of wearable electronics and human interface technologies. Wall Street Transcript, May 26, 2014, 2–6. https://www.twst.com/interview /opportunities-in-next-generation-of-wearable-electronics-and-human-interface-technologies

U.S. Department of Health and Human Services. (2013). Usability.gov: Task analysis. http://www .usability.gov/how-to-and-tools/methods/task-analysis.html

Vincent, D., Hastings-Tolsma, M., & Effken, J. (2010). Data visualization and large nursing datasets. *Online Journal of Nursing Informatics, 14*(2). http://ojni.org/14_2/Vincent.pdf

Vicente, K. J. (1999). *Cognitive work analysis: Toward safe, productive, and healthy computer-based work.* Mahwah, NJ: Lawrence Erlbaum Associates.

Vicente, K. (2004). *The human factor.* New York: Routledge.

Walsh, T., & Beatty, P. C. W. (2002). Human factor error and patient monitoring. *Physiological Measurement, 23*, R111–R132.

Watson, G., & Gill, T. (2004). Earcon for intermittent information in monitoring environments. In *Proceedings of the 2004 Conference of the Computer–Human Interaction Special Interest Group of the Human Factors and Ergonomics Society of Australia* (OzCHI2004), Wollonggong, New South Wales, November 22–24, 1994.

Wharton, C., Rieman, J., Lewis, C., & Polson, P. (1994). The cognitive walkthrough: A practitioner's guide. In J. Nielsen & R. L. Mack (Eds.), *Usability inspection methods* (pp. 105–139). New York: Wiley.

Zhang, Y., Drews, F. A., Westenskow, D. R., Foresti, S., Agutter, J., Burmedez, J. C., et al. (2002). Effects of integrated graphical displays on situation awareness in anaesthesiology. *Cognition, Technology & Work, 4*, 82–90.

Electronic Security

Lisa Reeves Bertin, Dee McGonigle,
and Kathleen Mastrian

OBJECTIVES

1. Assess processes for securing electronic information in a computer network.
2. Identify various methods of user authentication and relate authentication to security of a network.
3. Explain methods to anticipate and prevent typical threats to network security.

Introduction

In addition to complying with federal guidelines of the Health Insurance Portability and Accountability Act (HIPAA) and Health Information Technology for Economic and Clinical Health (HITECH) regarding the privacy of patient information, health care systems need to be vigilant in the way that they secure information and manage network security. Mowry and Oakes (n.d.) discuss the vulnerability of electronic health records to data breaches. They suggest that as many as 77 persons could view a patient's record during a hospital stay. It is critical for information technology (IT) policies and procedures to ensure appropriate access by clinicians and to protect private information from inappropriate access. However, authentication procedures can be cumbersome and time consuming, thus reducing health care professional performance efficiency.

Physicians spend on average 7 minutes per patient encounter, with nearly 2 minutes of that time being devoted to managing logins and application navigation. Likewise, an average major health care provider must deal with more than 150 applications—most requiring different user names and passwords—making it difficult for caregivers to navigate and receive contextual information. Health care organizations must strike the right balance in terms of simplifying access to core clinical data sets while maximizing the time providers can interact with patients without jeopardizing data integrity and security.

Key Terms

Antivirus software
Authentication
Biometrics
Brute force attack
Confidentiality
Electronic protected
    health information
Firewalls
Flash drives
Hackers
Integrity
Intrusion detection
    devices
Intrusion detection
    systems
Jump drives
Malicious code
Malicious insiders
Malware
Mask
Negligent insider
Network
Network accessibility
Network availability
Network security
Password

(continues)

This chapter explores use of information and processes for securing information in a health system computer network.

Securing Network Information

Typically, a health care organization has computers linked together to facilitate communication and operations within and outside the facility. This is commonly referred to as a **network**. The linking of computers together and to the outside world creates the possibility of a breach of network security and exposes the information to unauthorized use. With the advent of smart devices, managing all of these risks has become a nightmare for some institutions' security processes. In the past, stationary devices or computers resided within health care facilities. Today, smart devices travel in and out of health care organizations with patients, family members, and other visitors as well as employees—both staff and health care providers alike. According to Sullivan (2012), "Even as they promise better health and easier care delivery, wireless medical devices (MDs) carry significant security risks. And the situation is only getting trickier as more and more MDs come with commercial operating systems that are both Internet-connected and susceptible to attack" (para. 1).

The three main areas of secure network information are (1) **confidentiality**, (2) availability, and (3) **integrity**. An organization must follow a well-defined policy to ensure that private health information remains appropriately confidential. The confidentiality policy should clearly define which data are confidential and how those data should be handled. Employees also need to understand the procedures for releasing confidential information outside the organization or to others within the organization and know which procedures to follow if confidential information is accidentally or intentionally released without authorization. In addition, the organization's confidentiality policy should contain consideration for elements as basic as the placement of monitors so that information cannot be read by passersby. **Shoulder surfing**, or watching over someone's back as that person is working, is still a major way that confidentiality is compromised.

Availability refers to network information being accessible when needed. This area of the policy tends to be much more technical in nature. An accessibility policy covers issues associated with protecting the key hardware elements of the computer network and the procedures to follow in case of a major electric outage or Internet outage. Food and drinks spilled onto keyboards of computer units, dropping or jarring hardware, and electrical surges or static charges are all examples of ways that the hardware elements of a computer network may be damaged. In the case of an electrical outage or a weather-related disaster, the network administrator must have clear plans for data backup, storage, and retrieval. There must also be clear procedures and alternative methods of ensuring that care delivery remains largely uninterrupted.

Another way organizations protect the availability of their networks is to institute an acceptable use policy. Elements covered in such policy could include which types of activities are acceptable on the corporate network. For example, are employees permitted to download music at work? Restricting downloads is a very common way for organizations to prevent viruses and other malicious code from entering their networks. The policy should also clearly define which activities are not acceptable and identify the consequences for violations.

The last area of information security is integrity. Employees need to have confidence that the information they are reading is true. To accomplish this, organizations need clear policies to clarify how data are actually input, determine who has the authorization to change such data, and track how and when data are changed. All three of these areas use authorization and authentication to enforce the corporate policies. Access to networks can easily be grouped into areas of authorization (e.g., users can be grouped by job title). For example, anyone with the job title of "floor supervisor" might be authorized to change the hours worked by an employee, whereas an employee with the title of "patient care assistant" cannot make such changes.

Authentication of Users

Authentication of employees is also used by organizations in their security policies. The most common ways to authenticate rely on something the user knows, something the user has, or something the user is (**Figure 9-1**).

Something a user knows is a **password**. Most organizations today enforce a strong password policy because free software available on the Internet can break a password from the dictionary very quickly. Strong password policies include using combinations of letters, numbers, and special characters, such as plus signs and ampersands. Policies typically include the enforcement of changing passwords every 30 or 60 days.

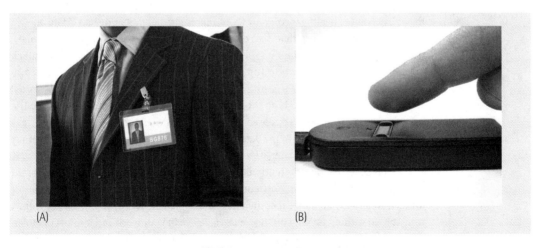

(A)   (B)

Figure 9-1 Ways to Authenticate Users: A: An ID Badge. B: A Finger on a Biometric Scanner
Sources: Part A: © Photos.com. Part B: © Gary James Calder/ShutterStock, Inc.

Passwords should never be written down in an obvious place, such as a sticky note attached to the monitor or under the keyboard.

The second area of authentication is something the user has, such as an identification (ID) card. ID cards can be magnetic, similar to a credit card, or have a **radio frequency identification chip** embedded into the card.

The last area of authentication is **biometrics**. Devices that recognize thumb prints, retina patterns, or facial patterns are available. Depending on the level of security needed, organizations commonly use a combination of these types of authentication.

Threats to Security

The largest benefit of a computer network is the ability to share information. However, organizations need to protect that information and ensure that only authorized individuals have access to the network and the data appropriate to their role. Threats to data security in health care organizations are becoming increasingly prevalent. A 2003 nationwide survey by the Computing Technology Industry Association found that human error was the most likely cause of problems with **security breaches**. The survey indicated that only 8% of such breaches were caused by purely technical errors, whereas more than 63% were caused by some type of human error (Gross, 2003). According to Degaspari (2010), "Given the volume of electronic patient data involved, it's perhaps not surprising that breaches are occurring. According to the Department of Health and Human Services' Office of Civil Rights (OCR), 146 data breaches affecting 500 or more individuals occurred between December 22, 2009, and July 28, 2010. The types of breaches encompass theft, loss, hacking, and improper disposal; and include both electronic data and paper records" (para. 4). The Fifth Annual Benchmark Study on Privacy & Security of Healthcare Data (Ponemon Institute, 2015) reported that "more than 90 percent of healthcare organizations represented in this study had a data breach, and 40 percent had more than five data breaches over the past two years" (para. 3). Interestingly, the most common type of data breach was related to a criminal attack on the health care organization (up 125% in the last 5 years). Key terms related to criminal attacks are **brute force attacks** (software used to guess network passwords) and **zero day attacks** (searching for and exploiting software vulnerabilities). Of the intentional data breaches (as opposed to unintentional), "45 percent of healthcare organizations say the root cause of the data breach was a criminal attack and 12 percent say it was due to a malicious insider" (Ponemon Institute, para. 4). That leaves nearly 43% of data breaches in the unintentional category. The HIMSS (2015) survey reported the negligent insider as the most common source of a security breach. Examples of unintentional/negligent breaches include lost or stolen devices or walking away from a workstation without logging off. If you use a device in your work and it is lost or stolen or you violate policy by walking away from a workstation without logging off, this may be considered negligence, and you may be subject to discipline or even lose your job. An interesting example of an unintentional data breach was reported on the OCR website— a company leased photocopier equipment and returned it without erasing the health care data stored on the copier hard drive, resulting in a settlement of over $1.2 million

(U.S. Department of Health and Human Services, n.d.). Health care organizations need to be proactive in anticipating the potential for and preventing security breaches.

The first line of defense is strictly physical. The power of a locked door, an operating system that locks down after 5 minutes of inactivity, and regular security training programs are extremely effective in this regard. Proper workspace security discipline is a critical aspect of maintaining security. Employees need to be properly trained to be aware of computer monitor visibility, shoulder surfing, and policy regarding the removal of computer hardware. A major issue facing organizations is removable storage devices (**Figure 9-2**). CD/DVD burners, **jump drives**, **flash drives**, and **thumb drives** (which use USB port access) are all potential security risks. These devices can be slipped into a pocket and, therefore, are easily removed from the organization. One way to address this physical security risk is to limit the authorization to write files to a device. Organizations are also turning off the CD/DVD burners and USB ports on company desktops.

The most common threats a corporate network faces are **hackers**, **malicious code** (**spyware**, **viruses**, **worms**, and **Trojan horses**), and **malicious insiders**. Acceptable use policies help to address these problems. For example, employees may be restricted from downloading files from the Internet. Downloaded files, including e-mail attachments, are the most common way viruses and other malicious codes enter a computer

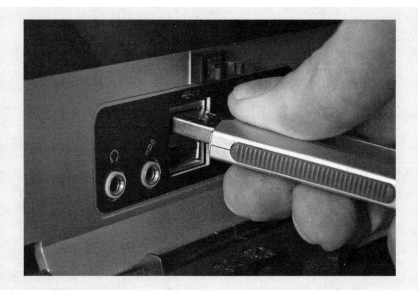

Figure 9-2 A Removable Storage Device
Sources: © Alex Kotlov/ShutterStock, Inc.

network. Network security policies typically prohibit employees from using personal CDs/DVDs and USB drives, thereby preventing the transfer of malicious code from a personal computer to the network.

Spyware is normally controlled by limiting functions of the browser used to surf the Internet. For example, the browser privacy options can control how cookies are used. A cookie is a very small file written to the hard drive of a computer whose user is surfing the Internet. This file contains information about the user. For example, many shopping sites write cookies to the user's hard drive containing the user's name and preferences. When that user returns to the site, the site will greet her by name and list products in which she is possibly interested. Weather websites send cookies to users' hard drives with their ZIP code so that when each user returns to that site, the local weather forecast is immediately displayed. On the negative side, cookies can follow the user's travels on the Internet. Marketing companies use spying cookies to track popular websites that could provide a return on advertising expenditures. Spying cookies related to marketing typically do not track keystrokes in an attempt to steal user IDs and passwords. Instead, they simply track which websites are popular and are used to develop advertising and marketing strategies. Spyware that does steal user IDs and passwords contains malicious code that is normally hidden in a seemingly innocent file download. This threat to security explains why health care organizations typically do not allow employees to download files. The rule of thumb to protect the network and one's own computer system is to download only files from a reputable site that provides complete contact information. Organizations may also use such devices as firewalls (covered in the next section) and **intrusion detection devices** to protect from hackers.

Another huge threat to corporate security is **social engineering**, or the manipulation of a relationship based on one's position in an organization. For example, someone attempting to access a network might pretend to be an employee from the corporate IT office who simply asks for an employee's digital ID and password. The outsider can then gain access to the corporate network. Once this access has been obtained, all corporate information is at risk. A second example of social engineering is a hacker impersonating a federal government agent. After talking an employee into revealing network information, the hacker has an open door to enter the corporate network.

An important security threat to a corporate network is the malicious insider. This person can be a disgruntled employee or a recently fired employee whose rights of access to the corporate network have not yet been removed. In the case of a recently fired employee, his or her network access should be suspended immediately on notice of termination. To avoid the potentially hazardous issues created by malicious insiders, health care organizations need some type of policy to monitor employee activity to ensure that employees carry out only those duties that are part of their normal job. Separation of privileges is a common security tool; no one employee should be able to complete a task that could cause a critical event without the knowledge of another employee. For example, the employee who processes the checks and prints them should not be the same person who signs those checks. Similarly, the employee who alters pay rates and hours worked should be required to submit a weekly report to a supervisor before the changes take effect. Software that can track and monitor employee activity is also available. This software can log which files an employee accesses, whether changes were made to files, and whether the files were copied. Depending on the number of employees, organizations may also employ a full-time electronic auditor who does nothing but monitor activity logs. More than half of health care organizations have hired full-time employees to provide network security (HIMSS, 2015). Additional strategies suggested in the most recent HIMSS survey were mock cyber defense exercises, sharing information between and among health care organizations, monitoring vendor intelligence feeds, and subscribing to security alerts and tips from US_CERT (United States Computer Emergency Readiness Team).

Security Tools

A wide range of tools are available to an organization to protect the organizational network and information. The 2015 HIMSS Cybersecurity Survey results indicate that an average of 11 different software tools were used by respondents to provide network security. These tools can be either a software solution, such as **antivirus software**, or a hardware tool, such as a proxy server. Such tools are effective only if they are used along with employee awareness training.

For example, e-mail scanning is a commonly used software tool. All incoming e-mail messages are scanned to ensure that they do not contain a virus or some other malicious code. This software can find only viruses that are currently known, so it is important that the virus software be set to search for and download updates automatically. Organizations can further protect themselves by training employees to never open an e-mail attachment unless they are expecting the attachment and know the sender. Even IT managers have fallen victim to e-mail viruses and sent infected e-mails to everyone in their address book. Employees should be taught to protect their organization from new viruses that may not yet be included in their scanning software by never opening an e-mail attachment unless the sender is known and the attachment is expected. E-mail scanning software and antivirus software should never be turned off, and updates should be installed at least weekly—or, ideally, daily. Software is also available to scan instant messages and to delete automatically any spam e-mail.

Many antivirus and adware software packages are available for fees ranging from free to more than $25 per month for personal use and several thousands of dollars per month to secure an organization's network. The main factors to consider when purchasing antivirus software are its effectiveness (i.e., the number of viruses it has missed), the ease of installation and use, the effectiveness of the updates, and the help and user support available. Numerous websites compare and contrast the most recent antivirus software packages. Be aware, however, that some of these sites also sell antivirus software, so they may present biased information.

Firewalls are another tool used by organizations to protect their corporate networks when they are attached to the Internet. A firewall can be either hardware or software or

---

BOX 9-1   SOURCES OF INFORMATION ON INTERNET SECURITY AND FIREWALLS

Check out YouTube for the following videos on the Internet and firewalls:

- "Warriors on the Net (Full Version)": http://www.youtube.com/watch?v=RhvKm0RdUY0
- "What Is a Firewall?": http://www.youtube.com/watch?v=0_EVfWpL6L4
- "Firewalls: An Introduction": http://www.youtube.com/watch?v=klAu7mvjBUU&feature=related

---

a combination of both that examines all incoming messages or traffic to the network. The firewall can be set up to allow only messages from known senders into the corporate network. It can also be set up to look at outgoing information from the corporate network. If the message contains some type of corporate secret, the firewall may prevent the message from leaving. In essence, firewalls serve as electronic security guards at the gate of the corporate network. **Box 9-1** contains links to short videos explaining Internet security and firewalls.

Proxy servers also protect the organizational network. Proxy servers prevent users from directly accessing the Internet. Instead, users must first request passage from the proxy server. The server looks at the request and makes sure the request is from a legitimate user and that the destination of the request is permissible. For example, organizations can block requests to view a website with the word "sex" in the title or the actual uniform resource locator of a known pornography site. The proxy server can also lend the requesting user a **mask** to use while he or she is surfing the Web. In this way, the corporation protects the identity of its employees. The proxy server keeps track of which employees are using which masks and directs the traffic appropriately.

With hacking becoming more common, health care organizations must have some type of protection to avoid this invasion. **Intrusion detection systems** (both hardware and software) allow an organization to monitor who is using the network and which files that user has accessed. Detection systems can be set up to monitor a single computer or an entire network. Corporations must diligently monitor for unauthorized access of their networks. Anytime someone uses a secured network, a digital footprint of all of the user's travels is left, and this path can be easily tracked by electronic auditing software.

Off-Site Use of Portable Devices

Off-site uses of portable devices, such as laptops, personal digital assistants (PDAs), home computing systems, smartphones, smart devices, and portable data storage devices, can help to streamline the delivery of health care. For example, physical or occupational therapists may need to access **electronic protected health information** (EPHI) via a wireless laptop connection during a home visit. These mobile devices are invaluable to health care efficiency and responsiveness to patient need in such cases. At the very least, however, agencies should require data encryption when EPHI is being transmitted over unsecured networks or transported on a mobile device as a way of protecting sensitive information. Hot spots provided by companies, such as local coffee shops and by airports, are not secured networks. Virtual private networks must be used to ensure that all data transmitted on unsecured networks are encrypted. The user must log into the virtual private network to reach the organization's network.

Only data essential for the job should be maintained on the mobile device; other nonclinical information, such as Social Security numbers, should never be carried outside the secure network. Some institutions make use of thin clients, which are basic interface portals that do not keep **secure information** stored on them. Essentially, users must log in to the network to get the data they need. Use of thin clients may be problematic in patient care situations where the user cannot access the network easily. For example, some rural areas of the United States do not have wireless coverage. In these instances, private health information may need to be stored in a clinician's laptop or PDA to facilitate a home visit. This is comparable to health care professionals carrying paper charts in their cars to make home visits, and it entails the same responsibilities accompanying such use of private information outside the institution's walls.

What happens if one of these devices is lost or stolen? The agency is ultimately responsible for the integrity of the data contained on these devices and is required by HIPAA regulations (U.S. Department of Health and Human Services, 2006) to have policies in place covering such items as appropriate remote use, removal of devices from their usual physical location, and protection of these devices from loss or theft. Simple rules, such as covering laptops left in a car and locking car doors during transport of mobile devices containing EPHI, can help to deter theft. If a device is lost or stolen, the agency must have clear procedures in place to help ensure that sensitive data are not released or used inappropriately. Software packages that provide for physical tracking of the static and mobile computer inventory including laptops and PDAs are being used more widely and can assist in the recovery of lost or stolen devices. In addition, some software that allows for remote data deletion in the event of theft or loss of a mobile device can be invaluable to the agency in preventing the release of EPHI.

If a member of an agency is caught accessing EPHI inappropriately or steals a mobile device, the sanctions should be swift and public. Sanctions may range from a warning or suspension with retraining to termination or prosecution, depending on the severity of the security breach. The sanctions must send a clear message to all that protecting EPHI is serious business.

The U.S. Department of Health and Human Services (2006) has identified potential risks and proposed risk management strategies for accessing, storing, and transmitting EPHI. Visit the following website for detailed tabular information (pp. 4–6) on potential risks and risk management strategies: http://its.syr.edu/infosec/docs/standards /remoteaccess-standard.pdf.

To protect our patients and their data, health care professionals must consider the impact of wireless mobile devices. Data can be stolen by an employee very easily through the use of e-mail or file transfers. **Malware** that infiltrates a network can collect easily accessible data. One of the evolving issues is lost or stolen devices that can provide a gateway into a health care organization's network and records. When the device is owned by the employee, other issues arise as to how the device is used and secured.

The increase in cloud computing has also challenged our personal and professional security and privacy. According to Jansen and Grance (2011), cloud computing "promises to have far reaching effects on the systems and networks of federal agencies and other organizations. Many of the features that make cloud computing attractive, however, can also be at odds with traditional security models and controls" (p. vi).

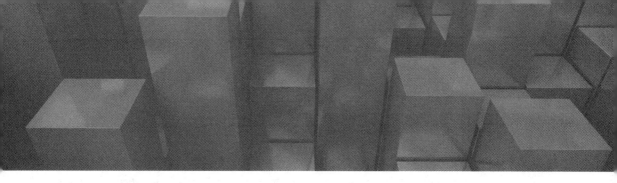

Summary

Technology changes so quickly that even the most diligent user will likely encounter a situation that could constitute a threat to his or her network. Organizations must provide their users with the proper training to help them avoid known threats and—more importantly—be able to discern a possible new threat. Consider that 10 years ago wireless networks were the exception to the rule, whereas today access to wireless networks is almost taken for granted. How will computer networks be accessed 10 years from now? The most important concept to remember from this chapter is that the only completely safe network is one that is turned off. **Network accessibility** and **network availability** are necessary evils that pose security risks. The information must be available to be accessed yet remain secured from hackers, unauthorized users, and any other potential security breaches. As the cloud expands, so do the concerns over security and privacy. In an ideal world, everyone would understand the potential threats to **network security** and would diligently monitor and implement tools to prevent unauthorized access of their networks, data, and information.

Thought-Provoking Questions

1. Sue is a respiratory therapist in the chronic obstructive pulmonary disorder clinic and enrolled in a master's education program. She is interested in writing a paper on the factors that are associated with poor compliance with medical regimens and associated repeat hospitalization of chronic obstructive pulmonary disorder patients. She downloads patient information from the clinic database to a thumb drive that she later accesses on her home computer. Sue understands rules about privacy of information and believes that because she is a licensed health care professional and needs this information for a graduate school assignment, she is entitled to the information. Is Sue correct in her thinking? Describe why she is or is not correct.

2. The employee education department of a large hospital system has been centralized; as a consequence, the educators are no longer assigned to one hospital but must now travel among all of the hospitals. They use their smartphones to interact and share data and information. What are the first steps you would take to secure these transactions? Describe why each step is necessary.

3. Research cloud computing in relation to health care. What are the major security and privacy challenges? Choose three and describe them in detail.

Apply Your Knowledge

Robert, a physical therapist, has decided to create a listserv from his own Internet service at home for his various patients' rehabilitation needs. He establishes one list for each of the following conditions: total knee replacements, total hip replacements, chronic back pain, and traumatic knee injuries. He automatically enrolls all of his patients that he has e-mail addresses for into their appropriate list with the intention that they can share information and support among themselves as well as making it easier for him to share general information and tips and pointers with his patients. Everything is going well for the first month of the listserv exchange. However, a virus is introduced to the lists, and everyone is contaminated. This virus has damaged the patients' hard drives on their home computers, and some patients' work computers have been harmed. The patients contact Robert's employer and demand to be reimbursed for all damages to their machines and are very upset that these lists were created in the first place. Robert's employer was unaware of the lists.

1. What is the difference between a virus and a worm?
2. How do viruses and worms damage computer systems?
3. What rules from Chapter 5 has Robert violated?
4. Develop a safe plan for using listservs to provide support and encouragement to patients that conforms to privacy and security rules.

Additional Resources

Syracuse University Information Technology Services
http://its.syr.edu/infosec/docs/standards/remoteaccess-standard.pdf

References

Degaspari, J. (2010). Staying ahead of the curve on data security. *Healthcare Informatics, 27*(10), 32–36. http://www.healthcare-informatics.com/ME2/dirmod.asp?sid=9B6FFC446FF748698 1EA3C0C3CCE4943&nm=Articles%2FNews&type=Publishing&mod=Publications%3A%3 AArticle&mid=8F3A7027421841978F18BE895F87F791&tier=4&id=35F1496AE0B144D3A 9716D5D9C2D03CF

Gross, G. (2003). Human error causes most security breaches. *InfoWorld.* http://www.infoworld .com/article/03/03/18/HNhumanerror_1.html

HIMSS. (2015). 2015 HIMSS Cybersecurity Survey. http://files.himss.org/FileDownloads/2015 -cybersecurity-executive-summary.pdf

Jansen, W., & Grance, T. (2011). National Institute of Standards and Technology (NIST): Guide- lines on security and privacy in public cloud computing. https://cloudsecurityalliance.org /wp-content/uploads/2011/07/NIST-Draft-SP-800-144_cloud-computing.pdf

Mowry, M., & Oakes, R. (n.d.). Not too tight, not too loose. *Healthcare Informatics, Healthcare IT Leadership, Vision & Strategy.* http://www.healthcare-informatics.com/ME2/dirmod.asp?nm =&type=Publishing&mod=Publications%3A%3AArticle&mid=8F3A7027421841978F18BE 895F87F791&tier=4&id=B7823E299AC64041AC3F253CE19DF298

Ponemon Institute. (2015, May). *Fifth Annual Benchmark Study on Privacy & Security of Health- care Data.* https://www2.idexpertscorp.com/fifth-annual-ponemon-study-on-privacy -security-incidents-of-healthcare-data (free download)

Sullivan, T. (2012). Government health IT: DHS lists top 5 mobile medical device security risks. http://www.govhealthit.com/news/dhs-lists-top-5-mobile-device-security-risks

U.S. Department of Health and Human Services. (2006). HIPAA security guidance. http://its.syr .edu/infosec/docs/standards/remoteaccess-standard.pdf

U.S. Department of Health and Human Services. (n.d.). HHS settles with health plan in pho- tocopier breach case. http://www.hhs.gov/ocr/privacy/hipaa/enforcement/examples/affinity -agreement.html

Work Flow and Meaningful Use

Denise Hammel-Jones, Dee McGonigle,
and Kathleen Mastrian

OBJECTIVES

1. Provide an overview of the purpose of conducting work flow analysis and design.
2. Deliver specific instructions on work flow analysis and redesign techniques.
3. Cite measures of efficiency and effectiveness that can be applied to redesign efforts.
4. Explore meaningful use from the health professional's perspective.

Key Terms
American Recovery and Reinvestment Act
Bar-code medication administration
Clinical transformation
Computerized provider order entry
Electronic health record
Events
Health information exchanges
Health information technology
Information systems
Interactions
Lean
Meaningful use
Medical home models
Metrics
Process analysis
Process owners
(continues)

Introduction

The health care environment has grown more complex and continues to evolve every day. Unfortunately, the complexities that help clinicians to deliver better care and improve patient outcomes also take a toll on the clinicians themselves. This toll is exemplified through hours spent learning new technology, loss in productivity as the user adjusts and adapts to new technology, and unintended work flow consequences from the use of technology.

Despite the perceived negative downstream effects to end users and patients as a result of technology, this very same technology can improve efficiency and yield a leaner health care environment. The intent of this chapter is to outline the driving forces that create the need to redesign work flow as well as to elucidate what the health care professional needs to know about how to conduct work flow redesign, measure the impact of work flow changes, and assess the impact of meaningful use.

Work Flow Analysis Purpose

According to the American Association for Justice (2013), "Preventable medical errors kill and seriously injure hundreds of thousands of Americans every year" (para. 1). Not only is there an impact on patients from these errors, but there is also a significant financial impact on health care organizations. Clearly, we must minimize these errors, and one of the most important tools for this purpose is the use of electronic records and **information systems** to provide point-of-care decision support and automation. The key point is that many of these errors are preventable and we must find ways to prevent them.

Technology can provide a mechanism to improve care delivery and create a safer patient environment, provided it is implemented appropriately and considers the surrounding work flow. In an important article by Campbell, Guappone, Sittig, Dykstra, and Ash (2009), the authors suggested that technology implemented without consideration of work flow can provide greater patient safety concerns than no technology at all. **Computerized provider order entry** (CPOE) causes us to focus more specifically on work flow considerations. These work flow implications are referred to as the unintended consequences of CPOE implementation; they are just some of the effects of poorly implemented technology. The Healthcare Information Management Systems Society (HIMSS, 2010) ME-PI Toolkit addresses work flow redesign and considers why it is so critical to successful technology implementations.

Technology is recognized to have a potentially positive effect on patient outcomes. Nevertheless, even with the promise of improving how care is delivered, adoption of technology has been slow. The cost of technology solutions such as CPOE, **bar-code medication administration** (BCMA), and **electronic health records** (EHR) remain staggeringly high. The cost of technology, coupled with the lengthy time lines required to develop and implement such technology, has put this endeavor out of reach for many health care organizations. In addition, upgrades or enhancements to the technology are often necessary either mid-implementation or shortly after a launch, leaving little time to focus efforts on the optimization of the technology within the current work flow. Furthermore, the existence of technology does not in itself guarantee that it will be used in a manner that promotes better outcomes for patients.

Given the sluggish adoption of technology, in 2009, the U.S. government took an unprecedented step when it formally recognized the importance of **health information technology** (HIT) for patient care outcomes. As a result of the provisions of **American Recovery and Reinvestment Act** (ARRA), health care organizations can qualify for financial incentives based on the level of meaningful use achieved. **Meaningful use** (MU) refers to the rules and regulations established by the ARRA. The three stages of meaningful use are part of an EHR incentive program. During stage 1, the focus is on data capturing and sharing (Centers for Medicare and Medicaid Services [CMS], 2013a, 2013b). Stage 2 focuses on advanced clinical processes, and stage 3 seeks improved outcomes (CMS, 2013b). Stage 1 was initiated during 2011–2012, stage 2 began in 2014, and stage 3 will be launched in 2016 (Sherman, 2013). Follow developments related to meaningful use at this site: http://www.cms.gov/Regulations-and-Guidance /Legislation/EHRIncentivePrograms/Meaningful_Use.html.

For an organization that seeks to use the 25 meaningful use measures to qualify for the incentives, the data to support these measures must be gathered and reported on electronically—necessitating the use of technology in all patient care areas. Additionally, a fundamental aspect of meaningful use is the assurance that a significant number of health care providers have adopted technology. Health care professionals who use EHRs in their practice setting, for example, will collect higher-quality data. Many of the **quality** reporting measures rely on health care professional's documentation. Those health care personnel who do not use EHRs should soon see their organizations moving in that direction. Meaningful use measures will push health care organizations to reexamine the use of clinical technologies within their organization and approach implementations in a new way.

Not only is there a potential for patient safety and quality issues to arise from technology implementations that do not address work flow, but a financial impact to the organization is possible as well. All organizations, regardless of their industry, must operate efficiently to maintain profits and continue to provide services to their customers. For hospitals, which normally have significantly smaller profit margins than other organizations, the need to maintain efficient and effective care is essential for survival. Given that hospital profit margins are diminishing, never has there been a more crucial time to examine the costs of errors and poorly designed work flows and the financial burden they present to an organization than now. Moreover, what are the costs to an organization that fails to address the integration of technology? This is an area where few supporting data exist to substantiate the claim that technology without work flow considerations can, in fact, impact the bottom line.

Today, many health care organizations are experiencing the effects of poorly implemented clinical technology solutions. These effects may be manifested in the form of redundant documentation, non–value-added steps, and additional time spent at the computer rather than in direct care delivery. Technology ought not to be implemented for the sake of automation unless it promises to deliver gains in patient outcomes and proper work flow. Examining the work flow surrounding the use of technology enables better use of the technology and more efficient work. It also promotes safer patient care delivery. The need to focus on work flow and technology is attracting increasing recognition, although there remains a dearth of literature that addresses the importance of this area. As more organizations work to achieve a level of technology adoption that will enable them to receive ARRA financial incentives, we will likely see more attention paid to the area of work flow design and, therefore, a greater body of research and evidence (Agency for Healthcare Research and Quality, n.d.; Qualis Health, 2011; Yuan, Finley, Long, Mills, & Johnson, 2013).

Work Flow and Technology

Work flow is a term used to describe the action or execution of a series of tasks in a prescribed sequence. Another definition of work flow is a progression of steps (**tasks**, **events**, and **interactions**) that constitute a **work process**, involve two or more persons, and create or add value to the organization's activities. In a sequential work flow, each step depends on the occurrence of the previous step; in a parallel work flow, two or more steps can occur concurrently. The term *work flow* is sometimes used interchangeably with *process* or *process flows*, particularly in the context of implementations. Observation and documentation of work flow to better understand what is happening in the current environment and how it can be altered is referred to as process or **work flow analysis**. A typical output of work flow analysis is a visual depiction of the process, called a process map. The process map ranges from simplistic to fairly complex and provides an excellent tool to identify specific steps. It also can provide a vehicle for communication and a tool on which to build educational materials as well as policies and procedures.

One school of thought suggests that technology should be designed to meet the needs of clinical work flow (Yuan et al., 2013). This model implies that system analysts have a high degree of control over screen layout and data capture. It also implies that technology is malleable enough to allow for the flexibility to adapt to a variety of work flow scenarios. Lessons learned from more than three decades of clinical technology implementations suggest that clinical technologies still have a long way to go on the road to maturity to allow this to be possible. The second and probably most prevalent thought process is that work flow should be adapted to the use of technology. Today, this is by far the most commonly used model given the progress of clinical technology.

A concept that has gained popularity in recent years relative to work flow redesign is clinical transformation. **Clinical transformation** is the complete alteration of the clinical environment, and, therefore, this term should be used cautiously to describe redesign efforts. Earl, Sampler, and Sghort (1995) define transformation as "a radical change approach that produces a more responsive organization that is more capable of performing in unstable and changing environments that organizations continue to be faced with" (p. 31). Many work flow redesign efforts are focused on relatively small changes and not the widespread change that accompanies transformational activities. Moreover, clinical transformation would imply that the manner in which work is carried out and the outcomes achieved are completely different from the prior state—which is not always true when the change simply involves implementing technology. Technology can be used to launch or in conjunction with a clinical transformation initiative, although the implementation of technology alone is not perceived as transformational.

Before undertaking transformative initiatives, the following guidelines should be understood:

- Leadership must take the lead and create a case for transformation.
- Establish a vision for the end point.
- Allow those persons with specific expertise to provide the details.
- Think about the most optimal experience for both the patient and the clinician.
- Do not replicate the current state.
- Focus on those initiatives that offer the greatest value to the organization.
- Recognize that small gains have no real impact on transformation.

Optimization

Most of what has been and will be discussed in this chapter is related to work flow analysis in conjunction with technology implementations. Nevertheless, not all work flow analysis and redesign occurs prior to the implementation of technology. Some analysis and redesign efforts may occur weeks, months, or even years following the implementation. When work flow analysis occurs post-implementation, it is often referred to as optimization. Optimization is the process of moving conditions past their current state and into more efficient and effective method of performing tasks. The *Merriam-Webster Online Dictionary* (2010) considers optimization to be the act, process, or methodology of making something (as a design, system, or decision) as fully perfect, functional, or effective as possible. Some organizations will routinely engage in optimization efforts following an implementation, whereas other organizations may undertake this activity in response to clinician concerns or marked change in operational performance.

Furthermore, work flow analysis can be conducted either as a stand-alone effort or as part of an operational improvement event. When the process is addressed alone, the effort is termed process improvement. Health informatics professionals should always be included in these activities to represent the needs of clinicians and to serve as a liaison for technological solutions to process problems. The National Consortium for Health Science Education's (2012) health informatics pathway was last updated in 2012; in Standard 6, Operations, health informaticists "demonstrate the use of systems used to capture, retrieve and maintain confidential health information from internal and external sources (para. 15). Additionally, informaticists will likely become increasingly operationally focused and will need to transform their role accordingly to address work flow in an overall capacity as well as respective to technology. As mentioned earlier, hospitals and practices tend to operate with smaller profit margins than other industries, and these profits will likely continue to diminish, forcing organizations to work smarter, not harder—and to use technology to accomplish this goal.

If optimization efforts are undertaken, the need to revisit work flow design should not be considered a flaw in the implementation approach. Even a well-designed future-state work flow during a technology implementation must be reexamined post-implementation to ensure that what was projected about the future state remains valid and to incorporate any additional work flow elements into the process redesign.

Exploring the topic of work flow analysis with regard to clinical technology implementation will yield considerably fewer literature results than searching for other topical areas of implementation. More research is needed in the area of the financial implications of work flow inefficiencies and their impact on patient care. Time studies require an investment of resources and may be subject to patient privacy issues as well as the challenges of capturing time measurements on processes that are not exactly replicable. Another confounding factor affecting the quality and quantity of work flow research is the lack of standardized terminology for this area. What all organizations ultimately strive for is efficient and effective delivery of patient care. The terms *efficient* and *effective* are widely known in quality areas or **Six Sigma** and **Lean** departments but are not necessarily known or used in informatics. Effective delivery of care or work flow suggests that the process or end product is in the most desirable state. An efficient delivery of care or work flow would mean that little waste—that is, unnecessary motion, transportation, overprocessing, or defects—was incurred. Health systems such as Virginia Mason University Medical Center, among others, have experienced significant quality and cost gains from the widespread implementation of Lean development throughout their organization.

Work Flow Analysis and Informatics Practice

The functional area of analysis identifies the specific functional qualities related to work flow analysis. Particularly, health informatics should develop techniques necessary to assess and improve human–computer interaction. Work flow analysis, however, is not relevant solely to analysis but rather is part of every functional area that the informatics support personnel engage in. Support personnel need to understand work flow and appreciate how lack of efficient work flow for health care professionals affects patient care.

A critical aspect of the informatics support role is work flow design. Health informatics is uniquely positioned to engage in the analysis and redesign of processes and tasks surrounding the use of technology. Work flow redesign is one of the fundamental skills sets that make up the discipline of this specialty. Moreover, work flow analysis should be part of every technology implementation, and the role of the informaticist within this team is to direct others in the execution of this task or to perform the task directly.

Unfortunately, many health care professionals find themselves in an informatics support capacity without sufficient preparation for a **process analysis** role. One area of practice that is particularly susceptible to inadequate preparation is the ability to facilitate process analysis. Work flow analysis requires careful attention to detail and the ability to moderate group discussions, organize concepts, and generate solutions. These skills can be acquired through a formal academic informatics program or through courses that teach the discipline of Six Sigma or Lean, by example. Regardless of where these skills are acquired, it is important to understand that they are now and will continue to remain a vital aspect of the informatics role.

CASE STUDY

In my experience consulting, I have seen several examples of organizations that engage in the printing of paper reports that replicate information that has been entered and is available with the electronic health record. These reports are often reviewed, signed, and acted on instead of using the electronic information. Despite the knowledge that the information contained in these reports was outdated the moment the report was printed and that the very nature of using the report for work flow is an inefficient practice, this method of clinical work flow remains prevalent in many hospitals across the United States.

There is an underlying fear that drives the decisions to mold a paper-based work flow around clinical technology. There is also a lack of the appropriate amount of integration that would otherwise allow this information to be available in an electronic form.

Denise Hammel-Jones

Some organizations have felt strongly enough about the need for work flow analysis that departments have been created to address this very need. Whether the department carries the name of clinical excellence, organizational effectiveness, or Six Sigma/Lean, it is critical to recognize the value this group can offer technology implementations and clinicians.

As we examine how work flow analysis is conducted, note that while the health informaticist is an essential member of the team to participate in or enable work flow analysis, a team dedicated to this effort is necessary for its success.

Building the Design Team

The work flow redesign team is an interdisciplinary team consisting of "process owners." **Process owners** are those persons who directly engage in the work flow to be analyzed and redesigned. These individuals can speak about the intricacy of process, including process variations from the norm. When constructing the team, it is important to include individuals who are able to contribute information about the exact current-state work flow and offer suggestions for future-state improvement. Members of the work flow redesign team should also have the authority to make decisions about how the process should be redesigned. This authority is sometimes issued by managers, or it could come from participation of the managers directly. Such a careful blend of decision makers and "process owners" can be difficult to assemble but is critical for forming the team and enabling them for success. Often, individuals at the manager level will want to participate exclusively in the redesign process. While having management participate provides the advantage of having decision makers and management-level buy-in, these individuals may also make erroneous assumptions about how the process should be versus how the process is truly occurring. Conversely, including only process owners who do not possess the authority to make decisions can slow down the work of the team while decisions are made outside the group sessions.

Team focus needs to be addressed at the outset of the team's assembly. Early on, the team should decide which work flow will be examined to avoid confusion or spending time unnecessarily on work flow that does not ultimately matter to the outcome. In the early stages of work flow redesign, the team should define the beginning and end of a process and a few high-level steps of the process. Avoid focusing on process steps in great detail in the beginning, as the conversation can get sidetracked or team members may get bogged down by focusing on details and not move along at a good pace. Six Sigma expert George Eckes uses the phrase "Stay as high as you can as long as you can"—a good catchphrase to remember to keep the team focused and at a high level. The pace at which any implementation team progresses ultimately affects the overall time line of a project; therefore, focus and speed are skills that the informatics expert should develop and use throughout every initiative, but particularly when addressing work flow redesign.

The work flow redesign team will develop a detailed process map after agreement is reached on the current-state process's beginning and end points and a high-level map depicting the major process steps is finalized. Because work flow crosses many different care providers, it may be useful to construct the process map using a swim-lane technique (**Figure 10-1**). A swim-lane technique uses categories such as functional work groups and roles to visually depict groups of work and to indicate who performs the work. The resulting map shows how work flow and data transition to clinicians and can demonstrate areas of potential process and information breakdowns.

It may take several sessions of analysis to complete a process map as details are uncovered and work-arounds discussed. There is a tendency for individuals who participate in process redesign sessions to describe work flow as they believe it to be occurring rather than not how it really is. The informatics expert and/or the process team facilitator should determine what is really happening, however, and capture that information accurately. Regardless of whether a swim-lane or simplistic process map design is used, the goal is to capture enough details to accurately portray the process as it is happening today.

Other techniques (aside from process mapping) may be used to help the team understand the work flow as it exists in the current state. The future-state work flow planning will be only as good as the reliability of the current state; thus, it is crucial to undertake whatever other actions are needed to better understand what is happening in the current state. Observation, interviews, and process or waste walks are also helpful in understanding the current state.

Value Added Versus Non–Value Added

Beyond analysis of tasks, current-state mapping provides the opportunity for the process redesign team to distinguish between value-added and non–value-added activities. A value-added activity or step is one that ultimately brings the process closer to completion or changes the product or service for the better. An example of a value-added step would be placing a name tag on a specimen sample. The name tag is necessary for the laboratory personnel to identify the specimen, and, therefore, its placement is an essential or value-added step in the process. Some steps in a process do not necessarily add value but are necessary for regulatory or compliance reasons. These steps are still considered necessary and need to be included in the future process. A non–value-added step, in contrast, does not alter the outcome of a process or product. Activities such as handling, moving, and holding are not considered value-added steps and should be evaluated during work flow analysis. Manipulating papers, moving through computer screens, and walking or transporting items are all considered non–value-added activities.

The five whys represent one technique to drive the team toward identifying value-added versus non–value-added steps. The process redesign facilitator will query the group about why a specific task is done or done in a particular way through a series of questions asking "why?" The goal is to uncover tasks that came about due to work-arounds or for other unsubstantiated reasons. Tasks that are considered non–value added and are not necessary for the purpose of compliance or regulatory reasons should be eliminated from the future-state process. The team's purpose in redesigning work flow is to eliminate steps in a process that do not add value to the end state or that create waste by their very nature.

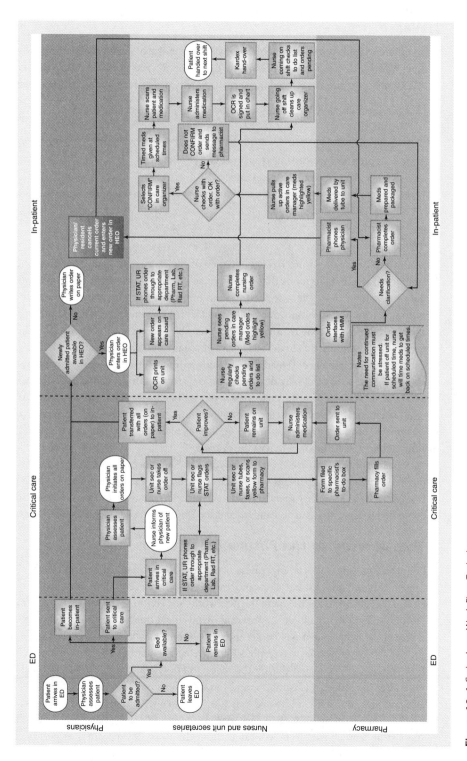

Figure 10–1 Swim Lane Work Flow Technique

Source: Greencastle Associates Consulting and Atlantic Health. Reprinted by permission.

Waste

A key underpinning of the Lean philosophy is the removal of waste activities from work flow. Waste is classified as unnecessary activities or an excess of products to perform tasks. The seven categories listed here are the mostly widely recognized forms of waste:

- Overproduction: pace is faster than necessary to support the process
- Waiting
- Transport
- Inappropriate processing: overprocessing
- Unnecessary inventory: excess stock
- Unnecessary motion: bending, lifting, moving, and so on
- Defects: reproduction

Variation

Health professionals do not have the luxury of single-focused care. There are often interruptions and disruptions that pull them away and distract them from their work flow and patient care. The more you have to multitask, the more chance you have of making errors. Variation in work flow is considered the enemy of all good processes and, therefore, should be eliminated when possible. Variation occurs when workers perform the same function in different ways. It usually arises because of flaws in the way a process was originally designed, lack of knowledge about the process, or inability to execute a process as originally designed due to disruption or disturbances in the work flow. Examining the process as it exists today will help with identifying variation. A brief statement about variation that cannot be eliminated: Processes that involve highly customized products or services are generally not conducive to standardization and the elimination of variation inherent to the process.

Some argue that delivery of care is subject to variation because of its very nature and the individual needs of patients. There is little doubt that each patient's care should be tailored to meet his or her specific needs. Nevertheless, delivery of care involves some common processes that can be standardized and improved on without jeopardizing care.

Transitioning to the Future State

Following redesign efforts, regardless of whether they occurred during or after an implementation or as a stand-alone process improvement event, steps must be taken to ensure that change takes hold and the new work flow continues after the support team has disbanded. Management support and involvement during the transition phase is essential, as management will be necessary to enforce new work flow procedures and further define/refine roles and responsibilities. Documentation of the future-state work flow should have occurred during the redesign effort but is not completely finished until after the redesign is complete and the work flow has become operational. Policies and procedures are addressed and rewritten to encompass the changes to work flows and role assignments. Help desk, system analyst, education personnel, and other support personnel need to be educated about the work flow specifics as part of the post-improvement effort. It is considered good practice to involve the operational staff in the future process discussions and planning so as to incorporate specifics of these areas and ensure the buy-in of the staff.

When work flow changes begin to fail and work-arounds develop, they signal that something is flawed about the way in which the new process was constructed and needs to be evaluated further. The work flow redesign team is then brought together to review and, if necessary, redesign the process.

The future state is constructed with the best possible knowledge of how the process will ideally work. To move from the current state to the future state, gap analysis is necessary. Gap analysis zeros in on the major areas most affected by the change—namely, technology. What often happens in redesign efforts is an exact or near-exact replication of the current state using automation. The gap analysis discussion should generate ideas from the group about how best to utilize the technology to transform practice. A prudent step is to consider having legal and risk representatives at the table when initiating future-state discussions to identify the parameters within which the group should work; nevertheless, the group should not assume the existing parameters are its only boundaries.

Future-state process maps become the basis of educational materials for end users, communication tools for the project team, and the foundation of new policies and procedures. Simplified process maps provide an excellent schematic for communicating change to others.

Informatics as a Change Agent

Technology implementations represent a significant change for clinicians, as does the work flow redesign that accompanies adoption of technology. Often, the degree of change and its impact are underappreciated and unaccounted for by leadership and staff alike. A typical response to change is anger, frustration, and a refusal to accept the proposed change. All of these responses should be expected and need to be accounted for; thus, a plan to address the emotional side of change is developed early on. Every work flow redesign effort should begin with a change management plan. Engagement of the end user is a critical aspect of change management and, therefore, technology adoption. Without end-user involvement, change is resisted and efforts are subject to failure. Users may be engaged and brought into the prospective change through question-and-answer forums, technology demonstrations, and frequent communications regarding change and as department-specific representatives in working meetings.

Many change theories have been developed. No matter which change theory is adopted by the informatics specialist, however, communication, planning, and support are key factors in any change management strategy. Informaticists should become knowledgeable about at least one change theory and use this knowledge as the basis for change management planning as part of every effort. John Kotter (1996), one of the most widely recognized change theorists, suggested that the following conditions must be addressed to deal with change in an organization:

- Education and communication
- Participation and involvement

- Facilitation and support
- Negotiation and agreement
- Manipulation and co-optation
- Explicit and implicit coercion

Health informaticists make up the most significant resource in a project team that influences adoption and change management. Health informaticists interact with various clinicians, gather data about their practice area and patient care, and help them appreciate the impact work flow changes that improve patient care. Nevertheless, no matter which change management techniques are employed by the informatics specialist and the project team, adoption of technology and work flow may be slow to evolve. Change is often a slow process that requires continual positive reinforcement and involvement of supporting resources. Failure to achieve strong adoption results early on is not necessarily a failure of the methods utilized but rather may be due to other factors not entirely within the control of the informaticist.

Perhaps a complete alteration in behavior is not possible, but modifications to behaviors needed to support a desired outcome can be realized. This situation is analogous to the individual who stops smoking; the desire for the cigarette remains, but the behavior has been modified to no longer sustain smoking. To manage change in an organization, health care professionals must modify behavior to produce the intended outcome.

Change takes hold when strong leadership support exists. This support manifests itself as a visible presence to staff, clear and concise communications, an unwavering position, and an open-door policy to field concerns about change. Too often, leadership gives verbal endorsement of change and then fails to follow through with these actions or withdraws support when the going gets tough. Inevitably, if leadership wavers, so too will staff. Refer to **Box 10-1**.

Measuring the Results

Metrics provide understanding about the performance of a process or function. Typically within clinical technology projects, we identify and collect specific metrics about the performance of the technology or metrics that capture the level of participation or adoption. Equally important is the need for process performance metrics. Process metrics are collected at the initial stage of project or problem identification. Current-state metrics are then benchmarked against internal indicators. When there are no internal indicators to benchmark against, a suitable course of action is to benchmark against an external source, such as a similar business practice within a different industry. Consider examining the hotel room changeover strategy or the customer service approach of Walt Disney Company or Ritz Carlton hotels, for example, to determine suitable metrics for a particular project or focus area.

The right work flow complement will provide the organization with the data it needs to understand operational and clinical performance. This area is highlighted through the need for health care organizations to capture meaningful use measures. Good

BOX 10-1 HEALTH CARE PROFESSIONS AND MEANINGFUL USE

NueMD (2015) reminds us that

incentive payments for eligible professionals are based on individual practitioners and not the practice as a whole. Each eligible professional in a practice must demonstrate meaningful use of certified EHR technology to qualify for an incentive payment. The number of individual incentive payments will not exceed one per year, regardless of how many practices or locations at which the individual provides service. (para. 12)

Miliard (2015) stated, "The clock is ticking on clinical quality improvement. If hospitals and practices want to be paid in the years to come, it's incumbent on them to show they're delivering better care" (para. 6).

The Academy of Nutrition and Dietetics and HIMSS (2013) called for "a multidisciplinary framework focused on thought leadership that is supported by membership programs for nutritionists, physicians, pharmacists, dietitians, clinical engineers and nurses" (slide 4).

According to Lung (2014),

By 2015, facilities are expected to enter at least 30 percent of radiology orders into their EHRs. Facilities that do not meet this expectation will face a 1 percent reduction in Medicare reimbursement rates per year, up to a maximum of 5 percent. The incentive program stipulates that only "licensed health care professionals and credentialed medical assistants" should enter electronic orders for radiology services. Determination of who is "licensed" is up to the Medicare administrative contractor who pays the reimbursement claim for the service. Facilities in states that have statutory or regulatory provisions to issue radiologic technologists a license shouldn't experience any problems complying with the requirement. (p. 56)

Bohnett (2015) reflected,

Well, 2015 hit. The deadline—at least for Stage 1—came and went. So, what happened? How did all those eligible professionals do with their mission? Before we examine the HITECH Act AD (after deadline), let me first calm all you PTs, OTs and SLPs who are reading this: You did not miss any deadlines; you never needed to demonstrate meaningful use. Physical therapists, occupational therapists, and speech-language pathologists are not considered "eligible professionals" per the ARRA (para. 2). . . . That's not to say, however, that PTs, OTs and SLPs won't ever be considered eligible professionals or that the federal government won't enact new legislation with more inclusive or intense mandates. That's why it's important that all medical professionals, regardless of eligibility, keep the HITECH Act on their radar. (para. 3)

Buckley (2015) asked,

How about smoking cessation? RTs have long been involved in the delivery of smoking cessation services to their patients and communities. Besides their understanding of the pulmonary impact of tobacco products, RTs are also experts in patient education and assessment, as well as proper medication use. Talk about adding value! Our system uses smoking cessation provided by RTs as support for the Medicare Meaningful Use program. Our patient education efforts and documentation alone have earned our health system a payment of $2 million for meeting the program targets. (para. 16)

(continues)

metrics should tell the story of accomplishment. The presence of technology alone does not guarantee an organization's ability to capture and report on these measures without also addressing the surrounding work flow. Metrics should focus on the variables of time, quality, and costs. **Table 10-1** provides examples of relevant metrics.

The ARRA highlights the need for health care organizations to collect information that represents the impact of technology on patient outcomes. Furthermore, data are necessary to demonstrate how a process is performing in its current state. In spite of the ARRA mandates, the need to collect data to demonstrate improvement in work flow— though it remains strong—is all too often absent in implementation or redesign efforts. A team cannot demonstrate improvements to an existing process without collecting information about how the process is performing today. Current-state measures also help the process team validate that the correct area for improvement was identified. Once a process improvement effort is over and the new solution has been implemented, post-improvement measures should be gathered to demonstrate progress.

In some organizations, the informatics professional reports to the director of operations, the chief information officer, or the chief operations officer. In this relationship, the need to demonstrate operational measures is even stronger. Operational measures, such as turnaround times, throughput, and equipment or technology availability, are some of the measures captured.

Future Directions

Work flow analysis is not an optional part of clinical implementations but rather a necessity for safe patient care supported by technology. The ultimate goal of work flow analysis is not to "pave the cow path" but rather to create a future-state solution that maximizes

TABLE 10-1 EXAMPLES OF METRICS		
Turnaround times	Cycle times	Throughput
Change-over time	Set-up time	System availability
Patient satisfaction	Employee satisfaction	

the use of technology and eliminates non–value-added activities. Although many tools to accomplish work flow redesign are available, the best method is the one that complements the organization and supports the work of clinicians. Redesigning how people do work will evidentially create change; thus, the health informaticist will need to apply change management principles for the new way of doing things to take hold.

Work flow analysis has been described in this chapter within the context of the most widely accepted tools that are fundamentally linked to the concepts of Six Sigma/Lean. Other methods of work flow analysis exist and may become commonly used to assess clinical work flow. An example of an alternative work flow analysis tool is the use of radio frequency badges to detect movement within a defined clinical area. Clinician and patient movements may be tracked using these devices, and corresponding actions may be documented, painting a picture of the work flow for a specific area (Vankipuram, 2010).

Another example of a work flow analysis tool involves the use of modeling software. An application such as ProModel provides images of the clinical work area where clinician work flows can be plotted out and reconfigured to best suit the needs of a specific area. Simulation applications enable decision makers to visualize realistic scenarios and draw conclusions about how to leverage resources, implement technology, and improve performance. Other vendors that offer simulation applications include Maya and Autodesk.

Health care organizations need to consider how other industries have analyzed and addressed work flow to their streamlined business practices and improved quality outputs to glean best practices that might be incorporated into the health care industry's own clinical and business approaches. First, however, each health care organization must step outside itself and recognize that not all aspects of patient care are unique; consequently, many aspects of care can be subjected to standardization. Many models of work flow redesign from manufacturing and the service sector can be extrapolated to health care. The health care industry is facing difficult economic times and can benefit from performance improvement strategies used in other industries.

Although work flow analysis principles have been described within the context of acute and ambulatory care in this chapter, the need to perform process analysis on a macro level will expand as more organizations move forward with **health information exchanges** (HIE) and **medical home models**. Health information exchanges require the health informaticist to visualize how patients move through the entire continuum of care and not just a specific patient care area.

Technology initiatives will become increasingly complex in the future. In turn, health informaticists will need greater preparation in the area of process analysis and improvement techniques to meet the growing challenges that technology brings and the operational performance demands of fiscally impaired health care organizations.

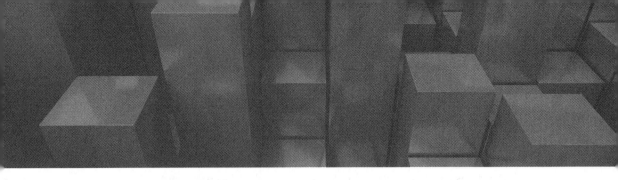

Summary

Meaningful use reflects the rules and regulations arising from ARRA. Health care professionals must lead the charge in this area because they play an important part in organizations' ability to meet the meaningful use criteria based on their documentation. EHR adoptions "represent a small step rather than a giant leap forward" (Murphy, 2013, para. 1). Work flows integrating technology provide the health care professional with the data necessary to make informed decisions. This quality data must be collected and captured to meet meaningful use criteria. Health care professionals must be involved in meaningful data collection and reporting. Insightful documentation by health care professionals can describe the patient's situational context and help the patient relate his or her story to other health care team members. In the health informatics pathway, Standard 5 deals with documentation: "Health informatics professionals will understand the content and diverse uses of health information. They will accurately document and communicate appropriate information using legal and regulatory processes" (National Consortium for Health Science Education, 2012, para. 11).

Work flow redesign is a critical aspect of technology implementation. When done well, it yields technology that is more likely to achieve the intended patient outcomes and safety benefits. Health informatics professionals are taking on a greater role with respect to work flow design, and this aspect of practice will grow in light of meaningful use–driven objectives. Other initiatives that impact hospital performance will also drive informatics professionals to influence how technology is used in the context of work flow to improve the bottom line for their organizations. In an ideal world, health informaticists who are experts at work flow analysis will be core members of every technology implementation team.

Thought-Provoking Questions

1. What do you perceive as the current obstacles to redesigning work flow within your clinical settings?
2. Thinking about your last implementation, were you able to challenge the policies and practices that constitute today's work flow, or were you able to create a work flow solution that eliminated non–value-added steps?
3. Is the work flow surrounding technology usage providing the health care organization with the data it needs to make decisions and eventually meet meaningful use criteria?
4. How does the current educational preparation need to change to address the skills necessary to perform work flow analysis and redesign clinical processes?

Apply Your Knowledge

Work flow analysis is not an optional part of clinical implementations but rather a necessity for safe patient care supported by technology. The ultimate goal of work flow analysis is not to "pave the cow path" but rather to create a future-state solution that maximizes the use of technology and eliminates non–value-added activities. Apply concepts learned in this chapter to create a work flow analysis of a procedure common to your practice.

1. Diagram the work flow for the procedure you chose.
2. Have you included all of the steps?
3. Assess each of the steps in the diagram and determine if they are value-added steps or non–value-added steps. Are the non–value-added steps necessary (i.e., required by accreditors or by law)?

Are there any aspects of the work flow that could be redesigned to achieve the same quality results?

Additional Resources

Centers for Medicare and Medicaid Services
http://www.cms.gov/Regulations-and-Guidance/Legislation/EHRIncentivePrograms/Meaningful _Use.html

References

Academy of Nutrition and Dietetics & HIMSS. (2013). Meaningful use in action—Exploring the possibility of nutrition informatics. Presented for the Nutrition Informatics Community. http://files.himss.org/FileDownloads/Nutrition_Informatics_MeaningfulUseNutritionEHRs Webinar.pdf

Agency for Healthcare Research and Quality. (n.d.). Workflow assessment for health IT toolkit. http://healthit.ahrq.gov/health-it-tools-and-resources/workflowassessment-health-it-toolkit

American Association for Justice. (2013). Preventable medical errors: The sixth biggest killer in America. http://www.justice.org/cps/rde/justice/hs.xsl/8677.htm

Bohnett, C. (2015). WebPT: 3 newsworthy notes about the HITECH ACT in 2015. https://www .webpt.com/blog/post/3-newsworthy-notes-about-the-hitech-act-in-2015

Buckley, T. (2015). Shift from measuring volume to measuring value. Winter 2015 Respiratory Care Management Bulletin. https://www.aarc.org/aarc-membership/community/specialty -sections/management/management-section-bulletins/winter-2015-management-bulletin

Campbell, E., Guappone, K., Sittig, D., Dykstra, R., & Ash, J. (2009). Computerized provider order entry adoption: Implications for clinical workflow. *Journal of General Internal Medicine, 24*(1), 21–26.

Centers for Medicare & Medicaid Services. (2013a). CMS.gov: Meaningful use. http://www.cms .gov/Regulations-and-Guidance/Legislation/EHRIncentivePrograms/Meaningful_Use.html

Centers for Medicare & Medicaid Services. (2013b). What is meaningful use? http://www.cms .gov/eHealth/downloads/Webinar_eHealth_July2_IntroEHRProgram.pdf

Earl, M., Sampler, J., & Sghort, J. (1995). Strategies for business process reengineering: Evidence from field studies. *Journal of Management Information Systems, 12*(1), 31–56.

Federal Register. (2015). Medicare and Medicaid programs: Electronic health record incentive program—Stage 3. Action: Proposed rule. *Federal Register, 80*(60), 16732–16804.

Healthcare Information Management Systems Society. (2010). ME-PI toolkit: Process management, workflow & mapping: Tools, tips and case studies to support the understanding, optimizing and monitoring of processes. Retrieved November 2010 from http://www.himss.org/ASP/topics_FocusDynamic.asp?faid=322

Kotter, J. P. (1996). *Leading change.* Cambridge, MA: Harvard Business Press.

Lung, C. (2014, June/July). A sticky "meaningful use" requirement. *ASRT Scanner,* 56.

Merriam-Webster Online Dictionary. (2010). Optimization. http://www.merriam-webster.com/dictionary/optimization

Miliard, M. (2015). Clinical decision support: No longer just nice to have. http://www.healthcareitnews.com/news/clinical-decision-support-no-longer-just-nice-have

Murphy, K. (2013). Nursing approach to meaningful use, EHR adoption: CIO series. http://ehrintelligence.com/2013/02/21/nursing-approach-to-meaningful-use-ehr-adoption-cioseries

National Consortium for Health Science Education. (2012). National Health Science Career Cluster Model. Health informatics pathway. Standards & accountability criteria. http://www.healthscienceconsortium.org/docs/health_info_pathway.pdf

NueMD. (2015). Meaningful use: Qualifying for EHR incentive programs. http://www.nuemd.com/white-papers/qualify-ehr-incentive-programsQualis Health. (2011). Workflow analysis. http://www.qualishealthmedicare.org/healthcare-providers/improvement-fundamentals/workflow-analysis

Sherman, R. (2013). What nurse leaders need to know about meaningful use. http://www.emergingrnleader.com/nurseleaderdevelopment-2

Vankipuram, K. (2010). Toward automated workflow analysis and visualization in clinical environment. *Journal of Biomedical Informatics.* doi: 10.1016/jbi.2010.05.015

Yuan, M., Finley, G., Long, J., Mills, C., & Johnson, R. (2013). Evaluation of user interface and workflow design of a bedside nursing clinical decision support system. http://www.ncbi.nlm.nih.gov/pmc/articles/PMC3628119

Section III

Informatics Applications for Care Delivery

Health care information systems must support professionals as they fulfill their roles in delivering quality patient care. Such systems must be responsive to health care professionals' needs, allowing them to manage their data and information as needed and providing access to necessary references, literature sources, and other networked departments. Health care professionals have always practiced in fields where they have needed to use their ingenuity, resourcefulness, creativity, initiative, and skills. To improve patient care and advance the disciplinary science, professionals, as knowledge workers, must apply these same abilities and skills to become astute users of available information systems.

In this section, the reader learns about clinical practice tools, electronic health records, and clinical information systems; informatics tools to enhance patient safety, engage and connect patients, provide consumer information, and meet education needs; and population and community health tools. Information systems, electronic documentation, and electronic health records are changing the way health care professionals practice. Health informatics systems are also changing how patients enter and receive data and information. Some institutions, for example, are permitting patients to access their own records electronically via the Internet or a dedicated patient portal. Confidentiality and privacy issues loom with these new electronic systems. Regulations of the Health Insurance Portability and Accountability Act and professional ethics principles (covered in the *Building Blocks of Health Informatics* section) must remain at the forefront when clinicians interact electronically with private patient data and information.

The material within this book is placed within the context of the Foundation of Knowledge model (**Figure III-1**) to meet the needs of health care delivery systems, organizations, patients, and professionals. Readers should continue to assess where they are in this model. The Foundation of Knowledge model reflects the fact that knowledge is powerful; for that reason, professionals must focus on information as a key resource. This section addresses the information systems with which clinicians interact in their health care environments as affected by legislation, professional codes of ethics, consumerism, and reconceptualization of practice paradigms, such as in telehealth.

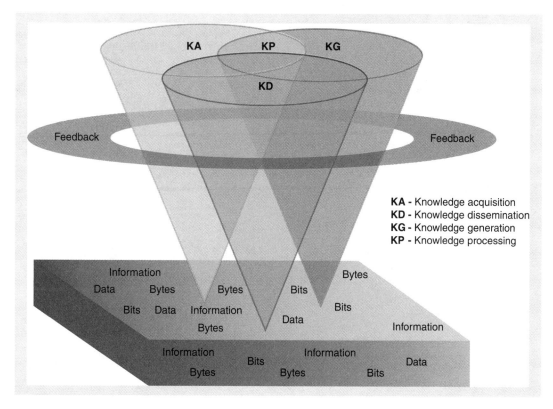

Figure III–1 Foundation of Knowledge Model
Source: Designed by Alicia Mastrian.

The Electronic Health Record and Clinical Informatics

Emily B. Barey, Kathleen Mastrian, and Dee McGonigle

OBJECTIVES

1. Describe the common components of an electronic health record.
2. Assess the benefits of implementing an electronic health record.
3. Explore the ownership of an electronic health record.
4. Evaluate the flexibility of the electronic health record in meeting the needs of clinicians and patients.

Introduction

The significance of **electronic health records** (EHRs) to health care cannot be underestimated. Although EHRs on the surface suggest a simple automation of clinical documentation, in fact their implications are broad, ranging from the ways in which care is delivered, to the types of interactions providers have with patients in conjunction with the use of technology, to the research surrounding EHRs that will inform disciplinary practice for tomorrow. A basic knowledge of EHRs and health informatics is now considered by many to be an entry-level health care professional competency.

This drive to adopt EHRs was underscored with the passage of the **Health Information Technology for Economic and Clinical Health Act of 2009** (HITECH). It is essential that EHR competency be developed if health care professionals are to participate fully in the changing world of health care information technology.

Key Terms
Administrative processes
American Recovery and Reinvestment Act of 2009
Connectivity
Decision support
Electronic communication
Electronic health record
Health information
Health Information Technology for Economic and Clinical Health Act of 2009
Interoperability
Meaningful use
Order entry management
Patient support
Population health management
Reporting
Results management

This chapter has four goals. First, it describes the common components of an EHR. Second, it reviews the benefits of implementing an EHR. Third, it provides an overview of successful ownership of an EHR, including the provider's role in promoting the safe adoption of EHRs in day-to-day practice. Fourth, it discusses the flexibility of an EHR in meeting the needs of both professionals and patients, including an introduction to interoperability.

Setting the Stage

The U.S. health care system faces the enormous challenge of improving the quality of care while simultaneously controlling costs. EHRs were proposed as one solution to achieve this goal (Institute of Medicine [IOM], 2001). In January 2004, President George W. Bush raised the profile of EHRs in his State of the Union address by outlining a plan to ensure that most Americans have an EHR by 2014. He stated that "by computerizing health records we can avoid dangerous medical mistakes, reduce costs, and improve care" (Bush, 2004). This proclamation generated an increased demand for understanding EHRs and promoting their adoption, but relatively few health care organizations were motivated at that time to pursue adoption of EHRs. The Healthcare Information and Management Systems Society (HIMSS) has been tracking EHR adoption since 2005 through its "Stage 7" award and in 2013 reported that most U.S. health care organizations (77%) are in Stage 3, reflecting only implementation of the basic EHR components of laboratory, radiology, and pharmacy ancillaries; a clinical data repository, including a controlled medical vocabulary; and simple nursing documentation and clinical decision support (HIMSS, 2013). Higher stages of the electronic medical record adoption model include more sophisticated use of clinical decision support tools (CDSS) and medication administration tools, with HIMSS Stage 7—the highest level—consisting of EHRs that have data sharing and warehousing capabilities and that are completely interfaced with emergency and outpatient facilities (HIMSS Analytics, 2013). Real progress is being made on the adoption of more robust EHRs. HIMSS Analytics (2015) reports that 1,313 hospitals in the United States have achieved Stage 6 with full physician documentation, a robust CDSS, and electronic access to medical images. Healthcare IT News (2015) reports that, to date, over 200 hospitals have achieved Stage 7 and are totally paperless and that more organizations are added every day.

In President Barack Obama's first term in office, Congress passed the **American Recovery and Reinvestment Act of 2009** (ARRA). This legislation included the HITECH Act, which specifically sought to incentivize health organizations and providers to become meaningful users of EHRs. These incentives came in the form of increased reimbursement rates from the Centers for Medicare and Medicaid Services (CMS); ultimately, the HITECH Act resulted in payment of a penalty by any health care organization that had not adopted an EHR by January 2015. The final rule was published by the Department of Health and Human Services (HHS) in July 2010 for the first phase of implementation. Stage 1 **meaningful use** criteria focus on data capture and sharing (HHS, 2010). Stage 2 criteria, slated for implementation by 2014, advanced several clinical processes and promoted health information exchange (HIE) and more patient control over personal data. Stage 3, which has a target implementation date of 2016, focuses on improved outcomes for individuals and populations and introduction of patient self-management tools (HealthIT.gov, 2013).

Components of Electronic Health Records

Overview

Before enactment of the ARRA, several variants of EHRs existed, each with its own terminology and each developed with a different audience in mind. The sources of these records included, for example, the federal government (Certification Commission for Healthcare Information Technology, 2007), the IOM (2003), the HIMSS (2007), and the National Institutes of Health (2006; Robert Wood Johnson Foundation [RWJF], 2006). Under ARRA, there is now an explicit requirement for providers and hospitals to use a certified EHR that meets a set of standard functional definitions to be eligible for the increased reimbursement incentive. Initially, HHS granted two organizations the authority to accredit EHRs: the Drummond Group and the Certification Commission for Healthcare Information Technology. In 2015, there are five recognized bodies for testing and certifying EHRs (HealthIT.gov, 2015a). These bodies are authorized to test and certify EHR vendors against the standards and test procedures developed by the National Institute of Standards and Technology (NIST) and endorsed by the Office of the National Coordinator for Health Information Technology for EHRs.

The initial NIST test procedure included 45 certification criteria, ranging from the basic ability to record patient demographics, document vital signs, and maintain an up-to-date problem list to more complex functions, such as electronic exchange of clinical information and patient summary records (Jansen & Grance, 2011; NIST, 2010). **Box 11-1** lists the 45 initial certification criteria outlined by NIST (2010). These criteria have been updated several times since 2010, with a 2015 version currently being developed after going out for public comment (HealthIT.gov, 2015b). Each iteration of testing procedures seeks to make the EHR more robust and functional to meet the needs of patients and users.

Despite the points articulated in the ARRA, the IOM definition of an EHR also remains a valid reference point. This definition is useful because it has distilled all the possible features of an EHR into eight essential components with an emphasis on functions that promote patient safety—a universal denominator that everyone in health care can accept. The eight components are (1) health information and data, (2) results management, (3) order entry management, (4) decision support, (5) electronic communication and connectivity, (6) patient support, (7) administrative processes, and (8) reporting and population health management (IOM, 2003). Each of these components is described in more detail here. With the exception of EHR infrastructure functions, such as security and privacy management, controlled medical vocabularies, and interoperability standards, the 45 initial NIST standards easily map into the IOM categories (Jansen & Grance, 2011).

BOX 11-1 EHR CERTIFICATION CRITERIA

Criteria #	Certification Criteria
§170.302 (a)	Drug–drug, drug–allergy interaction checks
§170.302 (b)	Drug formulary checks
§170.302 (c)	Maintain up-to-date problem list
§170.302 (d)	Maintain active medication list
§170.302 (e)	Maintain active medication allergy list
§170.302 (f)(1)	Vital signs
§170.302 (f)(2)	Calculate body mass index
§170.302 (f)(3)	Plot and display growth charts
§170.302 (g)	Smoking status
§170.302 (h)	Incorporate laboratory test results
§170.302 (i)	Generate patient lists
§170.302 (j)	Medication reconciliation
§170.302 (k)	Submission to immunization registries
§170.302 (l)	Public health surveillance
§170.302 (m)	Patient-specific education resources
§170.302 (n)	Automated measure calculation
§170.302 (o)	Access control
§170.302 (p)	Emergency access
§170.302 (q)	Automatic log-off
§170.302 (r)	Audit log
§170.302 (s)	Integrity
§170.302 (t)	Authentication
§170.302 (u)	General encryption
§170.302 (v)	Encryption when exchanging electronic health information
§170.302 (w)	Accounting of disclosures (optional)
§170.304 (a)	Computerized provider order entry
§170.304 (b)	Electronic prescribing
§170.304 (c)	Record demographics
§170.304 (d)	Patient reminders
§170.304 (e)	Clinical decision support
§170.304 (f)	Electronic copy of health information
§170.304 (g)	Timely access
§170.304 (h)	Clinical summaries
§170.304 (i)	Exchange clinical information and patient summary record

BOX 11-1 EHR CERTIFICATION CRITERIA (continued)	
§170.304 (j)	Calculate and submit clinical quality measures
§170.306 (a)	Computerized provider order entry
§170.306 (b)	Record demographics
§170.306 (c)	Clinical decision support
§170.306 (d)(1)	Electronic copy of health information
§170.306 (d)(2)	Electronic copy of health information
	Note: For discharge summary
§170.306 (e)	Electronic copy of discharge instructions
§170.306 (f)	Exchange clinical information and patient summary record
§170.306 (g)	Reportable lab results
§170.306 (h)	Advance directives
§170.306 (i)	Calculate and submit clinical quality measures

Data from National Institute of Standards and Technology (NIST). (2010). Meaningful use test measures: Approved test procedures. Retrieved October 2010 from http://healthcare.nist.gov/use_testing/finalized_ requirements.html.

Health Information and Data

Health information and data comprise the patient data required to make sound clinical decisions, including demographics, medical and nursing diagnoses, medication lists, allergies, and test results (IOM, 2003).

Results Management

Results management is the ability to manage results of all types electronically, including laboratory and radiology procedure reports, both current and historical (IOM, 2003).

Order Entry Management

Order entry management is the ability of a clinician to enter medication and other care orders, including laboratory, microbiology, pathology, radiology, nursing, supply orders, ancillary services, and consultations, directly into a computer (IOM, 2003).

Decision Support

Decision support entails the use of computer reminders and alerts to improve the diagnosis and care of a patient, including screening for correct drug selection and dosing; screening for medication interactions with other medications; preventive health reminders in such areas as vaccinations, health risk screening and detection; and clinical guidelines for patient disease treatment (IOM, 2003).

Electronic Communication and Connectivity

Electronic communication and connectivity include the online communication among health care team members, their care partners, and patients, including e-mail, Web messaging, and an integrated health record within and across settings, institutions, and telemedicine (IOM, 2003).

Patient Support

Patient support encompasses patient education and self-monitoring tools, including interactive computer-based patient education, home telemonitoring, and telehealth systems (IOM, 2003).

Administrative Processes

Administrative processes are activities carried out by the electronic scheduling, billing, and claims management systems, including electronic scheduling for inpatient and outpatient visits and procedures, electronic insurance eligibility validation, claim authorization and prior approval, identification of possible research study participants, and drug recall support (IOM, 2003).

Reporting and Population Health Management

Reporting and population health management are the data collection tools to support public and private reporting requirements, including data represented in a standardized terminology and machine-readable format (IOM, 2003).

NIST has not provided an exhaustive list of all possible features and functions of an EHR. Consequently, different vendor EHR systems combine different components in their offerings, and often a single set of EHR components may not meet the needs of all clinicians and patient populations. For example, a pediatric setting may demand functions for immunization management, growth tracking, and more robust order entry features to include weight-based dosing (Spooner & Council on Clinical Information Technology, 2007). These types of features may not be provided by all EHR systems, and it is important to consider EHR certification to be a minimum standard.

Advantages of Electronic Health Records

Measuring the benefits of EHRs can be challenging. Possible methods to estimate EHR benefits include using vendor supplied data that have been retrieved from their customers' systems, synthesizing and applying studies of overall EHR value, creating logical engineering models of EHR value, summarizing focused studies of elements of EHR value, and conducting and applying information from site visits (HealthIT.gov, 2012; Thompson, Osheroff, Classen, & Sittig, 2007).

Early on, the four most common benefits cited for EHRs were (1) increased delivery of guidelines-based care, (2) enhanced capacity to perform surveillance and monitoring for disease conditions, (3) reduction in medication errors, and (4) decreased use of care (Chaudhry et al., 2006; HealthIT.gov, 2012). These findings were echoed by two similar literature reviews. The first review focused on the use of informatics systems for managing patients with chronic illness. It found that the processes of care most positively impacted were guidelines adherence, visit frequency (i.e., a decrease in emergency department visits), provider documentation, patient treatment adherence, and screening and testing (Dorr et al., 2007).

The second review was a cost–benefit analysis of health information technology completed by the Agency for Healthcare Research and Quality (AHRQ) that studied the value of an EHR in the ambulatory care and pediatric settings, including its overall economic value. The AHRQ study highlighted the common findings already described but also noted that most of the data available for review came from six leading health care organizations in the United States, underscoring the challenge of generalizing these results to the broader health care industry (Shekelle, Morton, & Keeler, 2006). As noted previously by the HIMSS Stage 7 Awards, the challenge to generalize results persists in the hospital arena, with fewer than 1% of U.S. hospitals or eight leading organizations providing most of the experience with comprehensive EHRs (HIMSS, 2010a).

Finally, all three literature reviews cited here indicated that there are a limited number of hypothesis-testing studies of EHRs and even fewer that have reported cost data.

The descriptive studies do have value, however, and should not be hastily dismissed. Although not as rigorous in their design, they do describe the advantages of EHRs well and often include useful implementation recommendations learned from practical experience. As identified in these types of reviews, EHR advantages include simple benefits, such as no longer having to interpret poor handwriting and handwritten orders, reduced turnaround time for laboratory results in an emergency department, and decreased time to administration of the first dose of antibiotics in an inpatient nursing unit (HealthIT.gov, 2012; Husk & Waxman, 2004; Smith et al., 2004). In the ambulatory care setting, improved management of cardiac-related risk factors in patients with diabetes and effective patient notification of medication recalls have been demonstrated to be benefits of the EHR (Jain et al., 2005; Reed & Bernard, 2005). Two other unique advantages that have great potential are the ability to use the EHR and decision support functions to identify patients who qualify for research studies or who qualify for prescription drug benefits offered by pharmaceutical companies at safety-net clinics and hospitals (Embi et al., 2005; Poprock, 2005).

The HIMSS Davies Award may be the best resource for combined quantitative and qualitative results of successful EHR implementation. The Davies Award recognizes health care organizations that have achieved both excellence in implementation and value from health information technology (HIMSS, 2010b). One winner demonstrated a significant avoidance of medication errors because of bar-code scanning alerts, a $3 million decrease in medical records expenses as a result of going paperless, and a 5% reduction of duplicate laboratory orders by using computerized provider order entry alerting (HIMSS, 2010c). Another winner noted a 13% decrease in adverse drug reactions through the use of computerized physician order entry; it also achieved a decrease in methicillin-resistant *Staphylococcus aureus* (MRSA) nosocomial infections from

9.8 per 10,000 discharges to 6.4 per 10,000 discharges in less than a year using an EHR flagging function, which made clinicians immediately aware that contact precautions were required for MRSA-positive patients (HIMSS, 2009). At both organizations, there was qualitative and quantitative evidence of high rates of end-user adoption and satisfaction with use of the EHR.

A 2011 study of the effects of EHR adoption on nurse perceptions of quality of care, communication, and patient safety documented that nurses report better care outcomes and fewer concerns with care coordination and patient safety in hospitals with a basic EHR (Kutney-Lee & Kelly, 2011). In this study, nurses perceived that in hospitals with a functioning EHR, there was better communication among staff, especially during patient transfers, and fewer medication errors. Bayliss et al. (2015) demonstrated that an integrated care system utilizing an EHR resulted in fewer hospital readmissions and emergency room visits for over 12,000 seniors with multiple health challenges.

Without an EHR system, any of these benefits would be very difficult and costly to accomplish. Thus, despite limited standards and published studies, there is enough evidence to embrace widespread implementation of the EHR (Halamka, 2006; HealthIT.gov, 2012) and certainly enough evidence to warrant further study of the use and benefits of EHRs. **Box 11-2** describes some of the specific clinical information system (CIS) functions of an EHR.

BOX 11-2   THE EHR AS A CLINICAL INFORMATION SYSTEM

Denise Tyler

A clinical information system (CIS) is a technology-based system applied at the point of care and designed to support care by providing instant access to information for clinicians. Early CISs implemented prior to the advent of EHRs were limited in scope and provided such information as interpretation of laboratory results or a medication formulary and drug interaction information. With the implementation of EHRs, the goal of many organizations is to expand the scope of the early CISs to become comprehensive systems that provide clinical decision support, an electronic patient record, and in some instances professional development and training tools. Benefits of such a comprehensive system include easy access to patient data at the point of care, structured and legible information that can be searched easily and lends itself to data mining and analysis; and improved patient safety, especially the prevention of adverse drug reactions and the identification of health risk factors, such as falls.

TRACKING CLINICAL OUTCOMES

The ability to measure outcomes can be enhanced or impeded by the way an information system is designed and used. Although many practitioners can paint a very good picture of the patient by using a narrative (free text), employing this mode of expression in a clinical system without the use of a coded entry makes it difficult to analyze the care given or the patient's response. Free-text reporting also leads to inconsistencies of reporting from clinician to clinician and patient information that is fragmented or disorganized. This can limit the usefulness of patient data to other clinicians and interfere with the ability to create reports from the data for quality assurance and measurement purposes. Moreover, not all clinicians are equally skilled at the free-text form of communication, yielding inconsistent quality of documentation. Integrating standardized terminologies into computerized documentation systems enhances the ability to use the data for reporting and further research.

BOX 11-2 THE EHR AS A CLINICAL INFORMATION SYSTEM (continued)

According to the IOM (2012), "Payers, healthcare delivery organizations and medical product companies should contribute data to research and analytic consortia to support expanded use of care data to generate new insights" (para. 2). McLaughlin and Halilovic (2006) described the use of clinical analytics to promote medical care outcomes research. The use of a CIS in conjunction with standardized codes for patient clinical issues helps to support the rigorous analysis of clinical data. Outcomes data produced as part of these analyses may include length of stay, mortality, readmissions, and complications. Future goals include the ability to compare data and outcomes across various institutions as a means of developing clinical guidelines or best practices guidelines. With the implementation of a comprehensive CIS, similar analyses of clinicians' outcomes could also be performed and shared. Likewise, such a system could aid administrators in cross-unit comparisons and staffing decisions, especially when coupled with acuity systems data. In addition, clinical analytics can support required data reporting functions, especially those required by accreditation bodies.

SUPPORTING EVIDENCE-BASED PRACTICE

Evidence-based practice (EBP) can be thought of as the integration of clinical expertise and best practices based on systematic research to enhance decision making and improve patient care. References supporting EBP, such as clinical guidelines, are available for review at the click of a mouse or the press of a few keystrokes. The CIS's prompting capabilities can also reinforce the practice of looking for evidence to support patient care interventions rather than relying on how things have been done historically. This approach enhances processing and understanding of the information and allows the health care professional to apply the information to other areas, increasing the knowledge obtained about why certain conditions or responses result in prompts for additional questions or actions.

To incorporate EBP into the practice of professional clinical care, the information needs to be embedded in the computerized documentation system so that it is part of the work flow. The most typical way of embedding this timely information is through clinical practice guidelines. The resulting interventions and clinical outcomes need to be measurable and reportable for further research. The supporting documentation for the EBP needs to be easily retrievable and meaningful. Links, reminders, and prompts can all be used as vehicles for transmission of this information. The format needs to allow for rapid scanning, with the ability to expand the amount of information when more detail is required or desired. Balancing a consistency in formatting with creativity can be difficult but is worth the effort to stimulate an atmosphere for learning.

EBP is supported by translational research, an exciting movement that has enormous potential for the sharing and use of EBP. The use of translational research to support EBP may help to close the gap between what is known (research) and what is done (practice).

THE CIS AS A STAFF DEVELOPMENT TOOL

Joy Hilty, a registered nurse from Kaweah Delta, came up with a creative way to provide staff development or education without taking staff away from the bedside to a classroom setting. She created pop-up boxes on the opening charting screens for all staff who chart on the computer. These pop-ups vary in color and content and include a short piece of clinical information, along with a question. Staff can earn vacations from these pop-ups for as long as 14 days by e-mailing the correct answer to the question. This medium has provided information, stimulation, and a definite benefit: the vacation from the pop-up boxes. The pop-up box education format has also encouraged staff to share their answers, thereby creating interaction, knowledge dissemination, and reinforcement of the education provided.

(continues)

BOX 11-2 THE EHR AS A CLINICAL INFORMATION SYSTEM (continued)

Embedding EBP into the health care professional's documentation can also increase the compliance with Joint Commission core measures, such as providing information on influenza and pneumococcal vaccinations to at-risk patients. In the author's experience at Kaweah Delta, educating staff via classes, flyers, and storyboards was not successful in improving compliance with the documentation of immunization status or offering education on these vaccinations to at-risk patients. Embedding the prompts, information, and related questions in the nursing documentation with a link to the protocol and educational material, however, improved the compliance to 96% for pneumococcal vaccinations and to 95% for influenza vaccinations (Hettinger, 2007).

As more information is stored electronically, informaticists must translate the technology so that the input and retrieval of information are developed in a manner that is easy for clinicians to learn and use. A highly usable product should decrease errors and improve information entry and retrieval. Informaticists must be able to work with staff and expert users to design systems that meet the needs of the staff who will actually use the systems. The work is not done after the system is installed; the system must continue to be developed and improved because as staff use the system, they will be able to suggest changes to improve it. This ongoing revision should result in a system that is mature and meets the needs of the users.

In an ideal world, all clinical documentation will be shared through a national database, in a standard language, to enable evaluation of health care professionals' care, increase the body of evidence, and improve patient outcomes. With minimal effort, the information will be translated into new research that can be analyzed and linked to new evidence that will be intuitively applied to the CIS. Alerts will be meaningful and will be patient and provider specific. The steps required of the clinician to find current, reliable information will be almost transparent, and the information will be presented in a personalized manner based on user preferences stored in the CIS.

REFERENCES

Hettinger, M. (2007, March). *Core measure reporting: Performance improvement.* Visalia, CA: Kaweah Delta Health Care District.

McLaughlin, T., & Halilovic, M. (2006). Clinical analytics, rigorous coding bring objectivity to quality assertions. *Medical Staff Update Online, 30*(6). http://med.stanford.edu/shs/update/archives/JUNE2006/analytics.htm

The most recent description of the benefits of an EHR by HealthIT.gov (2014) emphasizes that EHRs hold the promise of transforming health care. Specifically, EHRs will lead to the following:

- *Better health care* by improving all aspects of patient care, including safety, effectiveness, patient centeredness, communication, education, timeliness, efficiency, and equity
- *Better health* by encouraging healthier lifestyles in the entire population, including increased physical activity, better nutrition, avoidance of behavioral risks, and wider use of preventative care
- *Improved efficiencies and lower health care costs* by promoting preventative medicine and improved coordination of health care services as well as by reducing waste and redundant tests
- *Better clinical decision making* by integrating patient information from multiple sources (para. 4)

Ownership of Electronic Health Records

The implementation of an EHR has the potential to affect every member of a health care organization. The process of becoming a successful owner of an EHR has multiple steps and requires integrating the EHR into the organization's day-to-day operations and long-term vision as well as into the clinician's day-to-day practice. All members of the health care organization—from the executive level to the clinician at the point of care—must feel a sense of ownership to make the implementation successful for themselves, their colleagues, and their patients. Successful ownership of an EHR may be defined in part by the level of clinician adoption of the tool, and this section reviews key steps and strategies for the selection, implementation and evaluation, and optimization of an EHR in pursuit of that goal.

Historically, many systems were developed locally by the information technology department of a health care organization. It was not unusual for software developers to be employed by the organization to create needed systems and interfaces between them. As commercial offerings were introduced and matured, it became less and less common to see homegrown or locally developed systems.

As this history suggests, the first step of ownership is typically a vendor selection process for a commercially available EHR. During this step, it is important to survey the organization's level of interest, identify possible barriers to participation, document desired functions of an EHR, and assess the willingness to fund the implementation (Holbrook, Keshavjee, Troyan, Pray, & Ford, 2003). Although clinicians should drive the project, the assessment should also include the needs and readiness of the executive leadership, information technology, and project management teams. It is essential that leadership understands that this type of project is as much about redesigning clinical work as it is about technically automating it and that they agree to assume accountability for its success (Goddard, 2000). In addition, this pre-acquisition phase should concentrate on understanding the current state of the health information technology industry to identify appropriate questions and the next steps in the selection process (American Organization of Nurse Executives, 2006). These first steps begin to identify any organizational risks related to successful implementation and pave the way for initiating a change management process to educate the organization about the future state of delivering health care with an EHR system.

The second step of the selection process is to select a system based on the organization's current and predicted needs. It is common during this phase to see a demonstration of several vendors' EHR products. Based on the completed needs assessment, the organization should establish key evaluation criteria to compare the different vendors and products. These criteria should include both subjective and objective items that cover such topics as common clinical work flows, decision support, reporting, usability, technical build, and maintenance of the system. Providing the vendor with these guidelines will ensure that the process meets the organization's needs; however, it is also essential to let the vendor demonstrate a proposed future state from its own perspective. This activity is critical to ensuring that the vendor's vision and the organization's vision are well aligned (Konschak & Shiple, n.d.). It also helps spark dialogue about the possible future state of clinical work at the organization and the change required in obtaining it. Such demonstrations not only enable the organization to compare and contrast the features and functions of different systems but also are a good way to engage the organization's members in being a part of this strategic decision.

Implementation planning should occur concurrently with the selection process, particularly the assessment of the scope of the work, initial sequencing of the EHR components to be implemented, and resources required. However, this step begins in earnest once a vendor and a product have been selected. In addition to further refining the implementation plan, this is the time to identify key metrics by which to measure the EHR's success. An organization may realize numerous benefits from implementing an EHR. It should choose metrics that match its overall strategy and goals in the coming years and may include expected improvements in financial, quality, and clinical outcomes. Commonly used metrics focus on reductions in the number of duplicate laboratory tests through duplicate orders alerting, reductions in the number of adverse drug events through the use of bar-code medication administration, meaningful use objectives and measures, and the EHR advantages mentioned earlier in this chapter. To ensure that the desired benefits are realized, it is important to avoid choosing so many that they become meaningless or unobtainable, to carefully and practically define those that are chosen, to measure before and after the implementation, and to assign accountability to a member of the organization to ensure the work is completed.

End-user adoption of the EHR is also essential to realizing its benefits. Clinicians must be engaged to use the EHR successfully in their practice and daily work flows so that data may be captured to drive the decision support that underlies so many of the advantages and metrics described. To promote adoption, a change management plan must be developed in conjunction with the EHR implementation plan. The most effective change management plans offer end users several exposures to the system and relevant work flows in advance of its use and continue through the go-live and post-live time periods. Successful pre-live strategies include end-user involvement as subject-matter experts to validate the EHR work flow design and content build, hosting end-user usability testing sessions, shadowing end users in their current daily work in parallel with the new system, and formal training activities. The goal of these pre-live activities is not only to ensure that the EHR implementation will meet end-user needs but also to assess the impact of the new EHR on current work flow and process. The larger the impact, the more change management is required above and beyond system training. For example, simulation laboratory experiences may be offered to more thoroughly dress rehearse a significant work flow change, executive leadership may need to convey their support and expectations of clinicians about a new way of working, and generally more anticipatory guidance is required to communicate to those impacted by the changes.

Training may be delivered in a variety of media. Often a combination of approaches works best, including classroom time, electronic learning, independent exercises, and peer-to-peer, at-the-elbow support. Training must be work flow based and reflect real clinical processes. It must also be planned and budgeted for through the post-live period to ensure that competency with the system is assessed at the go-live point and that any necessary retraining or reinforcements are made in the 30 to 60 days post-live. This not only promotes reliability and safe use of the system as it was designed but also can have a positive impact on end users' morale: Users will feel that they are being supported beyond the initial go-live period and have an opportunity to move from basic skills to advanced proficiency with the system.

Finally, the implementation plan should account for the long-term optimization of the EHR. This step is commonly overlooked and often results in benefits falling short of expectations because the resources are not available to realize them permanently. It also often means the difference between end users of EHRs merely surviving the change versus becoming savvy about how to adopt the EHR as another powerful clinical tool, to the same extent, for example, as the stethoscope (HealthIT.gov, 2012). Optimization activities of the EHR should be considered a routine part of the organization's operations, should be resourced accordingly, and should emphasize the continued involvement of clinician users to identify ways that the EHR can enable the organization to achieve its overall mission. Many organizations start an implementation of EHRs with the goal of transforming their care delivery and operations. An endeavor that differs from simply automating a previously manual or fragmented process, transformation often includes steps to improve the process so as to realize better patient care outcomes or added efficiency. Although some transformation is experienced with the initial use of the system, most of this work is done post-implementation and relies on widespread clinician adoption of the EHR. As such, it makes optimization a critical component to successful ownership of an EHR.

Box 11-3 reviews the barriers to and methods for successful acceptance of EHRs.

BOX 11-3   RESISTANCE TO IMPLEMENTATION

Julie A. Kenney and Ida Androwich
For an implementation to be successful, a few things need to happen. The health informatics specialist will need to understand and use change management theory to ensure that the implementation of the new EHR system will be successful. It is a well-known fact that health care professionals can make or break a system implementation. A staff that is involved early in the implementation process has been found to be a major determinant in a successful implementation. Assessing staff attitudes and concerns early in the process can aid the informatics specialist in determining the best way to proceed with staff education and implementation rollout. Staff may believe that the implementation that should be making their job easier will actually make it more challenging (Trossman, 2005). Professionals who feel that the system has been forced onto them are very likely to be highly resistant to the change. This is why it is imperative that health care professionals be involved in the design, development, and implementation of the EHR. Professionals who have been involved in the implementation process will ensure that the product meets the needs of the staff, which will result in high end-user satisfaction (McLane, 2005).

(continues)

Another challenge facing those wishing to implement an EHR is the issue that writing is nearly automatic for most, but using a computer is not. This potential problem can be overcome by ensuring that data entry and system navigation make for a system that is user friendly (Walsh, 2004). Voice data entry is an easy way to enter data into the system and may be a way for those who are not comfortable with computers to still use the system effectively (Walsh, 2004). Another way to encourage staff to accept the new EHR is to ensure that they have received adequate training prior to the implementation as well as to provide continued support and education after the implementation.

The implementation of a new EHR system requires the staff to make significant changes to how they work and how they handle patient information. The informatics specialist who is familiar with change management should have an integral role in the redesign of work flow processes to ensure a smooth transition from a paper record to an electronic record. Many excellent EHR systems fail after their installation due to poor implementation planning.

REFERENCES

McLane, S. (2005). Designing an EMR planning process based on staff attitudes toward and opinions about computers in health-care. *CIN: Computers, Informatics, Nursing, 23*(2), 85–92.

Trossman, S. (2005). Bold new world: Technology should ease nurses' jobs, not create a greater work load. *American Journal of Nursing, 105*(5), 75–77.

Walsh, S. (2004). The clinician's perspective on electronic health records and how they can affect patient care. *British Medical Journal, 328*(7449), 1184–1187.

Flexibility and Expandability of Electronic Health Records

Health care is as unique as the patients themselves. It is delivered in a variety of settings, for a variety of reasons, over the course of a patient's lifetime. In addition, patients rarely receive all their care from one health care organization; indeed, choice is a cornerstone of the American health care system. An EHR must be flexible and expandable to meet the needs of patients and caregivers in all these settings despite the challenges.

At a very basic level, there is as yet no EHR system available that can provide all functions for all specialties to such a degree that all clinicians would successfully adopt it. Consider oncology as an example. Most systems do not yet provide the advanced ordering features required for the complex treatment planning undertaken in this field. An oncologist could use a general system, but he or she would not find as many benefits without additional features for chemotherapy ordering, lifetime cumulative dose tracking, or the ability to adjust a treatment day schedule and recalculate a schedule for the remaining days of the plan. Some EHRs do a nice job of supporting the work of nursing staff and physicians but are not as supportive of the work of dieticians, physical and occupational therapists, and other health care personnel. These systems will continue to evolve as more health care professionals are exposed to the power of these systems to support their work and become better able to articulate their specific needs.

Further, most health care organizations do not yet have the capacity to implement and maintain systems in all care areas. As one physician stated, "Implementing an EMR is a complex and difficult multidisciplinary effort that will stretch an organization's skills and capacity for change" (Chin, 2004, p. 47).

These two conditions are improving every day at both vendor and health care organizations alike. Improvements in both areas were recently fueled by ARRA incentives (see **Box 11-4**).

ARRA has also set the expectation that despite the large number of settings in which a patient may receive care, a minimum set of data from those records must flow or "interoperate" between each setting and the unique EHR systems used in those settings. Today, **interoperability** exists through what is called a continuity-of-care document. This data set includes patient demographics, medication, allergy, and problem lists, among other things, and the formatting and exchange of the continuity-of-care document is required to be supported by EHR vendors and health care organizations seeking ARRA meaningful use incentives.

Despite this positive step forward, financial and patient privacy hurdles remain to be overcome to achieve an expansive EHR. Most health care is delivered by small community practices and hospitals, many of which do not have the financial or technical resources to implement EHRs. HHS recently loosened regulations so that physicians may now be able to receive health care information technology software, hardware, and implementation services from hospitals to alleviate the financial burden placed on individual providers and to foster more widespread adoption of the EHR.

Finally, patient privacy is a pivotal issue in determining how far and how easy it will be to share data across health care organizations. In addition to the Health Insurance Portability and Accountability Act privacy rules, many states have regulations in place related to patient confidentiality. An experience of the state of Minnesota foreshadows what all states will soon be facing. In 2007, Governor Tim Pawlenty announced the

BOX 11-4   CLOUDY EHRS

A paradigm shift from health care facility–owned, machine-based computing to off-site, vendor-owned cloud computing, Web browser–based login-accessible data, software, and hardware could link systems together and reduce costs. Hospitals with shrinking budgets and extreme information technology needs are exploring the successes in this area achieved in other industries, such as Amazon's S3. As providers strive to implement potent EHRs, they are looking for cloud-based models that offer the necessary functionality without having to assume the burden associated with all of the hardware, software, application, and storage issues. However, in the face of the HITECH Act and its associated penalties, how can we overcome the challenges to realize the benefits of this approach? Cloud computing has both advantages and disadvantages, and while they explore this new paradigm, health care providers must relinquish control as they continue to strive to maintain security. The vendors that are responsible for developing and maintaining this new environment are also facing challenges originating from both legislatures and health care providers. As the vendors and health care providers work together to improve the implementation and adoption of the cloud-based EHR, the sky is the limit!

creation of the Minnesota Health Information Exchange (State of Minnesota, 2007). Although the intentions of the exchange were to promote patient safety and increase health care efficiency across the state, it raised significant concerns about security and privacy. New questions arose about the definition of when and how patient consent is required to exchange data electronically, and older paper-based processes needed to be updated to support real-time electronic exchange (Minnesota Department of Health, 2007). For health exchanges such as these to reach their full potential, members of the public must be able to trust that their privacy will be protected, or else the health care industry risks that patients may not share a full medical history or, worse yet, may not seek care, effectively making the exchanges useless.

The Future

Despite the challenges, the future of EHRs is an exciting one for patients and clinicians alike. Benefits may be realized by implementing stand-alone EHRs as described here, but the most significant transformation will come as interoperability is realized between systems. As the former national information technology coordinator in HHS, David Brailer, noted about the potential of interoperability,

> For the first time, clinicians everywhere can have a longitudinal medical record with full information about each patient. Consumers will have better information about their health status since personal health records and similar access strategies can be feasible in an interoperable world. Consumers can move more easily between and among clinicians without fear of their information being lost. Payers can benefit from the economic efficiencies, fewer errors, and reduced duplication that arises from interoperability. Healthcare information exchange and interoperability (HIEI) also underlies meaningful public health reporting, bioterrorism surveillance, quality monitoring, and advances in clinical trials. In short, there is little that most people want from health care for which HIEI isn't a prerequisite. (Brailer, 2005, p. W 5-20)

The future also holds tremendous potential for EHR features and functions that will include not only more sophisticated decision support and clinical reporting capacity but also improved support for all health care professionals, biomedical device integration, ease of use and intuitiveness, and access through more hardware platforms.

Implementation of EHRs is becoming common, with ARRA putting pressure on health care organizations to move more quickly toward adoption of such records. More organizations adopting EHRs will facilitate broader dissemination of implementation best practices, with the hope of further shortening the time required to take advantage of advanced EHR features.

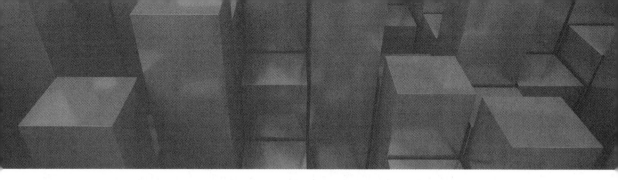

Summary

It is an important time for health care and technology. EHRs have come to the forefront and will remain central to shaping the future of health care. In an ideal world, all health care professionals from entry-level personnel to executives, will have a basic competency in health informatics that will enable them to participate fully in shaping the future use of technology in the practice at a national level and wherever care is delivered.

Thought-Provoking Questions

1. What are the implications for health care professional education as the EHR becomes the standard for caring for patients?
2. What are the ethical considerations related to interoperability and a shared EHR?
3. You are asked about a diagnosis with which you are unfamiliar. Where would you start looking for information? How would you determine the validity of the information?
4. Think about the documentation and knowledge management functions of your specialty. If you had the opportunity to create a wish list, what would you include in an EHR to support your work?

Apply Your Knowledge

One of the difficulties associated with intraprofessional collaboration using the EHR is that there is still not one universal system for health care terminology. Rather, terms and abbreviations are often related to specific organizational cultures and sometimes even differ by department in a single institution.

1. Brainstorm to think of an example of a condition where different terminologies exist. For example, some professionals use DOA to stand for Date of Admission, and others use DOA to indicate Dead on Arrival, clearly very different meanings and uses.
2. Reflect on the issues that differing terminologies for the same condition might create for interprofessional collaboration, transfers to other facilities, handoffs between units in a single facility, or the aggregation of data for research.

How does the use of an EHR help to mitigate this issues?

References

American Organization of Nurse Executives. (2006, September). *Defining the role of the nurse executive in technology acquisition and implementation*. Washington, DC: Author. http://www.aone.org/aone/pdf/Guiding%20Principles%20for%20Acquisition%20and%20Implementation%20of%20Information%20Technology.pdf

Bayliss, E. A., Ellis, J. L., Shoup, J. A., Chan, Z., McQuillan, D. B., & Steiner, J. F. (2015). Effect of continuity of care on hospital utilization for seniors with multiple medical conditions in an integrated health care system. *Annals of Family Medicine, 13*(2), 123–129. doi: 10.1370/afm.1739

Brailer, D. J. (2005, January). Interoperability: The key to the future healthcare system. *Health Affairs—Web Exclusive*, W 5-19–W 5-21. http://content.healthaffairs.org/cgi/reprint/hlthaff.w5.19v1

Bush, G. W. (2004). State of the Union address. http://www.whitehouse.gov/news/releases/2004/01/20040120-7.html

Certification Commission for Healthcare Information Technology. (2007). Certification Commission announces new work group members. http://www.cchit.org/about/news/releases/Certification-Commission-Announces-New-Work-Group-Members.asp

Chaudhry, B., Wang, J., Wu, S., Maglione, M., Mojica, W., Roth, E., et al. (2006). Systematic review: Impact of health information technology on quality, efficiency, and costs of medical care. *Annals of Internal Medicine, 144*(10), E-12–E-22.

Chin, H. L. (2004). The reality of EMR implementation: Lessons from the field. *Permanente Journal, 8*(4), 43–48.

Dorr, D., Bonner, L. M., Cohen, A. N., Shoai, R. S., Perrin, R., Chaney, E., et al. (2007). Informatics systems to promote improved care for chronic illness: A literature review. *Journal of the American Medical Informatics Association, 14*(2), 156–163.

Embi, P. J., Jain, A., Clark, J., Bizjack, S., Hornung, R., & Harris, C. M. (2005). Effect of a clinical trial alert system on physician participation in trial recruitment. *Archives of Internal Medicine, 165*, 2272–2277.

Goddard, B. L. (2000). Termination of a contract to implement an enterprise electronic medical record system. *Journal of American Medical Informatics Association, 7*, 564–568.

Halamka, J. D. (2006, May). Health information technology: Shall we wait for the evidence? [Letter to the editor]. *Annals of Internal Medicine, 144*(10), 775–776.

Healthcare Information and Management Systems Society. (2007). Electronic health record. http://www.himss.org/ASP/topics_ehr.asp

Healthcare Information and Management Systems Society. (2009). HIMSS Davies Organizational Award application: MultiCare. http://www.himss.org/davies/docs/2009_RecipientApplications/MultiCareConnectHIMSSDaviesManuscript.pdf

Healthcare Information and Management Systems Society. (2010a). Davies Award. http://www.himss.org/davies

Healthcare Information and Management Systems Society. (2010b). HIMSS Davies Award. http://apps.himss.org/davies

Healthcare Information and Management Systems Society. (2010c). Recipient list. http://www.himssanalytics.org/hc_providers/stage7Hospitals.asp

Healthcare Information and Management Systems Society. (2013). HIMSS 2013 iHIT Study: Executive summary. http://www.himss.org/library/clinical-informatics/2013-ihitstudy-executive-summary

Healthcare Information and Management Systems Society Analytics. (2013). Electronic medical record adoption model (EMRAM). http://www.himssanalytics.org/emram/index.aspx

Healthcare Information and Management Systems Society Analytics. (2015). Validated Stage 6 & 7 providers list. http://www.himssanalytics.org/case-study/validated-stage-6-7-providers-list

Healthcare IT News. (2015). 7 tips for EMR success from Stage 7 hospitals. http://www
.healthcareitnews.com/news/7-tips-emr-success-stage-7-hospitals

HealthIT.gov. (2012). Benefits of EHRs: Why adopt EHRs? http://www.healthit.gov/providers
-professionals/why-adopt-ehrs

HealthIT.gov. (2013). How to attain meaningful use. http://www.healthit.gov/providers
-professionals/how-attain-meaningful-use

HealthIT.gov. (2014). What are the advantages of electronic health records? http://www.healthit
.gov/providers-professionals/faqs/what-are-advantages-electronic-health-records

HealthIT.gov. (2015a). Certification bodies and testing laboratories. http://www.healthit.gov
/policy-researchers-implementers/certification-bodies-testing-laboratories

HealthIT.gov. (2015b). Test and testing methods. http://www.healthit.gov/policy-researchers
-implementers/2015-edition-draft-test-procedures

Holbrook, A., Keshavjee, K., Troyan, S., Pray, M., & Ford, P. T. (2003). Applying methodology to
electronic medical record selection. *International Journal of Medical Informatics, 71*, 43–50.

Husk, G., & Waxman, D. A. (2004). Using data from hospital information systems to improve
emergency care. *Academic Emergency Medicine, 11*(11), 1237–1244.

Institute of Medicine. (2001). *Crossing the quality chasm: A new health system for the 21st century.*
Washington, DC: National Academies Press.

Institute of Medicine. (2003). *Key capabilities of an electronic health record system: Letter report.*
Washington, DC: National Academies Press.

Institute of Medicine. (2012). Best care at lower cost. http://www.iom.edu/~/media/Files
/Report%20Files/2012/Best-Care/Best%20Care%20at%20Lower%20Cost_Recs.pdf

Jain, A., Atreja, A., Harris, C. M., Lehmann, M., Burns, J., & Young, J. (2005). Responding to the
rofecoxib withdrawal crisis: A new model for notifying patients at risk and their healthcare
providers. *Annals of Internal Medicine, 142*(3), 182–186.

Jansen, W., & Grance, T. (2011). National Institute of Standards and Technology (NIST): Guidelines on security and privacy in public cloud computing. https://cloudsecurityalliance.org
/wp-content/uploads/2011/07/NIST-Draft-SP-800-144_cloud-computing.pdf

Konschak, C., & Shiple, D. (n.d.). System selection: Aligning vision and technology. http://www
.divurgent.com/images/White%20Paper.Vendor%20Selection.vfinal.pdf

Kutney-Lee, A., & Kelly, D. (2011). The effect of hospital electronic health record adoption on
nurse-assessed quality of care and patient safety. *Journal of Nursing Administration, 41*(11),
466–472. doi: 10.1097/NNA.0b013e3182346e4b

Minnesota Department of Health. (2007, June). *Minnesota Health Records Act—HF 1078 fact
sheet.* Minneapolis: Author. http://www.health.state.mn.us/e-health/hras/hras050113facts.pdf

National Institute of Standards and Technology. (2010). Meaningful use test measures: Approved
test procedures. http://healthcare.nist.gov/use_testing/finalized_requirements.html

National Institutes of Health. (2006, April). *Electronic health records overview.* McLean, VA: Mitre
Corporation.

Poprock, B. (2005, September). *Using Epic's alternative medications reminder to reduce prescription
costs and encourage assistance programs for indigent patients.* Presented at the Epic Systems
Corporation user group meeting, Madison, WI.

Reed, H. L., & Bernard, E. (2005). Reductions in diabetic cardiovascular risk by community primary care providers. *International Journal of Circumpolar Health, 64*(1), 26–37.

Robert Wood Johnson Foundation. (2006). Health information technology in the United States:
The information base for progress. http://www.rwjf.org/programareas/resources/product
.jsp?id=15895&pid=1142&gsa=1

Shekelle, P. G., Morton, S. C., & Keeler, E. B. (2006). *Costs and benefits of health information technology. Evidence report/technology assessment*, No. 132. Prepared by the Southern California
Evidence-Based Practice Center under Contract No. 290-02-0003. Agency for Healthcare

Research and Quality Publication No. 06-E006. Rockville, MD: Agency for Healthcare Research and Quality.

Smith, T., Semerdjian, N., King, P., DeMartin, B., Levi, S., Reynolds, K., et al. (2004). *Nicholas E. Davies Award of Excellence: Transforming healthcare with a patient-centric electronic health record system*. Evanston, IL: Evanston Northwestern Healthcare. http://www.himss.org/content/files/davies2004_evanston.pdf

Spooner, S. A., & Council on Clinical Information Technology. (2007). Special requirements of electronic health record systems in pediatrics. *Pediatrics, 119*, 631–637.

State of Minnesota, Office of the Governor. (2007). New public–private partnership to improve patient care, safety and efficiency. http://www.governor.state.mn.us/mediacenter/pressreleases/2007/PROD008303.html

Thompson, D. I., Osheroff, J., Classen, D., & Sittig, D. F. (2007). A review of methods to estimate the benefits of electronic medical records in hospitals and the need for a national database. *Journal of Healthcare Information Management, 21*(1), 62–68.

U.S. Department of Health and Human Services. (2010). Medicare and Medicaid programs: Electronic health record incentive program. http://www.ofr.gov/OFRUpload/OFRData/2010-17202_PI.pdf

Informatics Tools to Promote Patient Safety, Quality Outcomes, and Interdisciplinary Collaboration

Dee McGonigle and Kathleen Mastrian

OBJECTIVES

1. Explore the characteristics of a safety culture.
2. Examine strategies for developing a safety culture.
3. Recognize how human factors contribute to errors.
4. Appreciate the impact of informatics technology on quality and patient safety.
5. Assess the interdisciplinary collaboration necessary to support quality patient care.

Introduction

Health care professionals have an ethical duty to ensure patient safety. Increasing demands on professionals in complex and fast-paced health care environments, however, may lead them to cut corners or develop work-arounds that deviate from accepted and expected practice protocols. These deviations are not carried out deliberately to put patients at risk but rather are often practiced in the interest of saving time or because the organizational culture is such that risky behaviors are common. Occasionally, these inappropriate actions or omissions of appropriate actions result in harm or significant risk of harm to patients. Consider the following case scenario:

Key Terms
Alarm fatigue
Bar-code medication administration
Clinical decision support
Computerized physician order entry
Failure modes and effects analysis
High-hazard drugs
Human factors engineering
Interdisciplinary collaboration
Interprofessional collaboration
(continues)

Key Terms (continued)
Radio-frequency identification
Root-cause analysis
Safety culture
Smart pump
Smart rooms
Wearable technology
Work-around

A 19-year-old obese woman who had recently undergone C-section delivery of a baby presented in the emergency department (ED) with dyspnea. Believing the patient had developed a pulmonary embolism, the physician prescribed an IV heparin bolus dose of 5,000 units followed by a heparin infusion at 1,000 units/hour. After administering the bolus dose, a nurse started the heparin infusion but misprogrammed the pump to run at 1,000 mL/hour, not 1,000 units/hour (20 mL/hour). By the time the error was discovered, the patient had received more than 17,000 units (5,000 unit loading dose and about 12,000 units from the infusion) in less than an hour since arrival in the ED. A smart pump with dosing limits for heparin had been used. Thus, the programming error should have been recognized before the infusion was started. However, the nurse had elected to bypass the dose-checking technology and had used the pump in its standard mode. It was quite fortunate that the patient did not experience adverse bleeding, as her aPTT values were as prolonged as 240 seconds when initially measured and 148 seconds two hours later. (Institute for Safe Medication Practices, 2007, para. 2)

The smart pump used in this scenario was equipped with dose calculation software that compares the programmed infusion rate to a drug database to check for dosing within safe limits. This technology is particularly important when high-alert or high-hazard drugs are being administered. In this case, however, the available dose-checking technology had been turned off, and the pump was operated in standard mode. A subsequent analysis of the error event revealed that many nurses in the institution were bypassing the safety technology afforded by the smart pump to save time. It is important to remember that "more than 200,000 people in the U.S. die in hospitals every year due to patient safety errors that could easily be fixed by implementing simple practices available to every hospital out there today" (Kallstrom, 2015, para. 1).

This chapter focuses on some of the recommended organizational strategies used to promote a culture of safety and some of the specific informatics technologies designed to reduce errors and promote patient safety.

What Is a Culture of Safety?

The Institute of Medicine (2000) report *To Err Is Human* is widely credited for launching the current focus on patient safety in health care. This report was followed by the Institute of Medicine's (2001) *Crossing the Quality Chasm* report, which brought to national attention health care quality and safety. This national attention resulted in a $50 million grant by Congress to the Agency for Healthcare Research and Quality (AHRQ) to launch initiatives focused on safety research for patients. Other initiatives prompted by these seminal reports were the Joint Commission's National Patient Safety Goals (2002), the National Quality Forum's adverse events and "never events" list (2002), the creation of the Office of National Coordinator for Health IT to computerize health care (2004), the formation of the World Health Organization's Alliance for Patient Safety (2004), the Institute for Healthcare Improvement's (IHI's) 100,000 Lives campaign (2005) and 5 Million Lives campaign (2008), congressional authorization of patient safety organizations created by the Patient Safety and Quality Improvement Act to promote blameless error reporting and shared learning (2005), the "no pay for errors" initiative launched by Medicare (2008), and the $19 billion congressional appropriation to support electronic health records (EHRs) and patient safety (Wachter, 2010).

The AHRQ (2012) safety culture primer suggested that organizations should strive to achieve high reliability by being committed to improving health care quality and preventing medical errors and to demonstrate an overall commitment to patient safety. That is, everyone and every level in an organization must embrace the safety culture. Key features of a **safety culture** identified by the AHRQ are as follows:

- Acknowledgment of the high-risk nature of an organization's activities and the determination to achieve consistently safe operations
- A blame-free environment where individuals are able to report errors or near misses without fear of reprimand or punishment
- Encouragement of collaboration across ranks and disciplines to seek solutions to patient safety problems
- Organizational commitment of resources to address safety concerns (AHRQ, 2012, para. 1)

An important part of the safety culture is cultivating a blame-free environment. Errors and near misses must always be reported so that they can be thoroughly analyzed. All organizations can learn from mistakes and change their organizational processes or culture to ensure patient safety. The Patient Safety and Quality Improvement Act of 2005 mandates the creation of a national database of medical errors and funded several organizations to analyze these data with the goal of developing shared learning to prevent medical errors. Organizations themselves can engage in **root-cause analysis** or **failure modes and effects analysis** to examine medical errors closely and to determine the system processes that need to be changed to prevent similar future errors (Harrison & Daly, 2009). A tool for implementing root-cause analysis developed by the National Center for Patient Safety is detailed at this website: http://www.patientsafety .gov/CogAids/RCA/index.html#page=page-1. Similarly, the IHI has a website dedicated to failure modes and effects analysis. "Failure Modes and Effects Analysis (FMEA) is a systematic, proactive method for evaluating a process to identify where and how it might fail, and to assess the relative impact of different failures in order to identify the parts of the process that are most in need of change" (IHI, 2011b, para. 1). This powerful tool and shared experiences from other organizations can be viewed at http://www.ihi .org/knowledge/Pages/Tools/FailureModesandEffectsAnalysisTool.aspx.

If one embraces a blame-free environment to encourage error reporting, then where does individual accountability fit in? According to the ARHQ, one way to balance these competing cultural values (blameless versus accountability) is to establish a "just culture" where system or process issues that lead to unsafe behaviors and errors are addressed by changing practices or work flow processes and a clear message is communicated that reckless behaviors are not tolerated. The "just culture" approach accounts for three types of behaviors leading to patient safety compromises: (1) human error (unintentional mistakes), (2) risky behaviors (**work-arounds**), and (3) reckless behavior (total disregard for established policies and procedures). According to the Organization for Safety, Asepsis and Prevention (2014),

> *Patient safety (PS) in dentistry is the delivery of safe dental care to patients. PS is rooted in establishing an overall Culture of Safety in the dental facility. This reflects the shared commitment of the employer and employees/students toward ensuring safety for patients and dental personnel. (p. 24)*

Strategies for Developing a Safety Culture

Strategies for achieving a safety culture have been addressed frequently in the literature. The focus here is limited to those strategies described by two key organizations: the AHRQ and the IHI. The AHRQ (2012) provides access to data from two validated surveys: the Patient Safety Culture Survey and the Safety Attitudes Questionnaire. The AHRQ suggests that teamwork training, executive walk-arounds, and unit-based safety teams have improved safety culture perceptions but have not led to a significant reduction in error rates. The IHI (2011a) stresses that organizational leaders must drive the culture change by making a visible commitment to safety and by enabling staff to share safety information openly. Some of the strategies suggested by the IHI include appointing a safety champion for every unit, creating an adverse event response team, and reenacting or simulating adverse events to better understand the organizational or procedural processes that failed.

A systems engineering approach to patient safety, in which technology manufacturers partner with organizations to identify risks to patient safety and promote safe technology integration, is advocated by Ebben, Gieras, and Gosbee (2008). They note that **human factors engineering** is "the discipline of applying what is known about human capabilities and limitations to the design of products, processes, systems, and work environments." Its application to system design improves "ease of use, system performance and reliability, and user satisfaction, while reducing operational errors, operator stress, training requirements, user fatigue, and product liability" (p. 327). For example, Ebben et al. describe the feel of an oxygen control knob that rotated smoothly between settings, suggesting to the user that oxygen flows at all points on the knob, when in fact oxygen flowed only at specifically designated liter flow settings. Human factors engineering testing would most likely reveal this design flaw, and the setting knob could be improved to include discrete audio or tactile feedback (click into place) to the user to indicate a point on the dial where oxygen flows. Ebben et al. emphasize that testing human use factors provides more objective safety data than the subjective responses gained from user preference testing. "Understanding how the equipment shapes human performance is as important as evaluating reliability or other technical criteria" (p. 329). Organizations that are purchasing medical technology devices should avail themselves of shared safety data on equipment maintained by several key organizations, including the Joint Commission, the Food and Drug Administration, and the Medical Product Safety Network(http://www.fda.gov/MedicalDevices/Safety /MedSunMedicalProductSafetyNetwork/default.htm).

Safety technologies are increasingly being implemented in various health care disciplines. Here are some examples. Dietitians are using databases and analytic software as well as calorimeters and glucose monitors in their practice. Their ability to provide proper nutrition and hydration is critical since poor nutrition and dehydration are major sources of mortality or severe morbidity (Association of UK Dietitians, 2015). Respiratory therapists rely on ventilator alarms to alert themselves or other health care personnel. According to Kallstrom (2015), "Patient safety has to be a number one priority for respiratory therapists as they care for and manage patients" (para. 7).

Providing individualized patient care requires dental professionals to think critically

about radiographic recommendations, rather than providing a one-size-fits-all approach. Informed dental patients often bring questions about new technology to their appointment. The ease with which the clinician can get results with digital imaging should not cloud the basics of radiology, which include taking the time to properly place the sensor, open the contacts, and produce a diagnostic image, all while following the guidelines of ALARA. By following proper technique, digital radiography can offer a safe and efficient alternative to traditional dental radiographs. (Francisco, Horlak, & Azevedo, 2010, para. 18)

Medical sonographers' computer skills are not keeping pace with the technological advances, according to Watson and Odle (2013). In order to safely and effectively use radiologic technologies, medical sonographers must enhance their skills and competencies. Physical therapists "frequently make use of technology such as computerized motion analysis and gait assessment to analyze problems, measure performance, and enhance potential" (American Physical Therapy Association, 2011, p. 54). The assistive technologies that occupational therapists and physical therapists use must be patient specific with a focus on patient education to make sure the devices help the patients rather than hurt them. Can you name additional examples of safety technologies?

Once the technology is integrated into the organization, biomedical engineers can become valuable partners in promoting patient safety through appropriate use of these technologies. For example, in one organization, the biomedical engineers helped to revamp processes associated with the new technology alarm systems after they discovered several key issues: slow response times to legitimate alarms and multiple false alarms (promoting **alarm fatigue**) created by alarm parameters that were too sensitive. Strategies for addressing these issues included improving the patient call system by adding Voice over Internet Protocol telephones that wirelessly receive alarms directly from technology equipment carried by all nurses, thus reducing response times to alarms; feeding alarm data into a reporting database for further analysis; and encouraging nurses to round with physicians to provide input into alarm parameters that were too sensitive and were generating multiple false alarms (Williams, 2009). The Research Brief describes a study of intelligent agent technology to improve the specificity of physiologic alarms.

Clearly, there is more work to be done to create safety cultures in complex health care organizations and to reduce the incidence of errors. Miller and Hoffman (2014) discussed the importance of patient safety beginning in our programs of study. "Teaching patient safety (PS) and quality improvement (QI) to health professions students is a relatively new concept but has been recognized as vital to the future of health care" (p. 17). Many organizations are looking to informatics technology to help manage these complex safety issues by using smart technologies that provide knowledge access to users, provide automated safety checks, and improve communication processes.

Informatics Technologies for Patient Safety

Health care technologies are frequently designed to improve patient safety, streamline work processes, and improve the quality and outcomes of health care delivery. Technology is not always the answer to patient safety, as the Joint Commission (2008) cautions: "the overall safety and effectiveness of technology in health care ultimately depends on its human users, and . . . any form of technology can have a negative impact on the quality and safety of care if it is designed or implemented improperly or is misinterpreted" (para. 2). Although technology may certainly help to prevent or reduce errors, one must always remember that technology is not a substitution for safety vigilance by the health care team in a safety culture.

Bates and Gawande (2003) urged the adoption of information technology (IT) processes to improve safety. They suggest that information technologies improve communication, reduce errors and adverse events, increase the rapidity of response to adverse events, make knowledge more accessible to clinicians, assist with decisions, and provide feedback on performance. They also describe the benefits of technology-based forcing functions that direct or restrict actions or orders implemented by computer technologies. For example, physicians may be forced to write complete and accurate medication orders, restricted from ordering an inappropriate dosing route for a medication, or prompted to write corollary orders that should be included in the care regimen as part of the standard of care.

The Wired for Health Care Quality Act of 2005 began a series of funding streams to promote health IT, promote sharing of best practices in health IT, and help organizations implement health IT (Harrison & Daly, 2009). Many early adopters opted to focus technology and safety initiatives on medication ordering and administration processes. Medication errors are the most frequent and the most visible errors because the medication administration cycle has many poorly designed work processes with several opportunities for human error. Thus, **computerized physician order entry** (CPOE), automated dispensing machines, **smart pump** technologies for intravenous drug administration, and **bar-code medication administration** (BCMA) frequently preceded the adoption of the EHR in many institutions because of the costs associated with implementing these technologies. In an ideal world, the EHR would be adopted concurrently as part of an interoperable health IT system. In the early EHR systems, clinicians were prompted by electronic alerts reminding them of important interventions that should be part of the standard of care, but these alerts tended to be generalized and not patient specific—for example, "Did you check the allergy profile?" or "Has the patient received a pneumonia immunization?" These early alert and care reminders are now evolving into more sophisticated **clinical decision support** (CDS) systems to promote accurate diagnoses and suggest appropriate interventions based on patient data.

The National Patient Safety Foundation (2013) listed the top patient safety issues as wrong-site surgery, hospital-acquired infections, falls, hospital readmissions, diagnostic errors, and medication errors. Many of these issues can be prevented or detected in their early stages using informatics technologies. Other technologies designed to promote patient safety include wireless technologies for patient monitoring, clinician alerts, point-of-care applications, and radio-frequency identification applications. Each of these is reviewed here, and the chapter concludes with a section discussing future technologies for patient safety.

Technologies to Support the Medication Administration Cycle

The steps in the medication administration cycle (assessment of need, ordering, dispensing, distribution, administration, and evaluation) have been relatively stable for many years. Each of the steps depends on vigilant humans to ensure patient safety, resulting in the five rights of medication administration: (1) the right patient, (2) the right time and frequency of administration, (3) the right dose, (4) the right route, and (5) the right drug. Human error can be related to many aspects of this cycle. Distractions, unclear thinking, lack of knowledge, short staffing, and fatigue are a few of the factors that cause humans to deviate from accepted safety practices and commit medication errors. Integration of technology into the medication administration cycle promises to reduce the potential for human errors in the cycle by performing electronic checks and providing alerts to draw attention to potential errors.

CPOE is an electronic prescribing system designed to support physicians and nurse practitioners in writing complete and appropriate medication and care orders for patients. When CPOE is part of an EHR with a CDS system, the medication order is electronically checked against specific data in the patient record to prevent errors, such as ordering a drug that might interact with a drug the patient is already taking, ordering a dose that is too large for the patient's weight, or ordering a drug that is contraindicated by the patient's allergy profile or renal function. Because it is impossible for and unreasonable to expect a clinician to remember each of the more than 600 drugs that require a dose adjustment in the case of renal dysfunction, for example, safe dosing parameters are provided by the CPOE (Bates & Gawande, 2003). In a stand-alone CPOE system without a CDS system, the medication orders are simply checked by the computer against the drug database to ensure that the dose and route specified in the order are appropriate for the medication chosen. Specific benefits of CPOE include the following:

- Prompts that warn against the possibility of drug interaction, allergy, or overdose
- Accurate, current information that helps physicians keep up with new drugs as they are introduced into the market
- Drug-specific information that eliminates confusion among drug names that look and sound alike
- Improved communication between physicians and pharmacists
- Reduced health care costs caused by improved efficiencies (LeapFrog Group, 2008)

CPOE solves the safety issues associated with poor handwriting and unclear or incomplete medication orders. Orders can be entered in seconds and from remote sites, eliminating the use of verbal orders that are especially subject to interpretation errors. Orders are then transmitted electronically to the pharmacy, reducing the potential for the transcription errors commonly encountered in the paper-based system, such as lost or misplaced orders, delayed dosing, or unreadable faxes. Thus CPOE changes work flows for all clinical staff and physicians as well as health care team communication patterns (Manor, 2010). As with any technology integration, introduction of CPOE was associated with a resistance to change and a learning curve to gain proficiency, and users must learn to trust the system. Manor urged careful planning and training during implementation with plenty of staff support. She also reported on the need for a paper-based backup system in the case of network or electrical outages or system maintenance.

The verification and dispensing functions of the pharmacy can also be assisted by technology. The pharmacist begins by verifying the allergy status of the patient and the medication reconciliation information to ensure that the new medication is compatible with other medication in the care regimen. This verification function is computer based, and the medication order is electronically checked via the knowledge database. If the order is verified as safe and appropriate, the pharmacist proceeds to the dispensing process. Bar-code medication labeling at a unit dose level was mandated by the Food and Drug Administration in 2004, with targeted compliance to be achieved by 2006.

A bar code is a series of alternating bars and spaces that represents a unique code that can be read by a special bar-code reader. Bar-code technology spans both the medication dispensing and the administration steps in the medication administration cycle. In the pharmacy, the bar code helps to ensure that the right drug and the right dose are dispensed by the pharmacy. Medications that are labeled with bar codes can also be dispensed by robots capable of reading the codes or by automated dispensing machines. In this way, bar-code technology helps with the processes of procurement, inventory, storage, preparation, and dispensing (Cohen, 2002).

The processes of drug storage, dispensing, controlling, and tracking are easily carried out via automated dispensing machines (also known as automated dispensing cabinets, unit-based cabinets, automated dispensing devices, and automated distribution cabinets). These devices have benefits for both the user and the organization, specifically in the areas of access security (especially with narcotics administration tracking), safety, supply chain, and charge functions (Institute for Safe Medication Practices, 2008).

Radio-frequency identification (RFID) technology is used in health care technology and maybe used in the medication administration cycle. Although more expensive than bar coding for packaging, the RFID tags are reprogrammable (Wicks, Visich, & Li, 2006), and issues associated with bar-code printing imperfections and bar-code scanner resolution can be mitigated (Snyder, Carter, Jenkins, & Frantz, 2010). As discussed later in this chapter, RFID technologies may be an important component of a medication compliance system for patients.

BCMA systems help to ensure adherence to the five rights of medication administration. Whether BCMA is part of the larger EHR or a free-standing electronic medication administration system (eMAR), bar-code technology provides a system of checks and balances to ensure medication safety. Although this example is specific to nursing, it is provided here to illustrate the potential of informatics technologies and their effectiveness in promoting patient safety. The nurse begins by scanning his or her name badge, thereby logging in as the person responsible for medication administration. Next, the bar code on the patient's identification bracelet is scanned, prompting the electronic system to pull up the medication orders. Next, the bar code on each of the medications to be administered is scanned. This technology check ensures that the five rights of medication administration are met. If there is a discrepancy between the order and the medication that was scanned or a contraindication for administration, an alert is generated by the system. For example, in an EHR system with CDS, the nurse may be prompted to check the most recent laboratory results for electrolytes before administering a potassium supplement. In a free-standing eMAR without CDS or EHR links, if the medication orders have recently been changed, the nurse is alerted to the change. When an alert is generated, the nurse must chart the action taken in response to that alert. For example, an early dose might need to be given if the patient is leaving the unit for a diagnostic test.

Despite the promising advances in patient safety afforded by this technology, it is not fail-safe (Cochran, Jones, Brockman, Skinner, & Hicks, 2007). Medications that are labeled individually by the in-house pharmacist increase the potential for human error if the medication is given an incorrect bar code, such as one signifying a wrong dose or even the wrong medication. In addition, the bar-code printers themselves may generate unreadable labels, leading to staff work-arounds in the interest of saving time. Cochran et al. make the following recommendations to reduce BCMA errors:

- Purchase unit-of-use medications with manufacturer bar codes whenever possible.
- Double-check all hospital-generated bar-code labels, including those for compounded injectable medications, before the product leaves the pharmacy.
- Carefully review all BCMA override reports. Address system work-arounds through process change and staff education.
- Minimize false-positive warnings to reduce the likelihood that staff will ignore warnings for real errors.
- Ensure that an urgent need exists for all "stat" orders, as pharmacy review and advantages of bar-code administration are usually circumvented in such cases.
- Establish institutional policies and procedures that can be easily implemented when products fail to scan. Processes in pharmacy will likely be different than processes at the point of care (p. 300).

Smart pump technologies are designed for safe administration of **high-hazard drugs** and to reduce adverse drug events during intravenous medication administration. Smart pumps have software that is programmed to reflect the facility's infusion parameters and a drug library that compares normal dosing rates with those programmed into the pump. Discrepancies generate an alarm alerting the clinician to a safety issue. A soft alarm can typically be overridden by a clinician at the bedside, but a hard alarm requires the clinician to reprogram the pump so that the dosing falls within the facility's intravenous administration guidelines for the drug to be infused. All alarms generated by the smart pump are tracked along with the clinician's responses to them (Dulak, 2005; University of Alabama at Birmingham, 2013). Smart pumps can be seamlessly integrated into BCMA systems, and data can be fed directly into the EHR. The IHI recommends the following steps to ensure safe implementation of smart pump technology:

- Prior to deploying these pumps, standardize concentrations within the hospital. Asking the nurse to choose among several concentrations increases the risk of selection error.
- Prior to deploying these pumps, standardize dosing units for a given drug (for example, agree to always dose nitroglycerin in terms of mcg/min or mcg/kg/min, but not both). Asking the nurse to choose among several dosing units increases the risk of selection error.
- Prior to deploying these pumps, standardize drug nomenclature (for example, agree to always use the term KCl, but not potassium chloride, K, pot chloride, or others). Asking the nurse to remember and choose among several possible drug names increases the risk of selection error.
- Perform a failure modes and effects analysis on the deployment of these devices.

- Ensure that the concentrations, dose units, and nomenclature used in the pump are consistent with that used on the medication administration record (MAR), the pharmacy computer system, and the EHR.
- Meet with all relevant clinicians to come to agreement on the proper upper and lower hard and soft dose limits.
- Monitor overrides of alerts to assess whether the alerts have been properly configured or whether additional quality intervention is required.
- Be sure the "smart" feature is utilized in all parts of the hospital. If the pump is set up volumetrically in the operating room but the "smart" feature is used in the ICU, an error may occur if the pump is not properly reprogrammed.
- Be sure there are upper and lower dose limits for bolus doses, when applicable.
- Engage the services of a human factors engineer to identify new opportunities for failure when the pumps are deployed.
- Identify a procedure for the staff to follow in the event a drug that is not in the library must be given or when its concentration is not standard.
- Deploy the pump in all areas of the hospital. If a different pump is used on one floor and the patient is later transferred, this will create new opportunities for failure. Also, there may be incorrect assumptions about the technology available to a given floor or patient.
- Consider using "smart" technology for syringe pumps as well as large-volume infusion devices (IHI, 2012, para. 7).

CDS can enhance the medication administration cycle by promoting safety and improving patient outcomes. Clinical decision making is guided by targeted information delivery ensuring that the five rights of CDS are implemented: the right information provided to the right person in the right format through the right channel at the right time in work flow. For example, during medication selection, a CDS helps a clinician select an appropriate medication based on client data, such as clinical condition, weight, renal function, concurrent medications, and cost. This system ensures that the order is complete by performing checks for drug interactions, duplications, or allergy contraindications and ensures that the right dose and right route are specified. During the verification and dispensing phase of the medication administration cycle, the CDS provides double checks for interactions, allergies, and appropriate dose orders. Consideration is also given to potential infusion pump programming issues, incompatibilities during infusion, and proper notation and dispensing when portions of a dose must be wasted. During the administration phase, the CDS assists with patient identification and current assessment parameters (i.e., blood pressure, glucose level) that may contraindicate the use of the medication at that point in time. In addition, checks for interactions with foods or other medications and timing and monitoring guidelines are provided to the clinician administering the medication. The CDS has patient education guidelines and printable handouts to assist clinicians in educating patients about their medications. The monitoring functions of the CDS provide a structured data reporting system to track side effects and adverse events across the population (Healthcare Information and Management Systems Society [HIMSS], 2009a).

Several promising technologies may become available in the future to assist patients with medication compliance after discharge. For example, eMedonline collects patient medication compliance data by scanning package bar codes or RFID medication tags and using personal digital assistant or smartphone technology to send compliance data to the server. Clinicians review the medication compliance data and provide education and feedback to patients to increase their compliance with proper medication administration (eMedonline, n.d.). The SIMpill Medication Adherence System uses web-based technology to monitor patient compliance and provide reminders about taking medications or refilling prescriptions by sending text messages to the patient or caregivers (SIMpill, 2008). Caps of pill bottles may contain RFID tags that monitor and collect data on when the bottle is opened or that contain flashing time reminders when a dose is due (Blankenhorn, 2010). Smart inhalers track asthma medication compliance using a microprocessor that records and stores medication compliance. They may also include visual and audio reminders to use the inhaler (Nexus 6, 2010). These are just a sampling of the newer technologies for medication adherence; more are expected to emerge in the future.

Additional Technologies for Patient Safety

CDS systems have safety uses beyond the medication administration cycle. The robust data collection and data management functions help to ensure quality approaches to patient health challenges based on research evidence and clinical guidelines. A CDS may also ensure cost-effectiveness by alerting clinicians to duplicate testing orders or by suggesting the most cost-effective diagnostic test based on specific patient data (HIMSS, 2009b). Consider this description of the features of a CDS based on screen captures performed by a CDS system:

> *The patient is a 75-year-old male with coronary artery disease (CAD), diabetes mellitus (DM), and elevated creatine kinase (CK). Assessment prompts and reminders on the screen for this patient include no recent low-density-lipoprotein (LDL) test; blood pressure (BP) is above goal; patient is due for pneumovax and influenza vaccines; patient is a current smoker, not thinking of quitting, last counseled with date; patient is overweight; patient is due for eye and ear checks. The patient management prompts include the following:*
>
> - *Lipid Management: "No Recent LDL Management" is printed red with a series of check boxes presenting choices to the clinician:*
>   - ☐ *Order lipid panel now*
>   - ☐ *Order lipid panel with direct LDL now*
>   - ☐ *Print instructions for fasting lipid panel (link)*
>   - ☐ *Print orders for outside lab request for lipid panel testing (link)*
> - *BP management: BP is above goal average over last 2 visits; goal is 130/80*
>   - ☐ *Choices on check boxes: Start another antihypertensive ("help me choose") link*
>   - ☐ *Series of links listing current medications with opportunities to adjust each*
> - *Order Chem 7 now or order Chem 7 in (drop-down menu for timing of order)*

- *Suggestions for referrals include: Refer to nutritionist*
  - *Refer to cardiac rehabilitation ("help me choose" link). Refer to BP specialist ("help me choose" link)*
  - *Prompts for patient education handouts include: Print "control high blood pressure" link*
  - *Print DASH diet instructions link*
  - *Print exercise prescription (White, Shiffman, Middleton, & Cabán, 2008)*

The prompts and instructions provided to the clinician by the system in this example are detailed and easy to navigate. As the example suggests, implementation of a CDS has the potential to optimize care by ensuring that all of the details of a patient's health issues are presented to the clinician for management, thereby promoting individualized approaches to the total health of the patient based on best available evidence and clinical guidelines (HealthIT.gov, n.d.).

RFID technologies have both supply chain and patient care applications to patient safety. An RFID system contains a tag affixed to an object or to a person that functions as a radio-frequency transponder and provides a unique identification code, a reader that receives and decodes the information contained on the tag, and an antenna that transmits the information between the tag and the reader. When RFID tags are embedded in patient identification bracelets, they can help with patient tracking during procedures and testing or function as part of the EHR communicating pertinent information to clinicians at the bedside. RFIDs may be part of the medication administration process, replacing bar-code technologies. They can be used to track medical supplies and equipment, thereby reducing staff time in locating such items. They may also be embedded into surgical supplies to automate supply-counting procedures, thereby reducing the likelihood that sponges or tools will be erroneously left in a patient. RFIDs may also reduce the likelihood of wrong-patient, wrong-site surgical procedures (Revere, Black, & Zalila, 2010). RFIDs used in the medication supply chain protect patients by reducing the potential that a counterfeit medication might be inadvertently introduced into the supply and by providing for efficient medication recalls. Potential terrorist manipulation of the medication supply is also thwarted by RFID supply chain tracking technology. Blood and blood products can be efficiently tracked by RFIDs because specialized tags can detect temperature fluctuations and, therefore, ensure that the blood or blood product was stored at the optimal temperature for safe administration (Wicks et al., 2006).

Smart rooms are being tested for wider use in health care facilities. As a caregiver enters the room, the RFID tag on his or her name badge announces to the patient on a monitor (typically mounted on the wall in the patient's line of sight) exactly who has entered the room and triggers "need to know" data based on caregiver status to be displayed on the monitor in the room. For example, when a dietary aide enters the room, only dietary information is displayed; when a physician or nurse enters, all of the pertinent medical data from the EHR are available. Clinicians can review patient data in real time and chart care at the bedside using touchscreen technology, thereby increasing productivity (Cronin, 2010). Some smart room technologies include work flow algorithms to alert clinicians as they enter the room about procedures that need to be implemented for the patient and can track individual clinician efficiency and effectiveness by aggregating data over time (Sharbaugh & Boroch, 2010).

New technologies to improve patient monitoring include **wearable technology** and wireless area networks, variously called "body area networks" or "patient area networks." The technologies provide the ability to wear a small unobtrusive monitor that collects and transmits physiologic data via a cell phone to a server for clinician review. Although most of these technologies are designed for monitoring patients with chronic diseases, they also have safety implications because they help to identify early warning physiologic signs of impeding serious health events (California Healthcare Foundation, 2007). A wireless chip on a disposable Band-Aid with a 5- to 7-day battery promises to be able to monitor the patient's heart rate and electrocardiogram, blood glucose, blood pH, and blood pressure, allowing for the collection of important clinical data outside the hospital (Miller, 2008). Wearable stress-sensing monitors detect electrical changes in the skin that may signal increased stress in autistic children who are unable to communicate an impending crisis; caregivers are alerted to the potential crisis via wireless transmission and can intervene to reduce the stress and prevent the crisis (Murph, 2010). Several new technologies promise to aid in early detection of falls in the elderly, including a wearable pendant that triggers a personal emergency response system (Aging in Place Technology Watch, 2012) and smart slippers with pressure sensors in the soles that transmit movement data wirelessly to a remote monitoring site (Mobihealthnews, 2009).

Robotics technologies are also being increasingly tested for safety and efficiency uses. Robotics has been used in minimally invasive surgery for some time; however, newer devices are including haptic (tactile) feedback to the surgeon, thereby increasing the sense of reality during the procedure and reducing the potential for unsafe manipulation (June, 2010). A robot designed to assist with patient lifting promises increased safety for both patients and clinicians (Melanson, 2010). Finally, laser-guided robots are performing such routine functions as emptying and disposing of trash, cleaning rooms, delivering supplies and meals, and dispensing drugs (Savoy, 2010).

Interdisciplinary Collaboration

Interdisciplinary collaboration or **interprofessional collaboration** are terms used to describe a cooperative relationship among actively engaged professionals where health care decision making is shared, combining their collective knowledge and skills to care for their patients. The professionals are all working toward the same goal: positive patient outcomes. Interprofessional collaboration is crucial when caring for patients since the open exchange of ideas, experience, and knowledge helps the professionals develop a comprehensive plan of care. Kuziemsky and Reeves (2012) stated,

Informatics and interprofessional collaboration are two fields where there is great potential for synergy. Importantly, information technology can assist communication between professionals in both a synchronous fashion (e.g. computer

conferencing and web-based interactions) and an asynchronous manner (e.g. email and Wikis). As a result, it can also overcome traditional limitations related to interprofessional work and its need for real-time interaction in a shared physical location. (p. 438)

It is important for educators and administrators to realize the potential for preparing collaborators by developing a collaborative approach and interprofessional educational activities and opportunities. This will foster their willingness to participate in interprofessional collaboration efforts on behalf of their patients. Refer to the website of the Center for the Advancement of Interprofessional Education for information on the principles, values, processes, and outcomes of interprofessional education (http://caipe.org.uk/about-us/the-definition-and-principles-of-interprofessional-education).

Informaticists must recognize their position on the team to promote interprofessional collaboration; so too, each professional must appreciate that this is his or her obligation to every patient. They must be willing to share, communicate, and deliberate with other professionals caring for the same patient to achieve the best outcome for the patient. We must all work together to enhance quality and secure the most positive patient outcomes for each and every patient we treat.

Role of the Health Informaticist

The human side of patient safety is paramount. As technologies that can help to reduce errors and increase safety are integrated into caregiving activities, health care professionals must also improve their ability to use and manage these technologies. Therefore, not only must the technology be scrutinized and tested routinely, but the users must also be maintained and nurtured so that they are able to use the tools to the patient's benefit, avoiding harm and keeping the patient safe. Even the best CDS systems can contribute to mistakes by providing meaningless or harmful information. Health informaticists and the IT team in the facility must ensure that all systems are properly configured and maintained. They should routinely monitor and check these systems while making sure that their human potential—that is, the user—is capable of using the systems accurately to avoid errors. A technology and its user can never be left to their own devices.

Human inputting activities must focus on patient safety to raise the appropriate issues and sound out solutions. Health informaticists must be involved in all stages of the system development life cycle while maintaining a focus on safety. Safety concerns and remedies need to be analyzed, synthesized, and integrated throughout the system development life cycle to have a robust tool that provides meaningful information and enhances patient care while preventing errors and promoting patient safety. According to Effken and Carty (2002), "Creating a safe patient environment is a very complex issue that will require the combined knowledge and skill of clinical informaticists, informatics faculty, researchers, and system designers" (para. 16). There are two Research Briefs. Research Brief 1 describes the results of a survey on the impact of nurse informaticists on patient safety, and Research Brief 2 describes the effect of a pleural checklist on patient safety in the ultrasound era.

RESEARCH BRIEF 1: IMPACT OF NURSE INFORMATICISTS ON PATIENT SAFETY

In 2009, HIMSS conducted an Informatics Nurse Impact Survey sponsored by McKesson (HIMSS, 2009c). This web-based survey yielded 432 acceptable responses over a 2-month period from December 2008 to February 2009.

One of the areas assessed was "value and impact of informatics nurse," on a scale of 1 to 7, with 7 being the highest rating:

Respondents believe that informatics nurses involved in system analysis, design, selection, implementation and optimization of IT have the greatest impact on patient safety (6.21), work flow (6.17), and user/clinician acceptance (6.15). The area with the least impact was integration with other systems (6.03). These findings suggest the informatics nurse is a driver of quality of care and enhanced patient safety within their organization (p. 2).

This demonstrates the belief that nurse informaticists can greatly improve patient safety. The nurse executives who responded rated the positive impact of nurse informaticists on patient safety at 6.36 out of 7.

In their conclusion, the researchers stated,

The role of informatics nurses is not limited to IT; this research also suggests that informatics nurses play an instrumental role with regard to patient safety, change management and usability of systems as evidenced by their impact on quality outcomes, workflow, and user acceptance. These additional areas highlight the value of informatics nurses—their expertise truly translates to the adoption of more effective, higher quality clinical applications in healthcare organizations. (p. 11)

Source: The full article appears in HIMSS (2009c).

RESEARCH BRIEF 2: THE EFFECT OF A PLEURAL CHECKLIST ON PATIENT SAFETY IN THE ULTRASOUND ERA

Safety checklists such as this can be easily implemented as part of the EHR.

Background and Objective: Bedside ultrasound allows direct visualization of pleural collections for thoracentesis and tube thoracostomy. However, there is little information on patient safety improvement methods with this approach. The effect of a checklist on patient safety for bedside ultrasound-guided pleural procedures was evaluated.

Methods: A prospective study of ultrasound-guided pleural procedures from September 2007 to June 2010 was performed. Ultrasound guidance was routine practice for all patients under the institution's care and the freehand method was used. All operators took a half-day training session on basic thoracic ultrasound and were supervised by more experienced operators. A 14-item checklist was introduced in June 2009. It included systematic thoracic scanning and a safety audit. Clinical and safety data are described before (Phase I) and after (Phase II) the introduction of the checklist.

Results: There were 121 patients in Phase I (58.7 ±18.9 years) and 134 patients in Phase II (60.2 ±19.6 years). Complications occurred for 10 patients (8.3%) in Phase I (six dry taps, three pneumothoraces, one haemothorax) and for 2 patients (1.5%) in Phase II (one significant bleed, one malposition of chest tube) (P = 0.015). There were no procedure-related deaths. The use of the checklist alone was associated with fewer procedure-related complications. This was independent of thoracostomy rate, pleural effusion size and pleural fluid ultrasound appearance.

Conclusions: A pleural checklist with systematic scanning and close supervision may further enhance safety of ultrasound-guided procedures. This may also help promote safety while trainees are learning to perform these procedures (See et al., 2013, p. 534).

According to Kuziemsky and Reeves (2012), "Informatics is more than just technology. Rather it is an interdisciplinary science" (p. 437). The informaticist can facilitate interprofessional collaboration to improve patient care by enhancing the capability for sharing data and information in both synchronous and asynchronous formats. Therefore, the informaticist's role is critical to facilitate data, information, and knowledge exchange in a safe, secure environment that affords professionals connectivity, access, and confidence in their ability to collaborate.

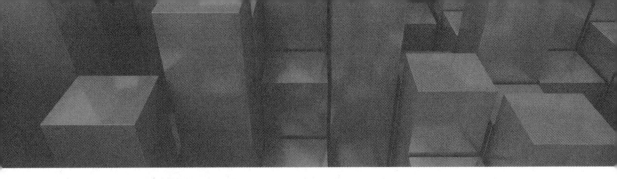

Summary

Patient safety is an important and ubiquitous issue in health care. This chapter explored the characteristics of a safety culture and technologies designed to promote patient safety. The need to evaluate errors carefully to determine why and how they occurred and how work flow processes might be changed to prevent future errors of the same type was emphasized. Technology is changing rapidly, and the culture of sharing related to technology implementation, error reporting, and troubleshooting should prompt continuous process improvements. The key for organizations is to invest in their users and choose wisely so that the technologies they are adopting will be interoperable and easily upgradable as technologies and safety practices evolve.

Organizations must make a commitment to a safety culture in which everyone at every level is committed to patient safety at every moment. In an ideal world, everyone would first stop and think "Is this safe?" before every action, work-arounds would not occur, and everyone would embrace rather than resist the technologies and work flow processes designed to promote patient safety. **Table 12-1** provides a list of websites to watch for updates on patient safety technologies. The informaticist with help professionals harness the evolving communications technologies to facilitate interprofessional collaboration and promote positive patient outcomes.

TABLE 12-1 PATIENT SAFETY WEBSITES	
Title	URL
AHRQ Patient Safety Network	http://www.psnet.ahrq.gov/primerHome.aspx
National Patient Safety Foundation	http://www.npsf.org/
National Center for Patient Safety	http://www.patientsafety.va.gov/
Institute for Healthcare Improvement	http://www.ihi.org/explore/patientsafety/Pages/default.aspx
Center for Patient Safety	http://www.centerforpatientsafety.org/
QSEN Institute (Quality and Safety Education for Nurses)	http://qsen.org/

Thought-Provoking Questions

1. What are the current patient safety characteristics of your organizational culture? Identify at least three aspects of your culture that need to be changed with regard to patient safety and suggest strategies for change.

2. Describe a current technology that you use in patient care that would benefit from human factors engineering concepts. What are some ways this technology should be improved?
3. Identify a work-around that you have used and analyze why you chose this risk-taking behavior over behavior that conforms to a safety culture.
4. Reflect on a patient situation where there was interprofessional collaboration. What was that experience like for you as the professional as well as for the patient?
5. Think about an encounter you have had with a professional who did not want to collaborate or share. What could you have done differently? What was the patient outcome?

Apply Your Knowledge

The AHRQ Patient Safety Primer on Disruptive and Unprofessional Behavior (https://psnet.ahrq.gov/primers/primer/15) offers the following insights on the effects of such behavior on patient safety:

> *Although there is no standard definition of disruptive behavior, most authorities include any behavior that shows disrespect for others, or any interpersonal interaction that impedes the delivery of patient care. Fundamentally, disruptive behavior by individuals subverts the organization's ability to develop a culture of safety. Two of the central tenets of a safe culture—teamwork across disciplines and a blame-free environment for discussing safety issues—are directly threatened by disruptive behavior. An environment in which frontline caregivers are frequently demeaned or harassed reinforces a steep authority gradient and contributes to poor communication, in turn reducing the likelihood of errors being reported or addressed. Indeed, a workplace culture that tolerates demeaning or insulting behavior is likely to be one in which workers are "named, blamed, and shamed" for making an error.*

1. If you have experienced disruptive or unprofessional behavior by another professional, share the scenario with your classmates. If you have not experienced such an event, develop a role-play scenario where one student is the aggressor and another the recipient of the disrespectful behavior.
2. Reflect on how this type of behavior impedes intraprofessional communication.
3. How is patient safety potentially compromised by disruptive or unprofessional behaviors?
4. If you were in charge, what strategies would you use to address such behaviors?

Additional Resources

Agency for Healthcare Research and Quality, Patient Safety Primer on Disruptive and Unprofessional Behavior
   https://psnet.ahrq.gov/primers/primer/15
Center for the Advancement of Interprofessional Education
   http://caipe.org.uk/about-us/the-definition-and-principles-of-interprofessional-education

Institute for Healthcare Improvement
http://www.ihi.org/knowledge/Pages/Tools/FailureModesandEffectsAnalysisTool.aspx
Medical Product Safety Network
http://www.fda.gov/MedicalDevices/Safety/MedSunMedicalProductSafetyNetwork/default.htm
National Center for Patient Safety
http://www.patientsafety.gov/CogAids/RCA/index.html#page=page-1

References

Agency for Healthcare Research and Quality. (2012). Patient safety primer: Safety culture. http://psnet.ahrq.gov/primer.aspx?primerID=5

Aging in Place Technology Watch. (2012). New more accurate fall detector helps seniors age in place safely. http://www.ageinplacetech.com/pressrelease/new-more-accurate-fall-detectorhelps-seniors-age-place-safely

American Physical Therapy Association. (2011). Today's physical therapist: A comprehensive review of a 21st-century health care profession. http://www.apta.org/uploadedFiles/APTAorg/Practice_and_Patient_Care/PR_and_Marketing/Market_to_Professionals/TodaysPhysicalTherapist.pdf

Association of UK Dietitians. (2015). How are nutrition and diet linked to patient safety? https://www.bda.uk.com/improvinghealth/yourhealth/patientsafety

Bates, D., & Gawande, A. (2003). Improving safety with information technology. *New England Journal of Medicine, 348*, 2526–2534.

Blankenhorn, D. (2010). Can better tools overcome the medical compliance crazy? http://www.zdnet.com/blog/healthcare/can-better-tools-overcome-the-medical-compliance-crazy/3925

Blum, J., Kruger, G., Sanders, K., Gutierrez, J., & Rosenberg, A. (2009). Specificity improvement for network distributed physiologic alarms based on a simple deterministic reactive intelligent agent in the critical care environment. *Journal of Clinical Monitoring and Computing, 23*(1), 21–30.

California Healthcare Foundation. (2007). Healthcare unplugged: The evolving role of wireless technology. http://www.chcf.org/~/media/Files/PDF/H/PDF%20HealthCareUnpluggedTheRoleOfWireless.pdf

Cochran, C., Jones, K., Brockman, J., Skinner, A., & Hicks, R. (2007). Errors prevented by and associated with bar-code administration systems. *The Joint Commission Journal on Quality and Patient Safety, 33*(5), 293–301. http://www.scribd.com/doc/12844778/Errors-Prevented-by-and-Associated-With-BCMA

Cohen, M. (2002). Bar code labeling for drug products. Proceedings of the Food and Drug Administration's July 26, 2002, public meeting. http://www.ismp.org/pressroom/viewpoints/FdaBarCoding.asp

Cronin, M. (2010). SmartRooms from IBM connect hospital staff to patient data. http://www.cerner.com/uploadedFiles/Content/Solutions/_White_Papers/Medical_Devices/NCH_Smart_Room_Whitepaper.pdf

Dulak, S. (2005). Technology today: Smart IV pumps. http://www.modernmedicine.com/modernmedicine/article/articleDetail.jsp?id=254828

Ebben, S., Gieras, I., & Gosbee, L. (2008). Harnessing hospital purchase power to design safe care delivery. *Biomedical Instrumentation & Technology, 42*(4), 326–331.

Effken, J., & Carty, B. (2002). The era of patient safety: Implications for nursing informatics curricula. *Journal of the American Medical Informatics Association, 9*(6, Suppl. 1). http://www.ncbi.nlm.nih.gov/pmc/articles/PMC419434

eMedonline. (n.d.). How eMedonline works. http://www.emedonline.com/about.asp?topic=howitworks

Francisco, E., Horlak, D., & Azevedo, S. (2010). The balance between safety and efficacy. *Journal of Professional Excellence Dimensions of Dental Hygiene, 8*(2), 26–27, 29–30. http://www.dimensionsofdentalhygiene.com/2010/02_February/Features/The_Balance_Between_Safety_and_Efficacy.aspx

Harrison, J., & Daly, M. (2009). Leveraging health information technology to improve patient safety. *Public Administration and Management, 14*(1), 218–237.

Healthcare Information and Management Systems Society. (2009a). Approaching CDS in medication management. http://healthit.ahrq.gov/images/mar09_cds_book_chapter/CDS_MedMgmnt_ch_1_sec_3_applying_CDS.htm

Healthcare Information and Management Systems Society. (2009b). Clinical decision support (CDS) fact sheet. http://www.himss.org/content/files/CDSFactSheet3-17-09.pdf

Healthcare Information and Management Systems Society. (2009c). Informatics nurse impact survey sponsored by McKesson. http://www.himss.org/files/HIMSSorg/content/files/HIMSS2009NursingInformaticsImpactSurveyFullResults.pdf

HealthIT.gov. (n.d.). CDS Implementation. http://www.healthit.gov/policy-researcher simplementers/cds-implementation

Institute of Medicine. (2000). *To err is human: Building a safer health system.* L. Kohn, Corrigan, & M. Donaldson (Eds.). Washington, DC: National Academies Press. http://psnet.ahrq.gov/resource.aspx?resourceID=1579

Institute of Medicine. (2001). *Crossing the quality chasm: A new health system for the 21st century.* Washington, DC: National Academies Press. http://psnet.ahrq.gov/resource.aspx?resourceID=1564

Institute for Healthcare Improvement. (2011a). Develop a culture of safety. http://www.ihi.org/knowledge/Pages/Changes/DevelopaCultureofSafety.aspx

Institute for Healthcare Improvement. (2011b). Failure modes and effects analysis tool. http://www.ihi.org/knowledge/Pages/Tools/FailureModesandEffectsAnalysisTool.aspx

Institute for Healthcare Improvement. (2012). Reduce adverse drug events (ADES) involving intravenous medications: Implement smart infusion pumps. http://www.ihi.org/knowledge/Pages/Changes/ReduceAdverseDrugEventsInvolvingIntravenousMedications.aspx

Institute for Safe Medication Practices. (2007, April 19). Smart pumps are not smart on their own. http://ismp.org/Newsletters/acutecare/articles/20070419.asp

Institute for Safe Medication Practices. (2008). Guidance on the interdisciplinary safe use of automated dispensing cabinets. http://www.ismp.org/tools/guidelines/ADC_Guidelines_Final.pdf

Joint Commission. (2008). Sentinel event alert #42: Safely implementing health information and converging technologies. http://www.jcrinc.com/Sentinel-Event-Alert-42

June, L. (2010). Sofie surgical robot gives haptic feedback for a more humane touch. http://www.engadget.com/2010/10/11/sofie-surgical-robot-gives-haptic-feedback-for-a-more/

Kallstrom, T. (2015). Putting patients first. http://www.aarc.org/putting-patients-first

Kuziemsky, C., & Reeves, S. (2012). The intersection of informatics and interprofessional collaboration. *Journal of Interprofessional Care, 26,* 437–439.

LeapFrog Group. (2008). Fact sheet: Computerized physician order entry. http://www.leapfroggroup.org/media/file/FactSheet_CPOE.pdf

Manor, P. (2010). CPOE: Strategies for success. *Nursing Management, 41*(5), 18.

Melanson, D. (2010). Yurina health care robot promises to help lift, terrify patients. http://www.engadget.com/2010/08/13/yurina-health-care-robot-promises-to-help-lift-terrify-patients

Miller, P. (2008). Wireless chip on a Band-Aid to monitor patients from home. http://www.engadget.com/2008/02/05/wireless-chip-on-a-band-aid-to-monitor-patients-from-home

Miller, R., & Hoffman, W. (2014, January). Building a whole new mind: An interprofessional experience in patient safety and quality improvement education using the IHI open school. *South Dakota Medicine,* 17–23.

Mobihealthnews. (2009). AT&T develops "smart slippers" for fall prevention. http://mobihealth news.com/5675/att-develops-smart-slippers-for-fall-prevention

Murph, D. (2010). Affectiva's Q Sensor wristband monitors and logs stress levels, might bring back the snap bracelet. http://www.engadget.com/2010/11/02/affectivas-q-sensor -wristbandmonitors-and-logs-stress-levels

National Patient Safety Foundation. (2013). Definitions and hot topics. http://www.npsf.org /for-healthcare-professionals/resource-center/definitions-and-hot-topics

Nexus 6. (2010). What are smart inhalers? http://www.smartinhaler.com

Organization for Safety, Asepsis and Prevention. (2014, November/December). Steering toward patient safety. CE course on establishing patient safety in the dental office. *The Dental Assistant*, 24–27.

Revere, L., Black, K., & Zalila, F. (2010). RFIDs can improve the patient care supply chain. *Hospital Topics, 88*(1), 26–31.

Savoy, V. (2010). Robots to invade Scottish hospital, pose as "workers." http://www.engadget .com/2010/06/21/robots-to-invade-scottish-hospital-pose-as-workers

See, K., Jamil, K., Chua, A., Phua, J., Khoo, K., & Keang, T. (2013). Effect of a pleural checklist on patient safety in the ultrasound era. *Respirology, 18*, 534–539.

Sharbaugh, D., & Boroch, M. (2010). Hospital smart rooms are ready for rollout. http://www .buildings.com/tabid/3413/ArticleID/9675/Default.aspx

SIMpill. (2008). The SIMpill medication adherence solution. http://www.simpill.com/thesimple solution.html

Snyder, M., Carter, A., Jenkins, K., & Frantz, C. (2010). Patient misidentifications caused by errors in standard barcode technology. *Clinical Chemistry, 56*(10), 1554–1561.

University of Alabama at Birmingham. (2013). UAB Medicine: The connected hospital. http:// www.uabmedicine.org/news/news-nursing-the-connected-hospital

Wachter, R. (2010). Patient safety at ten: Unmistakable progress, troubling gaps. *Health Affairs, 29*(1), 165–173.

Watson, L., & Odle, T. (2013). White paper: Patient safety and quality in medical imaging: The radiologic technologist's role. http://www.asrt.org/docs/default-source/whitepapers/asrt13 _patientsafetyqltywhitepaper.pdf?sfvrsn=6

White, J., Shiffman, R., Middleton, B., & Cabán, T. (2008). A national web conference on using clinical decision support to make informed patient care decisions. Slide 63: Partners CDS services: CAD/DM smart, Form Slides 63–65. Presented at Agency for Healthcare Research and Quality, September 19, 2008. http://healthit.ahrq.gov/images/sep08cdswebconference /textmostly

Wicks, A., Visich, J., & Li, S. (2006). Radio frequency identification applications in healthcare. *International Journal of Healthcare Technology and Management, 7*(6), 522–540.

Williams, J. (2009). Biomeds' increased involvement improves processes, patient safety. *Biomedical Instrumentation & Technology, 43*(2), 121–123.

Patient Engagement and Connected Health

Kathleen Mastrian and Dee McGonigle

OBJECTIVES

1. Define health literacy, e-health, and connected health.
2. Explore various technology-based approaches to consumer health education.
3. Assess the most common telehealth tools to engage patients at a distance.
4. Identify barriers and legal, ethical, and regulatory issues associated with technology-based connection and engagement strategies.
5. Imagine future approaches to technology-supported patient connection and engagement tools.

Introduction

Imagine that you have decided to take up running as your preferred form of exercise in a quest to get in shape. You start slowly by running a half mile and walking a half mile. You gradually build up your endurance and find yourself running nearly every day for longer distances and longer periods of time. But then you notice a nagging pain first in your right hip; over a few weeks, it gradually spreads to the center of your right buttocks and then down your right leg. You try rest and heat, but nothing seems to help. You visit your doctor, and she indicates that you have developed piriformis syndrome and prescribes physical therapy at a nearby clinic. Here, you are taught a series of stretching exercises, when and how to apply ice to the involved area, and the value of rest. You are intrigued by the diagnosis. On your return home, you log on to the Internet and begin a search for information about piriformis syndrome. When you type the words into your favorite search engine, you get 371,000 results in response to your query.

Your use of the Internet to seek health information mirrors the behavior of many consumers who are increasingly relying on the Internet for health-related

Key Terms

Blog
Central stations
Connected health
Digital divide
Domain name
E-brochure
E-health
eHealth Initiative
Empowerment
Gray gap
Health literacy
HONcode
Interactive technologies
Know–do gap
Medication management
    devices
Patient engagement
Peripheral biometric
    (medical) devices
Personal emergency
    response systems
Portals
Real-time telehealth
Sensor and activity-
    monitoring systems

(continues)

information. The challenge for consumers and health care professionals alike is the proliferation of information on the Internet and the need to learn how to recognize when information is accurate and meaningful to the situation at hand.

This chapter explores consumer information and education needs and considers how patient engagement and connected health technologies may help to meet those needs yet at the same time create ever-increasing demands for health-related information. It begins with a discussion of health literacy, e-health, and health education and information needs and explores various approaches by health care providers to using technology to promote health literacy. Also examined is the use of games, **Web quests**, and simulations as means of increasing health literacy among the school-age population. Issues associated with the credibility of web-based information and barriers to access and use are discussed. Finally, the use of telehealth technologies to engage patients at a distance and other future trends related to technology-supported consumer information are explored.

Consumer Demand for Health Information

This is the Knowledge Age; many people want to be in the know. People demand news and information, and they want immediate results and unlimited access. This is increasingly true with health information. More and more people, in trends known as consumer **empowerment**, **patient engagement**, and **connected health**, are interested in partnering with health care providers to take control of their health. They are not satisfied being dependent on a health care provider to supply them with the information they need to manage their health. Instead, they are increasingly embracing electronic technologies such as patient portals offering current and past health statuses, lab results, and secure messaging with providers; social media interactions; health-related games; wearable technologies for tracking health; apps; and remote monitoring and telehealth.

The most recent Pew Internet and American Life Project health online survey report (Fox & Duggan, 2013) indicates that 8 in 10 (comparable to the numbers in previous surveys conducted in 2006 and 2011) Americans who are online have searched for health information. The most frequent health topic searches (69%) are related to a specific disease or medical problem that the searcher or a member of the family is experiencing. Other frequent topics of health-related searches are weight, diet, and exercise (60%) and health indicators such as blood parameters or sleep patterns (33%). The 2011 survey ($n = 3,001$) reports that consumers also searched for information on food (29%) and drug safety (24%) (Fox, 2011). Just over half of "online diagnosers" (those who search online for information about medical conditions) reported that they shared their Internet findings with their health care providers, and 41% reported that their findings were confirmed by a clinician (Fox & Duggan, 2013). It is clear that patients are increasingly looking to be partners with health care providers in managing their health challenges and maintaining a level of wellness. All health care professionals need to be prepared to listen to the ideas of patients about their personal health and at the same time to provide direction toward credible health information supplied by electronic provider portals on the Internet. Here is some good news: In an attempt to improve the credibility of the results of online searches about health, in 2015 Google partnered with Mayo Clinic to fact-check the information in a database for 400 of the most commonly searched for health issues (Lapowsky, 2015). Mayo Clinic (2015) reported that Google

> *became part of our daily lives. There's no need to sift through mountains of data and endless links to find the few nuggets we need. So naturally, when people have health concerns, one of their first stops is Google. But anyone who has searched the Internet to self-diagnose knows the dizzying, and sometimes scary, array of results. To help give their users the best health information possible, Google now provides relevant medical facts upfront. (p. 4)*

Google intends to "surface these pre-vetted facts at the top of its search results in hopes of getting people to the right information faster" (Lapowsky, 2015, para 2).

It is important to note that the surveys of online health behaviors are limited to those individuals who are online and do not reflect the health information needs or demands of those persons who are not online. **Digital divide** is the term used to describe the gap between those who have and those who do not have access to online information. Health care professionals need to be aware of the various components of the digital divide to ensure that patients and clients are receiving the health information they need in a format that they are interested in and can comprehend. Notably, persons with chronic diseases are less likely to have Internet connectivity. Fox and Purcell (2010) explain the disparity in that having a chronic disease is associated with increased age, level of education, ethnicity, and income—all factors also associated with the digital divide. Persons living with a chronic disease who have Internet access are likely to use the Internet for blogging and online discussion forums, activities popularly referred to as peer-to-peer support.

Missen and Cook (2007) discuss the potential impact that technology-based health information dissemination can have on the know–do gap in developing countries. The **know–do gap** reflects the fact that solutions to global health problems exist but are not implemented in a timely fashion because of the lack of access to important health information. The Internet connections in developing countries are widely scattered and may not be efficient or sufficient for viewing health care information. Missen and Cook describe the use of a freestanding hard drive loaded with hundreds of CDs of health-related information in a webpage format that responds to a search command. This is a great example of providing technologies that work with the constraints of the situation. Another example of addressing the digital divide is the growing number of health-related websites that support a Spanish language format.

Health Literacy and Health Initiatives

The goal of **health literacy** for all is one that is widely embraced in many sectors of health care; it was a major goal of *Healthy People 2010* and is being continued in the health communication and health information technology objective of *Healthy People*

2020 (Office of Disease Prevention and Health Promotion & U.S. Department of Health and Human Services, 2009). Clinicians who have been practicing for some time recognize that informed patients have better outcomes and pay more attention to their overall health and changes in their health than those who are poorly informed. Some of the earliest formally developed patient education programs, which included postoperative teaching, diabetes education, cardiac rehabilitation, and diet education, were implemented in response to research that suggested the positive impact of patient education on health outcomes and satisfaction with care. Glassman (2008) updated the National Network Libraries of Medicine webpage on health literacy (http://nnlm.gov/outreach/consumer/hlthlit.html). She concluded from the research on the economic impact of health literacy that those persons with low health literacy have less ability to manage a chronic illness properly and tend to use more health care services than those who are more literate. In addition, she used results of health research to demonstrate the impact of low health literacy and the incidence of disease.

The site states that "Health Literacy is defined in the Institute of Medicine report *Health Literacy: A Prescription to End Confusion* as 'The degree to which individuals have the capacity to obtain, process, and understand basic health information and services needed to make appropriate health decisions'" (Glassman, 2008, para. 2). For example, health care providers depend on a patient's ability to understand and follow directions associated with dietary restrictions or exercising at home. It is also assumed, sometimes erroneously, that people will correctly interpret symptoms of a serious illness and act appropriately. The ability to locate and evaluate health information for credibility and quality, to analyze the various risks and benefits of treatments, and to calculate dosages and interpret test results are among the tasks Glassman identifies as essential for health literacy. Other important and less easily learned health literacy skills are the ability to negotiate complex health care environments and understand the economics of payment for services. Parker, Ratzan, and Lurie (2003) estimated that at least one-third of all Americans have health literacy problems and lament that in a time-is-money economic climate, health care practitioners are not always reimbursed for patient education activities. This is still true today. The National Institutes of Health (NIH) (2015) reported that many studies have been done concerning health literacy and that a variety of challenges remain on both the patient and the health care provider parts of the equation.

The **eHealth Initiative** was developed to address the growing need for managing health information and to promote technology as a means of improving health information exchange, health literacy, and health care delivery. The eHealth Initiative website provides more information (http://www.ehealthinitiative.org). Although the scope of the eHealth Initiative goes beyond health literacy, a major goal continues to be empowering consumers to understand their health needs better and to take action appropriate to those needs. Poor interoperability among health care systems and failure to embrace national data standards for health care continue to be identified as barriers to the eHealth Initiative. Further, concerns about privacy and security of information and the failure to invest appropriately in technology have slowed the development of this important initiative. Several states developed viable health information networks as part of the eHealth Initiative: the Utah Health Information Network (http://www.uhin .org) and the Vermont Health Information Technology Plan (http://hcr.vermont.gov /sites/hcr/files/pdfs/vermont_health_it_plan.pdf) are examples of attempts to implement **e-health** initiatives. The Centers for Disease Control and Prevention (CDC, 2012) maintains an interactive map of the United States that provides access to health literacy and e-health initiatives by state (http://www.cdc.gov/healthliteracy).

Health Care Organization Approaches to Engagement

Health care organizations (HCOs) use a wide variety of approaches and tools to engage patients and to promote patient education and health literacy. Although the old standby for disseminating information is the paper-based flyer, some HCOs are recognizing that today's consumers are more attracted to a dynamic rather than **static medium**. In addition, the cost of designing and printing pamphlets and flyers becomes prohibitive when one considers the rapidity of change of information; the brochure may be outdated almost as soon as it is printed. One approach to deal with these issues is to have patient education information stored electronically so that changes can be made as needed or information can be better tailored to the specific patient situation and then printed out and reviewed with the patient.

Another old standby approach that is still widely used is the group education class. These classes initially were developed to help people manage chronic health problems (e.g., diabetes) and were typically scheduled while people were hospitalized. Now, many HCOs also sponsor health promotion education classes as a way of marketing their facilities and showcasing some of their expert practitioners.

The movement from static to dynamic presentations began in many HCOs as DVDs and videotapes that were shown in groups or broadcast on demand over dedicated channels via television in patients' rooms. HCOs are now also taking advantage of the fact that patients and families are captive audiences in waiting rooms by promoting education via pamphlet distribution, health promotion programs broadcast on television, and health information kiosks in those locations. The kiosks are typically computer stations and often contain a variety of self-assessment tools (especially those related to risks for diabetes, heart disease, or cancer) and searchable pages of information about specific health conditions. The self-assessment tools represent yet another step forward in technological support for education: In addition to being dynamic, the kiosk is interactive. On the assessment page, the user is asked to respond to a series of questions, and then the health risk is calculated by the computer program. One caution, however, is that just because the information is made available does not mean that people will participate or that they will understand what they have experienced. Issues related to the level of health literacy, the digital divide, and the **gray gap** (differences in electronic connectivity by age) still exist in these situations.

Many HCOs have invested time and money in developing interactive websites and believe that Web presence is a critical marketing strategy. Sternberg (2002) suggests that many websites begin as an **e-brochure** and progress through various stages to reach a true e-care status. Most offer physician search capabilities, e-newsletters, and call-center tie-ins. As with all patient education materials, there must be a sincere commitment to keeping information current and easily accessible. Web designers must pay particular attention to the aesthetics of the site, the ease of use, and the literacy level of those in the intended audience.

A usability study conducted by Lauterbach (2010) provides some insights into how to measure website usability. This researcher compared the usability of the symptom checker functions of two popular websites by asking volunteers to navigate each using four different case scenarios. Users navigated the site to find the symptom checker and then entered the symptoms and evaluated site feedback. Users rated the ease of understanding for each site and completed a short comprehension quiz. Data were collected on descriptions of user site preferences, user satisfaction with the sites, results of the comprehension quiz, and efficiency, which was measured by tracking the number of webpage changes the user performed while navigating the site.

The rapid growth of electronic communication through increased use of computers and access to the Internet, particularly for medical purposes, empowers the clinician as well as the consumer of health care information. The integration of information and communication technologies (ICTs) and the growing trend of consumer empowerment have reshaped the delivery of health care. Many HCOs, as a result of meaningful use initiatives, have developed secure patient portals that allow patients to access their health records, including tracking laboratory results and reviewing the records. Most HCOs, however, do not allow patients to edit these records. Some people are interested in interacting with others who have the same or similar conditions, and some HCOs are

---

RESEARCH BRIEF

Case studies of educational videos used on six hospital websites were the focus of this qualitative study by Huang (2009). This researcher used both within-case and cross-case analyses to describe rationales for developing and using e-health videos. He identified six main reasons for implementing e-health videos:

1. The proliferation of high-speed Internet access has made online video a well-accepted culture in the United States.
2. Many online visitors, especially young people, like to watch videos rather than read lengthy articles.
3. Videos can draw online visitors' attention, thereby attracting online traffic and further attracting visitors to the hosting hospital.
4. A video, when well produced, is worth more than a thousand words.
5. Videos can relate not only to online visitors' minds but also, and more importantly, to their hearts to build trust and drive their decision making.
6. Videos empower and inform the visitors outside of the hospital visit time, and such self-driven homework is beneficial to both the visitor and the hospital (pp. 67–68).

Source: The full article appears in Huang, 2009.

providing the information necessary to help them connect. This so-called peer-to-peer support is especially popular with patients who have cancer diagnoses, diabetes, and other chronic and debilitating conditions (Lober & Flowers, 2011).

Some HCOs are using social media as health education tools to promote actual engagement of audiences rather than as means of one-way messaging. Neiger, Thackeray, Burton, Giraud-Carrier, and Fagen (2013) suggested "that the use of social media in health promotion must lead to engagement between the health promotion organization and its audience members, that engagement must provide mutual benefit, and that an engagement hierarchy culminates in program involvement with audience members in the form of partnership or participation (as recipients of program services)" (p. 158). The CDC (2011) has an excellent social media tool kit that can be used by health educators to guide the planning and implementation of social media strategies for health promotion. This tool kit can be accessed at the following website: http://www.cdc.gov /socialmedia/Tools/guidelines/pdf/SocialMediaToolkit_BM.pdf.

Promoting Health Literacy in School-Aged Children

Promoting health literacy in school-aged children presents special challenges to health educators. There is wide agreement that childhood obesity is a serious and growing issue that is related not only to poor choice of foods but also to the sedentary lifestyles promoted by video games and television. In addition, the time once devoted to health and physical education programs in schools has given way to more time spent on core subjects, such as math and science.

The Children's Nutrition Research Center responded early to these challenges by supporting the development of nutrition education programs as interactive computer games, video games, and cartoons referred to as "edutainment" (Flores, 2006). These e-health programs are developed specifically to appeal to the generational (highly connected and computer literate) and cultural needs of this group. Flores describes the Family Web project, which uses comic strips to impart nutrition information, and Squires Quest, where the students earn points by choosing fruits and vegetables to fight the snakes and moles that are trying to destroy the healthy foods in the Kingdom of SALot. These are great examples of health education programs that are designed to appeal to this connected generation of learners and their intuitive ability to use **interactive technologies.**

Donovan (2005) describes an interdisciplinary Web quest designed to appeal to older school-aged children. The quest is interdisciplinary in that it requires reading comprehension, critical thinking, presentation, and writing; thus, core skills and health literacy skills are learned in a single assignment. Students are directed to the Web to search for information on the pros and cons of low-carbohydrate diets and obesity prevention. Students learn along the way as they search for information, collect and interpret it, and then develop a presentation and final paper.

The Cancer Game (Oda & Kristula, n.d.) was developed by a young man who was taking a college class on Macromedia software and had previously undergone a bone marrow transplant. Subsequently, he and a professor collaborated and expanded the project to its present form. The game is designed as an arcade-style video game for cancer patients to relieve stress by visualizing the fighting of cancer cells. Although cancer victims of any age can access and play the game, it has a special appeal to children and adolescents. Find the game here: http://www.cancergame.org. Similarly, Ben's Game (http://www.makewish.org/site/pp.asp?c=cvLRKaO4E&b=64401) is a video game designed to help relieve the stress of cancer treatment for children (Anderson & Klemm, 2008).

Games have also been designed for other conditions, such as diabetes (Glymetrix Diabetes Game, 2009). You can access these newer games on the Internet by typing "health games" into a search engine. Be sure to review the information presented in the game for accuracy before you recommend it to parents and children. The National Library of Medicine maintains a site dedicated to health learning games for both children and adults (https://www.nlm.nih.gov/medlineplus/games.html). You can feel confident in recommending games from this trusted website, as they have been vetted for accuracy and credibility.

Supporting Use of the Internet for Health Education

Health care professionals need to embrace the Internet as a source of health information for patient education and health literacy. Patients are increasingly turning there for instant information about their health maladies. Health-related **blogs** (short for **weblog**, an online journal) and electronic patient and parent support groups are also proliferating at an astounding rate. Professionals need to be prepared to arm patients with the skills required to identify credible websites. They also need to participate in the development of well-designed, easy-to-use health education tools. Finally, they need to convince payers of the necessity of health education and the powerful impact education has on promoting and maintaining health. **Box 13-1** provides more information about patient education.

The Health on the Net (HON) Foundation (2005) survey describes the certifications and accreditation symbols that identify trusted health sites. The **HONcode** and **Trust-e** were identified as the two most common symbols that power users look for. The survey also indicated that Internet users look at the **domain name** and frequently gravitate toward university sites (.edu), government sites (.gov), and HCO sites (.org). Half of the survey respondents were in favor of the use of a domain name called .health to identify quality health information websites. In contrast, Pew/Internet (2006) indicates that nearly 75% of online searchers do not check the date or the source of information they are accessing on the Web and that 3% of online health seekers report knowing someone who was harmed by following health information found on the Web. Website developers can apply for HONcode certification of web-based materials. Initial certification is for 1 year, and then the site is reevaluated annually by experts. The HON Foundation also monitors site complaints and factors reported issues into the recertification process (HON Foundation, 2014).

BOX 13-1   CONSIDERATIONS FOR PATIENT EDUCATION

Julie A. Kenney and Ida Androwich

Health care professionals need to take many things into account when teaching patients. They need to assess patients' willingness to learn, their reading ability, the means by which they learn best, and their existing knowledge about the subject. Professionals also need to take cultural differences and language differences into account when teaching their patients. If the professional chooses to use an electronic method to educate the patient, digital natives (patients who have grown up with technology) need to be taught differently than digital immigrants (those who have been forced to learn technology) ("Educational Strategies," 2006). Digital natives are typically born after 1982 and may also be referred to as "Generation Y." This generation prefers to learn using technology. The younger group learns quite well if information is presented in a format to which they are accustomed, such as an interactive video game to introduce them to a topic. This group is also comfortable using information that they can access via their handheld devices, such as smartphones and tablets, as well as wearable devices, such as smartwatches. Those born before 1982 may have learning styles that range from preferring to learn in a classroom setting to reading a book about the topic to learning using a hands-on, interactive approach ("Educational Strategies," 2006).

REFERENCE

Educational strategies in generational designs. (2006). *Progress in Transplantation, 16*(1), 8–9.

PATIENT EDUCATION WEBSITE EXAMPLES

American Academy of Family Physicians: http://www.familydoctor.org

American Cancer Society: http://www.cancer.org

American Heart Association: http://www.americanheart.org

Centers for Disease Control and Prevention: http://www.cdc.gov

Krames (products to purchase): http://www.krames.com

Patient Education Center (provided by Harvard Medical School): http://www.patienteducationcenter.org

Patient Education Institute: http://www.patient-education.com

The U.S. National Library of Medicine and the National Institutes of Health jointly sponsor MedlinePlus, a website that has a tutorial for learning how to evaluate health information and an electronic guide to Web surfing that is available in both English and Spanish. This site is found at http://www.nlm.nih.gov/medlineplus/webeval/webeval.html. A similar guide explains the major things one should evaluate when accessing health-related resources on the Web (National Center for Complementary and Alternative Medicine, 2008) and can be accessed at http://nccam.nih.gov/health/webresources. Suggest that patients visit these sites to become more adept at identifying whether a website is credible before they adopt the recommendations provided.

Some health care professionals have partnered with their organizations to develop patient education materials. These materials must be carefully reviewed for accuracy and usability. The Agency for Healthcare Research and Quality (2013) published an assessment tool for both print and audio-visual patient education materials. Their tool is designed to assess both understandability and actionability by providing a series of review criteria for each of these domains. The tool can be accessed at http://www.ahrq .gov/professionals/prevention-chronic-care/improve/self-mgmt/pemat/index.html. Clearly, the health care professional is very important in engaging the patient to partner with them in the management of their health . Refer to Box 13-1 and **Box 13-2** to review effective education methods used in teaching patients and their families about their health challenges.

Some organizations and providers have developed a list of credible websites and apps that are shared with patients or family members. Recommendations for websites might include the U.S. Department of Health and Human Services–sponsored Healthfinder site (http://www.healthfinder.gov), a website dedicated to helping consumers find credible information on the Internet. Other excellent sources of reliable information are the National Institutes of Health (http://www.nih.gov), the Centers for Disease Control and Prevention (http://www.cdc.gov), Medline Plus (http://www.medlineplus.gov), NIH-SeniorHealth (http://www.nihseniorhealth.gov), and the National Health Information Center (http://www.health.gov/nhic). Some of the apps that might be recommended include Mayo Clinic on Pregnancy (https://itunes.apple.com/WebObjects/MZStore .woa/wa/viewSoftware?id=656908781&mt=8), WebMD Pain Coach (https://itunes .apple.com/us/app/webmd-pain-coach/id536303342?mt=8), and Understanding Diseases (https://itunes.apple.com/us/app/understanding-diseases/id530900371?mt=8). These are great examples of the wealth of patient information being developed as apps by hospitals and other health care providers. More apps are being developed every day to engage people in managing their health and to help them take control of their health. Perhaps the most important thing that health care professionals can stress is that not all of these have credible and valid information. We must encourage our patients to become savvy users of electronic information sources.

Future Directions for Engaging Patients

Predicting future directions for technology-based health education is somewhat difficult because one may not be able to completely envision the technology of the future. One can predict, however, that some current technologies will be used increasingly to support health literacy, and new technologies will be developed every day. For example, audio and video podcasts may become more common in health education and be provided as free downloads from the websites of HCOs.

Voice recognition software used to navigate the Web may reduce the frustration and confusion associated with attempting to spell complex medical terms. However, the confusion and frustration may increase if the patient or client is unable to pronounce the terms. Voice interactivity should help to reduce the digital access disparity associated with those who have limited keyboard or mouse skills. For those persons with visual impairments, some websites may provide both audio and text information and support increased text size for greater ease of reading (Anderson & Klemm, 2008).

BOX 13-2   CLINICIAN'S VIEW ON PATIENT EDUCATION

Denise D. Tyler

Knowledge dissemination in health care practice includes sharing information with patients and families so that they understand their health care needs well enough to participate in developing the plan of care, make informed decisions about their health, and ultimately comply with the plan of care, both during hospitalization and as outpatients.

There are several effective methods for educating patients and their families. Providing one-on-one and classroom instruction are traditional and valuable forms of education. One-on-one education is interactive and can be adjusted at any time during the process based on the needs of the individual patient or family; it can also be supplemented by written material, videos, and web-based learning applications. Classroom education can be beneficial because patients and families with similar needs or problems can network, thereby enhancing the individual experience. However, the ability to interact with each member of the group and to tailor the educational experience based on individual needs may be limited by the size and dissimilarities of the group. Individual follow-up should be available when possible.

Paper-based education that is created, printed, and distributed by individual institutions or providers can be very effective because materials can be distributed at any time and reviewed when the patient feels like learning. Many agencies, such as the CDC, have education for patients available on their websites. These documents can be reviewed online, or they can be printed out by health care providers or patients. Organizations can also develop and distribute information and instructions specific to their policies and procedures. In addition, printed educational material can be purchased from companies that employ experts in the subject matter and instructional design.

One of the most popular sources of patient education information is the Internet. Many hospitals and health care organizations provide proprietary information, such as directions to the facility, information on procedures, and instructions on what to expect during hospitalization, in this manner. Other health organizations, such as the National Institutes of Health, provide detailed information on their websites. Clinicians should be cautious when recommending websites to patients and families because not all sites are reliable or valid.

Many companies that provide clinical information systems or electronic health records also include patient education materials linked to the clinical system via an intranet. Thus, standardized instructions that are specific to a procedure or disease process can be printed from this computer-based application. Discharge instructions that are interdisciplinary and patient specific can often be modified via drop-down lists or selectable items that can be deleted or changed by the health care professionals caring for the patient. This ability to modify before printing provides more consistent and individualized instruction. The computer-based generation of instruction is preferable to free text and verbal instruction because it also allows the information to be linked to a coded language and, therefore, easily used for measurement and quality assurance reporting. Relevant triggers may be embedded in the clinical information systems. For example, when a patient answers "yes" to a question about current smoking, smoking cessation information should automatically be printed, or a trigger should remind the respiratory therapist or nurse to explore this topic with the patient and then provide the patient with preprinted information on smoking cessation.

Integration of standardized discharge instructions and patient education into the clinical system is another way to improve the compliance and documentation of education; it also streamlines the work flow of clinicians. Printing the information to give to the patient should be seamless to the clinician who is documenting in the electronic health record. The format should be logical and easy to read. The more transparent the process, the more efficient the system and the easier it is to use for the health care professional. What I envision for the future is a system that "remembers" the style of learning preferred by patients and their families, prompts the provider to print handouts, and programs the bedside computer/video education system based on previous selections and surveys. This interactive patient and family education will be integrated into the clinical system and the patient's personal health record.

Many websites associated with government and national organizations are also providing multiple-language access to health information and decision support tools. The multilanguage access broadens the population to whom education can be provided, and the decision support programs allow users to access results that are tailored to their age, risk factors, or disease state (Anderson & Klemm, 2008).

As patient engagement strategies become more common, we will also see a movement toward connected health. Those individuals who are frequent e-mail users may be interested in being able to communicate with physicians and other health care personnel via e-mail rather than the telephone. This idea may meet with some resistance from professionals who perceive the e-mail correspondence as bothersome and time consuming. However, it is possible that work efficiency might also increase if patients and their needs are screened via secure e-mail before an office or clinic visit. For example, as a result of an e-mail correspondence in lieu of an initial office visit, medications could be changed or diagnostic tests performed before the office visit. In addition, patients could be directed to an interactive screening form housed on a secure website where they would answer a series of questions that would help them make a decision about whether they should call for an appointment, head for the emergency room, or self-manage the issue. If self-management is the outcome of the screening tool, then the patient or caregiver could be directed to a credible website for more information. The idea is not to interfere with or replace the face-to-face visit but rather to supplement the provider–patient relationship and perhaps streamline the efficiency of health care delivery. McCray (2005) also suggests that physicians may be resistant to providing e-mail consultations and recommending health-related websites because of the potential for malpractice liability. Other health care professionals may share some of these same concerns. There is some evidence that text message reminders delivered via a cell phone are more effective and efficient as appointment reminders than traditional phone calls (Car, Gurol-Urganci, de Jongh, Vodopivec-Jamsek, & Atun, 2012). Similarly, in a descriptive research study by Dudas, Pumilia, and Crocetti (2013), it was found that parents of children who recently visited an emergency department were interested in receiving follow-up communication from health care providers by text messaging and/or e-mail. It is possible that text message reminders related to health behaviors, such as diet and exercise, might also be effective. A major barrier to widespread adoption of e-mail and text messaging among American health care providers is the fact that reimbursement mechanisms for electronic health care interventions are inadequate or nonexistent. This may be an issue that is resolved in the near future.

Other health care professionals may soon be a part of these patient engagement and connected health trends. Piette (2007) describes the use of interactive behavior change technology to improve the effectiveness of diabetes management. The goal of the interactive behavior change technology is to improve communication between patients and health care providers and to provide educational interventions that promote better disease management between office visits. The combination of electronic medication reminders, meters that track glycemic control longitudinally, and personal digital assistant–based calculators was found to support the behavioral interventions necessary to better manage the diabetes.

As a conclusion to their study, Watson, Bell, Kvedar, and Grant (2008) caution that even though patients are part of the digital divide (lacking access or skill in electronic communications and Internet use), one cannot assume that they will be resistant to using other forms of technology to support health. These authors compared Internet users to non-Internet users and found that both groups were willing to learn to use new technology to manage type 2 diabetes, including wireless communication devices for information sharing with physicians.

Health care practitioners may soon embrace the use of "information prescriptions" (D'Alessandro, 2010) that direct patients and families to credible websites, including government and HCO websites, and wikis and blogs that may help them understand their health issues or share information with and seek support from others who have similar issues. "Information prescriptions are prescriptions of focused, evidence-based information given to a patient at the right time to manage a health problem" (D'Alessandro, 2010, p. 81). The National Health Service in the United Kingdom has developed an information prescription generator that can be used by providers or the public to access web-based health information (http://www.nhs.uk/ipg/Pages/IPStart.aspx).

Telehealth: A Tool for Connected Health

Telehealth, a relatively new term in the health care provider vocabulary, refers to a wide range of health services that are delivered by telecommunications-ready tools, such as the telephone, videophone, computer, and other technologies. The most basic of telecommunications technology, the telephone, has been used by health professionals for many years. Because of these widespread uses, people are already somewhat familiar with the value of the direct, expedient contact that telecommunications-ready tools provide for health care professionals. A press release by IMS Research (2013) reported that telehealth monitoring was used for 308,000 patients in the United States in 2012 and that the demand for services on a worldwide basis is expected to reach 1.8 million patients by 2017. The growing field of telehealth will allow clinicians to improve the efficiency of care delivery services even more.

This capacity to supervise patients at a distance is predicted to continue to grow rapidly; indeed, "worldwide telemedicine markets at $7 billion in 2009 are expected to reach $24 billion by 2016" (Aarkstore Enterprise, 2010, para. 30). The ability to provide better health care access is the number one benefit of using telehealth. By reducing the need for face-to-face interaction with the patient, health care professionals can be much more efficient and productive. When information is collected in the home, it becomes much more convenient for patients, and the quality and timeliness of the information are improved dramatically. In addition, there is real value to home data collection in the normal environment rather than in a clinic, office, or hospital, where the patient's data may not be a true representation of their usual state (white coat syndrome). Home **telemonitoring** should be viewed as an enhancement to care because it allows more direct, physical intervention to occur only when it is actually needed. Care is not directed by prescheduled appointment or subjective perceptions of condition but instead can be determined by objective measures of physical status that are collected electronically at a distance. With telehealth, care can also be delivered at the most appropriate site of care, reducing reliance on emergency departments and inpatient facilities. Telehealth also helps to engage patients as partners in their care.

A significant increase is expected in the use of information technology tools in health care venues in the coming decades. This use is affected by a number of factors in all of Western society. The following factors are drivers of the growing trend toward telehealth and technology use and will influence health care professional practice significantly in the next decades: demographics (the population is aging); health care worker shortages; increased incidence of chronic diseases and conditions; the new, educated consumers who seek when-needed, as-needed care or care services delivered on their own terms and timing; and excessive costs of health care services that are increasing in need and kind.

When one connects the drivers of today's health care market—the demographics, professional shortages, and increased number of persons living with chronic conditions and their extensive use of health care services—with excessive costs of this health care, the critical need for solutions becomes obvious. The U.S. health care system spends $1.4 trillion per year on conventional medical care. Much more will be spent annually in the coming decades. One must ask, Taking all of the driving factors of today's health care market into account, what needs to be done to address health care issues in the United States and meet the burgeoning numbers and needs of patients?

One solution is to develop a new clinical model for American health care that includes technology. In particular, telehealth technology should be included to fill the gap resulting from an overabundance of patients and a scarcity of health care providers. This concept is indicated in **Figure 13-1**.

Consider the use of technology that might potentially fill the current gaps in the health care system. Tools of telehealth can, for example, help render needed services without requiring in-person professional care at all contacts. The remote or virtual visit made by skilled clinicians is just one approach to using the range of health technologies available today. More needs to be learned about what telehealth is, how it works, and which aspects have been successful so that clinicians can plan to incorporate its use into routine clinical care.

Health care professionals need to be aware of the specific legal, ethical, and regulatory issues associated with telehealth. In the United States, interstate practice of telehealth, for example, requires providers to be licensed to practice in all of the states in which they provide telehealth services by directly interacting with patients. This is particularly important when health care professionals work for health systems that are located near state borders and draw patients from both states. The Telehealth Resource Center provides a nice overview of Licensure and Scope of Practice issues; access it at http://www .telehealthresourcecenter.org/toolbox-module/licensure-and-scope-practice.

Patient confidentiality and the privacy and safety of clinical data must also be given special consideration. Informed consent releases to receive telehealth services are a critical first step. Follow the evolution of policies related to telehealth at the Center for Connected Health Policy (http://cchpca.org).

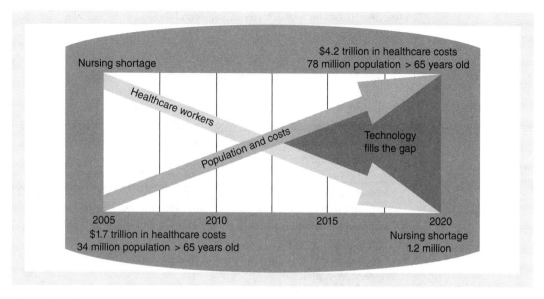

Figure 13-1 Technology Fills the Gap
Source: Courtesy of Honeywell International Inc.

Telehealth Care

Let us start with a basic definition of **telehealth care**. Keep in mind, however, that telehealth is an emerging field, and definitions are subject to change and improvement as technology evolves. The American Telemedicine Association (2010) provides the following definition:

> *Telemedicine is the use of medical information exchanged from one site to another via electronic communications to improve patients' health status. Closely associated with telemedicine is the term "telehealth," which is often used to encompass a broader definition of remote health care that does not always involve clinical services. Videoconferencing, transmission of still images, e-health including patient portals, remote monitoring of vital signs, continuing medical education and nursing call centers are all considered part of telemedicine and telehealth. (para. 1)*

Indeed, "telehealth" is generally used as an umbrella term to describe all of the possible variations of health care services that use telecommunications. Telehealth can refer to clinical and nonclinical uses of health-related contacts. Delivery of patient education, such as menu planning for patients with diabetes or the transmission of exercise reminders, is an example of the health-promoting aspects of telehealth.

A few clinical uses for telehealth technologies and some sample clinical applications include the following:

- Transmitting images for assessment or diagnosis. One example is transmission of digital images, such as images of wounds for assessment and treatment consults.
- Transmitting clinical data for assessment, diagnosis, or disease management. One example is remote patient monitoring and transmitting patients' objective or subjective clinical data, such as monitoring of vital signs and answers to disease management questions.
- Providing disease prevention and promotion of good health. One example is telephonic case management and patient education provided through asthma and weight management programs conducted in schools.
- Using telephonic health advice in emergent cases. One example is performing teletriage in call centers.
- Using real-time video. One example is exchanging health services or education live via videoconference.

Telehealth Transmission Formats and Their Clinical Applications

Nurses must become familiar with the many and varied clinical and nonclinical transmission formats and applications of telehealth technologies so that they can make informed choices about the tools that are available for their use, as needed. Among these applications are store-and-forward telehealth, real-time telehealth, remote monitoring, and telephony.

Store-and-Forward Telehealth

In a **store-and-forward telehealth transmission**, digital images, video, audio, and clinical data are captured and stored on the client computer or device; then, at a convenient time, the data are transmitted securely (forwarded) to a specialist or clinician at another location where they are studied by the relevant specialist or clinician. If indicated, the opinion of the specialist or clinician is then transmitted back. Based on the requirements of the participating health care entities, this round-trip interaction could take anywhere from a few minutes to 48 hours. In many store-and-forward specialties, such as teleradiology, an immediate response is not critical. Dermatology, radiology, and pathology are common specialties whose practices are conducive to store-and-forward technologies. Transmission of wound care images for assessment by specialty care nurses or other specialists has become a frequently used and important form of home telehealth nursing practice.

Real-Time (or Interactive) Telehealth

In **real-time telehealth**, a telecommunications link between the involved parties allows a real-time or live interaction to take place. Videoconferencing equipment is one of the most common forms of technologies used in synchronous telehealth. In addition, peripheral devices can be attached to computers or to the videoconferencing equipment to facilitate an interactive examination. Use of computers for real-time two-way audio and video streaming between centers over ever-improving and cheaper communication channels is becoming common. These developments have contributed to lowering of costs in telehealth.

Examples of real-time clinical telehealth applications include the following:

- Telemental health, which uses videoconferencing technology to connect a mental health specialist with a mental health client.
- Telerehabilitation, which uses videocameras and other technologies to assess patients' progress in home rehabilitation.
- Telehome care, which uses video technologies to observe, assess, and teach patients living in rural areas.
- Teleconsultations, which use a variety of technologies to enable collaborative exchanges or consultations between individuals or among groups that are involved with a case. These teleconsults may be transmitted live using videoconferencing technology. They may, for example, involve teaching a certain technique to a less experienced clinician, or they may provide several clinicians with an opportunity to discuss an appropriate approach to a difficult case.
- Telehospice or telepalliative care, which can use real-time or remote monitoring to provide psychological support to patients and caregivers. Telehealth devices can also play a role in symptom management, in effect helping end-of-life patients achieve an optimal quality of life.

Remote Monitoring (Telemonitoring or Remote Patient Monitoring)

In remote monitoring, devices are used to capture and transmit biometric data. For example, a tele-electroencephalogram device can monitor the electrical activity of a patient's brain and then transmit those data to a specialist assigned to the case. This interaction could occur either in real time or as a stored and then forwarded transmission. Examples of telemonitoring include the following:

- Monitoring patient parameters during home-based nocturnal dialysis
- Cardiac and multiparameter monitoring of remote intensive care units
- Home telehealth—for example, daily home telemonitoring of vital signs and weight by patients and subsequent transmission of those data that enables off-site professionals to track their patients regularly and precisely and address noticeable changes through education and information suggestions about diet or exercise
- Disease management

Tools of Home Telehealth

A wide and growing range of telecommunications-ready tools are available for health care professionals' and patients' use in the home. These tools are examined in more detail next.

Central Stations, Web Servers, and Portals

Central stations, Web servers, and portals are various terms for the technologies presently used as part of multifunctional telehealth care platforms and application servers. These clinical management software programs receive and display patients' vital signs and other information transmitted from a medical device, including blood pressure, weight, and glucose information. Such transmission is most commonly accomplished over plain old telephone system (POTS) lines; however, network access and wireless communication is gaining popularity as technology advances and access improves.

Central stations and Web servers are key components of telehealth that can be as minimal as a single screen display or as comprehensive as software applications that provide various functions, including triaging the data based on medical alerts, which allows clinicians to quickly identify those patients requiring immediate attention. Other features found in these packages allow clinicians to build personal medical records for patients and provide trended patient data and analysis reports supporting improved patient outcomes using telehealth. In addition, some of the software packages provide remote programming capabilities that allow the clinician to remotely program the medical device in the patient's home. Such an application can change monitoring report times for patients, individualize alert parameters, set up reminders, and send educational content to a patient.

Peripheral Biometric (Medical) Devices

Peripheral biometric (medical) devices can consist of fully integrated systems, such as a vital signs monitor, or they may be stand-alone telecommunications-ready devices, such as blood pressure cuffs and blood glucose meters. Many of these devices plug directly into the household telephone jack to send data to a central server location.

An ever-increasing number of peripheral devices are being introduced to the market. Examples of other peripheral devices seen in home telehealth today include pulse oximeters; prothrombin time, International Normalized Ratio meters; spirometers; peak flow meters; electrocardiogram monitors; and card readers and writers that use smart card technology and enable multiple users to use one device.

Telephones

Telephones are already the most familiar household communication tool used in telehealth care. A telephone device can be augmented for easier use by patients, as needed, with a lighted dial pad, an auto-dial system, or a louder ringer.

Videocameras and Videophones

Videocameras and videophones are readily available consumer items that can be used in telehealth for show-and-tell demonstrations by health care professionals for patients or to capture wound healing progress, among other applications. Typically, these products operate as a standard telephone or as a video picture telephone, using standard telephone lines to transmit information or interactions.

Currently, the image quality over a POTS is limited by the bandwidth of POTS technology, which favors use of such images for assessment rather than delivering diagnostic-quality images. These imaging capabilities will improve as integrated services digital network lines become more widely available in the home environment. Typically, medical centers and hospitals have access to larger bandwidth capabilities for image transmission and viewing, thus ensuring high-quality diagnostic images and point-to-point consultations in hospital- or medical center–based settings.

Personal Emergency Response Systems

Personal emergency response systems are signaling devices worn as a pendant or otherwise made easily accessible to patients to ensure their safety and to enable them to quickly access emergency care when needed, usually in case of a fall. A preset telephone number is alerted by the patient's pushing a button on the pendant; on this signal, predesignated emergency help is dispatched. Many newer sensor options for tracking patients at home are being incorporated into multifunctioning personal emergency response systems devices, such as alerting a central call center to water flooding or smoke in a patient's home. The next section provides details on these sensors and monitors.

Sensor and Activity-Monitoring Systems

Sensor and activity-monitoring systems can track activities of daily living of seniors and other at-risk individuals in their place of residence. These sensors and monitoring systems can provide insight into behavior changes that might signal changes or deterioration of health status. Such technologies consist of wireless motion sensors that are strategically placed around the residence and can detect motion on a 24-hour basis.

One authority on these technologies, David J. Stern (2007), describes their operation further. Data from these sensors are wirelessly sent to a receiver and base station that periodically transmits the information to a centralized server through standard telephone lines. Sophisticated algorithms analyze the data, compiling data on each individual's normal patterns of behavior, including bathroom usage, sleep disturbance, meal preparation, medication interaction, and general levels of activity including fall detection. Deviations from these norms can be important warning signs of emerging health problems and can enable caregivers to intervene early.

In addition to widely used fire, security, and home gas detectors, other sensors can monitor appliances to detect whether a household appliance is turned on or off and can sometimes switch the appliance on and off for the resident. Typical applications for affixing programmable sensors can include lamps, television sets, irons, and kitchen stoves. Such sensors might be very valuable for ensuring the safety of elderly, forgetful persons who live alone. One excellent example of today's sensor use for assistance with the elderly are sensors placed in or on stovetops to alert the user when he or she is standing too close to the equipment or when the kettle or pot has boiled over. Benefits realized from these technologies include enabling people to live independently with an improved quality of life. They can also provide peace of mind for other family members living at a distance.

Medication Management Devices

Medication management devices address a well-recognized major problem in health care: medication management and compliance. According to the American Heart Association (2007), 49% of Americans use prescription drugs. In fact, 32 million people are taking three or more medications daily, with even more medications typically being taken by those 65 years of age or older.

What has become a national problem in health care today is the failure of patients to take medications as prescribed. Failure to do so can have devastating consequences, particularly for those patients living with chronic illnesses. The National Pharmaceutical Council (2013) estimates that the cost of noncompliance with prescribed medications is $290 billion per year: three out of four people do not take their medications as prescribed, and one out of three people never fills his or her prescription.

To address some of these very pressing problems, a host of telecommunications-ready medication devices have become available, and many more are in development. Some are as simple as a watch that reminds a person to take medications, others are pill organizers with audible reminders, and some can be programmed to dispense prefilled containers with medications and alert a patient or caregiver of a missed dose. Furthermore, some of these medication tools send data from the device back to a central server so that patient's medication compliance can be tracked. These telecommunications-ready devices can organize, manage, dispense, or remind, and they will play an increasingly important role in helping people live independently and manage their disease processes through medication compliance.

Special Needs Telecommunications-Ready Devices

Special needs telecommunications ready-devices can include preprogrammed, multi-functional infusion pumps for meeting a range of infusion needs, including medications for pain management and other infusion delivery needs, such as hydration and nutrition, peak flow meters, electrocardiogram monitors, and so on. Many such tools are in development to meet the more demanding and challenging needs of today's at-home patients. The common goal of these tools is to increase communications between health care professionals and patients and to increase the professional's knowledge of the patient's status in a timely manner.

The Patient's Role in Telehealth

The range and sophistication of home telehealth tools are expanding regularly, and a concern of providers when choosing appropriate tools for their patients is to ask, Will my patient use this device? Elderly patients may find the monitoring technology that may speak to them in their homes and videocameras to assist in wound care tracking, for example, to be a daunting introduction to home health care. To assuage the possible discomfort, these and other such tools have undergone much iteration so that they are easier to use and patients' ability to turn them on and off is ensured. When patients are scheduled for a televisit, these devices can be turned on and used. This use by patients is critical, of course, so that the necessary information about them will be gathered and transmitted and so that their needs can be acted on by health care professionals.

Demiris, Doorenbos, and Towle (2009) emphasize consideration of usability issues when using telehealth applications with elders who may have sensory, cognitive, and motor disabilities. They suggest rigorous usability testing to maximize the quality of the user experience and special attention to design details for web-based interfaces, such as font choices and color schemes to improve readability. Similarly, Kaplan and Litweka (2008) emphasized the need for ethical design principles:

- How provider-centric or patient-centric is the technology?
- Does the shift to remote services promote rationality and efficiency at the expense of values traditionally at the heart of caregiving?
- How does the design affect home life and family dynamics?
- To what extent should technology usage involve attempts to manipulate users into different behaviors?
- How might the replacement of human contact by new technologies be ameliorated?
- To what extent is the deployment of technology an end in itself, aimed not toward the improvement of health or well-being but to create market needs?
- How do we identify the boundaries between genuine solutions and futility in light of technologies that may shift them? (p. 404)

The importance of ensuring patient satisfaction with home health service delivery was predicted to be a megatrend in 2007 (Remington, 2007). Data gathered from the Hospital Consumer Assessment of Health Providers and System survey tool will measure consumer satisfaction, which in turn will enable patient satisfaction to become a performance measurement for every provider across the health care delivery system. For this reason, health care providers must pay attention to the many examples of studies in home telehealth indicating a great deal of patient satisfaction with telehealth, particularly those that note a preference for telehealth, not conventional care. In one investigation, patients reported that the telehealth monitor helped them change the way they performed self-care (Chetney, 2006). Other studies have noted that patients seen with telehealth have a better understanding of their own disease process and describe the ease with which patients are able to manage self-care and so enjoy an improved quality of life (Sanderson, 2007). When patients achieve a good understanding of and perform self-care by the end of their home health admission periods, an important goal of home telehealth has been attained.

However, when one moves beyond issues of technical ease of use and looks more closely at patients' preferences for privacy or at their desires to use the telehealth devices according to their own schedules, the growing trend of consumer-directed health care becomes a concern. This is the new reality in health care. In part, the baby-boom generation, many of whom are educated and comfortable with technology, are driving this trend toward as-needed, when-wanted care. Challenges of scheduling and possibly even reengineering telehealth care services may be a concern (or an opportunity) for tomorrow's home telehealth care providers. Clinicians are only now beginning to learn how to care differently for this new generation of patients, who want telehealth care to be delivered on their own terms. Kaplan and Litweka (2008) stressed that we must consider cultural and community meanings associated with technology when we suggest telehealth as a care delivery model.

Health Care in the Future

Consumers will drive the way health care is delivered in the future. Consider that tomorrow's health care facility might have no walls. The evolving role of the Internet, personal health records, and telehealth all will support a more integrated health care model. This convergence of trends and solutions will continue to expand with the introduction of new business practice models, such as retail clinics and concierge care.

The care continuum will need to be supported by a clinical and caregiver structure that uses the data collected from patients to make better and more informed health care decisions. Health parameter data could be used by the end user for personal direct care decision making, or it may be used by a member of the health care community to determine appropriate health care interventions.

The technology of today will be different from the technology of tomorrow, as access to broadband communications systems, acceptance of technology, and mobility and data transfer continue to evolve. As a result of emerging needs, many companies will enter the market and offer a wide range of information technology tools, ranging from embedded and worn sensors to remote monitoring devices. There will continue to be different user interfaces to receive customized health services. Clearly, by making key information readily accessible, solutions across all areas (home health, hospitals, and a range of other settings) will facilitate collaboration in care delivery and support patient engagement in their care. Products that integrate into consumers' and patients' everyday lives to improve the quality of life will continue to emerge. Foremost, health care professionals must be open to change and willing to embrace ever-evolving practice models. Tools should always be used to improve care delivery models so as to make more targeted contact with and about patients. In an ideal world, there will be seamless integration of clinical data systems and robust data exchange to engage patients in their care and provide quality care for patients no matter their location.

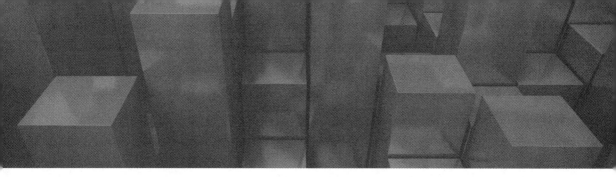

Summary

It is clear that the trends of consumer empowerment, patient engagement, and connected health will be an integral part of the evolving health care system. Health care professionals need to hone their health informatics skills and competencies to be prepared to practice in this new paradigm. In an ideal world, practitioners will embrace emerging technologies for patient engagement and connected health and will design practice interventions and educational materials that are technology enhanced, user friendly, culturally competent, interesting, dynamic, and interactive and that meet the skills, education needs, and interests of the user.

Thought-Provoking Questions

1. Choose two patient engagement or connectivity tools and discuss specifically how you would use these to deliver care in your specialty.
2. Formulate a patient education plan for a common chronic health challenge related to your specialty. Provide a rationale for each approach and describe a technology tool you would use to engage and educate the patient and his or her family.
3. Reflect on connected health from your specialty's perspective. What are you doing currently that connects your patients? Describe in detail what you plan to do in the next 6 months to 1 year.

Apply Your Knowledge

Pretend you are a member of the Health Professional-IT Innovation Council in a community hospital system. The council is exploring the use of smartphones as a support for recently discharged patients with chronic illnesses. You are asked to investigate the potential of such a system and to present your findings to the council. Use information from your text as well as information from scholarly and Internet sources. Define the main concepts of your presentation and provide an outline of the key points you will make. Be sure to include consideration of work flow and resistance that you learned about in Chapter 10.

Additional Resources

Agency for Healthcare Research and Quality
http://www.ahrq.gov/professionals/prevention-chronic-care/improve/self-mgmt/pemat/index
   .html
American Academy of Family Physicians
http://www.familydoctor.org

American Cancer Society
http://www.cancer.org
American Heart Association
http://www.americanheart.org
Center for Connected Health Policy
http://cchpca.org
Centers for Disease Control and Prevention
http://www.cdc.gov
Centers for Disease Control and Prevention Health Literacy
http://www.cdc.gov/healthliteracy
Centers for Disease Control and Prevention Social Media Tool Kit
http://www.cdc.gov/socialmedia/Tools/guidelines/pdf/SocialMediaToolkit_BM.pdf
eHealth Initiative
http://www.ehealthinitiative.org
Healthfinder
http://www.healthfinder.gov
Mayo Clinic on Pregnancy
https://itunes.apple.com/WebObjects/MZStore.woa/wa/viewSoftware?id=656908781&mt=8
Medline Plus
http://www.medlineplus.gov
National Health Information Center
http://www.health.gov/nhic
National Health Service, United Kingdom
http://www.nhs.uk/ipg/Pages/IPStart.aspx
National Institutes of Health
http://www.nih.gov
NIHSeniorHealth
http://www.nihseniorhealth.gov
Krames
http://www.krames.com
National Center for Complementary and Alternative Medicine
http://nccam.nih.gov/health/webresources
National Library of Medicine
https://www.nlm.nih.gov/medlineplus/games.html
National Network Libraries of Medicine
http://nnlm.gov/outreach/consumer/hlthlit.html
Patient Education Center
http://www.patienteducationcenter.org
Patient Education Institute
http://www.patient-education.com
Telehealth Resource Center
http://www.telehealthresourcecenter.org/toolbox-module/licensure-and-scope-practice.
The Cancer Game
http://www.cancergame.org
Understanding Diseases
https://itunes.apple.com/us/app/understanding-diseases/id530900371?mt=8
U.S. National Library of Medicine and National Institutes of Health
http://www.nlm.nih.gov/medlineplus/webeval/webeval.htmlUtah Health Information Network
http://www.uhin.org
Vermont Health Information Technology Plan
http://hcr.vermont.gov/sites/hcr/files/pdfs/vermont_health_it_plan.pdf

WebMD Pain Coach
https://itunes.apple.com/us/app/webmd-pain-coach/id536303342?mt=8

References

Aarkstore Enterprise. (2010). Telemedicine market shares, strategies, and forecasts, worldwide, 2010 to 2016. http://www.articlebuster.com/2010/03/telemedicine-market-shares-strategiesand-forecasts-worldwide-2010-to-2016-aarkstore-enterprise

Agency for Healthcare Research and Quality. (2013, October). The patient education materials assessment tool (PEMAT) and user's guide. http://www.ahrq.gov/professionals/prevention-chronic-care/improve/self-mgmt/pemat/index.html

American Heart Association. (2007). Statistics you need to know: Statistics on medication. http://www.americanheart.org/presenter.jhtml?identifier=107

American Telemedicine Association. (2010). Telemedicine defined. http://www.americantelemed.org/i4a/pages/index.cfm?pageid=3333

Anderson, A., & Klemm, P. (2008). The Internet: Friend or foe when providing patient education? *Clinical Journal of Oncology Nursing, 12*(1), 55–63.

Car, J., Gurol-Urganci, I., de Jongh, T., Vodopivec-Jamsek, V., & Atun, R. (2012). Mobile phone messaging reminders for attendance at healthcare appointments. *Cochrane Database of Systematic Reviews, 7.*

Centers for Disease Control and Prevention. (2011). The health communicator's social media toolkit. http://www.cdc.gov/socialmedia/Tools/guidelines/pdf/SocialMediaToolkit_BM.pdf

Centers for Disease Control and Prevention. (2012). Health literacy: Accurate, accessible and actionable health information for all. http://www.cdc.gov/healthliteracy

Chetney, R. (2006, July/August). What do patients really think about telehealth? In-depth interviews with patients and their caregivers. *Remington Report, 26,* 28–29.

D'Alessandro, D. (2010). Challenges and options for patient education in the office setting. *Pediatric Annals, 39*(2), 78–83.

Demiris, G., Doorenbos, A., & Towle, C. (2009). Ethical considerations regarding the use of technology for older adults: The case of telehealth. *Research in Gerontological Nursing, 2*(2), 128–136.

Donovan, O. (2005). The carbohydrate quandary: Achieving health literacy through an interdisciplinary WebQuest. *Journal of School Health, 75*(9), 359–362.

Dudas, R. A., Pumilia, J., & Crocetti, M. (2013). Pediatric caregiver attitudes and technologic readiness toward electronic follow-up communication in an urban community emergency department. *Telemedicine & E-Health, 19*(6), 493–496. doi: 10.1089/tmj.2012.0166

Flores, A. (2006). Using computer games and other media to decrease child obesity. *Agricultural Research, 54*(3), 8–9.

Fox, S. (2011, February 1). Health topics. http://www.pewinternet.org/Reports/2011/Health Topics.aspx

Fox, S., & Duggan, M. (2013). Health online 2013. http://www.pewinternet.org/2013/01/15/health-online-2013

Fox, S., & Purcell, K. (2010). Chronic disease and the Internet. http://www.pewinternet.org/Reports/2010/Chronic-Disease/Summary-of-Findings/Adults-living-with-chronic-diseaseare-disproportionately-offline-in-an-online-world.aspx

Glassman, P. (2008). Health literacy. http://nnlm.gov/outreach/consumer/hlthlit.html

Glymetrix Diabetes Game. (2009). http://www.diabetesgame.com

Health on the Net Foundation. (2005). Analysis of 9th HON survey of health and medical Internet users. http://www.hon.ch/Survey/Survey2005/res.html

Health on the Net Foundation. (2014). HONcode. http://www.hon.ch/HONcode/Pro/Visitor/visitor.html

Huang, E. (2009). Six cases of e-health videos on hospital web sites. *E-Service Journal, 6*(3), 56–72.

IMS Research. (2013). Telehealth to reach 1.8 million patients by 2017. http://www.imsresearch.com/press-release/Telehealth_to_Reach_18_Million_Patients_by_2017

Kaplan, B., & Litweka, S. (2008). Ethical challenges of telemedicine and telehealth. *Cambridge Quarterly of Healthcare Ethics, 17*(4), 401–416.

Lapwosky, I. (2015). Google will make health searches less scary with fact-checked results. *Wired.com/Business*. http://www.wired.com/2015/02/google-health-search

Lauterbach, C. (2010). Exploring the usability of e-health websites. *Usability News, 12*(2). http://psychology.wichita.edu/surl/usabilitynews/122/pdf/Usability%20News%20122%20-%20Lauterbach.pdf

Lober, W. B., & Flowers, J. L. (2011, August). Consumer empowerment in health care amid the Internet and social media. *Seminars in Oncology Nursing, 27*(3), 169–182. http://dx.doi.org/10.1016/j.soncn.2011.04.002

Mayo Clinic. (2015). Google works with Mayo. *Mayo Clinic Magazine, 29*(1), 4–5.

McCray, A. (2005). Promoting health literacy. *Journal of the American Medical Informatics Association, 12*(2), 152–163.

Missen, C., & Cook, T. (2007). Appropriate information-communications technologies for developing countries. http://www.who.int/bulletin/volumes/85/4/07-041475/en/index.html

National Center for Complementary and Alternative Medicine, National Institutes of Health. (2008). 10 things to know about evaluating medical resources on the Web. http://nccam.nih.gov/health/webresources

National Institutes of Health. (2015). Clear communication: Health literacy. http://www.nih.gov/clearcommunication/healthliteracy.htm

National Pharmaceutical Council. (2013). Medication compliance/adherence. http://www.npcnow.org/issue/medication-complianceadherence

Neiger, B. L., Thackeray, R., Burton, S. H., Giraud-Carrier, C. G., & Fagen, M. C. (2013). Evaluating social media's capacity to develop engaged audiences in health promotion settings: Use of Twitter metrics as a case study. *Health Promotion Practice, 14*(2), 157–162. doi: 10.1177/1524839912469378

Oda, Y., & Kristula, D. (n.d.). The Cancer Game: A side-scrolling, arcade-style, cancer-fighting video game. http://www.cancergame.org

Office of Disease Prevention and Health Promotion & U.S. Department of Health and Human Services. (2009). Proposed Healthy People 2020 objectives. http://www.healthypeople.gov/hp2020/Objectives/TopicAreas.aspx

Parker, R., Ratzan, C., & Lurie, N. (2003). Health literacy: A policy challenge for advancing high quality health care. *Health Affairs, 22*(4), 147.

Pew/Internet. (2006). The future of the Internet II. http://news.bbc.co.uk/1/shared/bsp/hi/pdfs/22_09_2006pewsummary.pdf

Piette, J. (2007). Interactive behavior change technology to support diabetes self-management: Where do we stand? *Diabetes Care, 30*(10), 2425–2432.

Remington, L. (2007, January/February). Healthcare megatrends, predictions and forecasts. *Remington Report, 15*, 5–10.

Sanderson, S. (2007, July/August). Cardiopulmonary disease management: A patient-focused approach to home health care. *Remington Report, 15*, 46–47.

Stern, D. J. (2007, January/February). Intuitive system monitors resident behavior patterns. *Assisted Living Consult, 3*(1), 21–25.

Sternberg, D. (2002). Building on your quick wins. *Marketing Health Services, 22*(3), 41–43.

Watson, A., Bell, A., Kvedar, J., & Grant, R. (2008). Reevaluating the digital divide: Current lack of Internet use is not a barrier to adoption of novel health information technology. *Diabetes Care, 31*(3), 433–435.

14

Using Informatics to Promote Community/ Population Health

Margaret Ross Kraft, Ida Androwich, Kathleen Mastrian, and Dee McGonigle

OBJECTIVES

1. Provide an overview of community and population health informatics.
2. Assess informatics tools for promoting community and population health.
3. Explore the roles of federal, state, and local public health agencies in the development of public health informatics.

Introduction

In the late fall of 2002, severe acute respiratory syndrome (SARS) appeared in China. By March 2003, SARS had become recognized as a global threat. According to World Health Organization (WHO) data, more than 8,000 people from 29 countries became infected with this previously unknown virus, and more than 700 people died. By 2004, the last SARS cases were caused by laboratory-acquired infections. Because of computerized global data collection, the potentially negative impact of a widespread global epidemic was averted.

Vong, O'Leary, and Feng (2014) reported that "heavy criticism of China's response in the early stages of the SARS outbreak led to huge investments in public health by the Chinese government" (p. 303). Post-SARS China had improved disease surveillance, preparing them to be able to quickly and effectively respond to future disease outbreaks.

Many **surveillance** systems, loosely termed "syndromic surveillance systems," use data that are not diagnostic of a disease but that might indicate the early stages

Key Terms

Behavioral Risk Factor
    Surveillance System
Bioterrorism
Centers for Disease
    Control and
    Prevention
Community risk
    assessment
Crowdsourcing
Epidemiology
National Center for Public
    Health Informatics
National Health
    Information Network
National Health
    and Nutrition
    Examination Survey
One health
Public health
Public health informatics

(continues)

of an outbreak. Outbreak detection is the overriding purpose of **syndromic surveillance** for terrorism preparedness. Enhanced case finding and monitoring the course and population characteristics of a recognized outbreak also are potential benefits of syndromic surveillance. In recent years, new data have been used by public health officials to enhance surveillance, such as patients' chief complaints in emergency departments, ambulance log sheets, prescriptions filled, retail drug and product purchases, school or work absenteeism, and medical signs and symptoms in persons seen in various clinical settings. With faster, more specific and affordable diagnostic methods and decision support tools, timely recognition of reportable diseases with the potential to lead to a substantial outbreak is now possible. Tools for pattern recognition can be used to screen data for patterns needing further public health investigation. During the 2003 epidemic, the **Centers for Disease Control and Prevention** (CDC) worked to develop surveillance criteria to identify persons with SARS in the United States, and the surveillance case definition changed throughout the epidemic to reflect increased understanding of SARS (CDC, 2007). China's commitment to improving its surveillance and quick response paid off:

On 31 March 2013, China's National Health and Family Planning Commission notified WHO of three human infections with A(H7N9): two in the city of Shanghai and one in Anhui province. By 7 November 2013, 139 confirmed cases of human infection with A(H7N9)—including 45 fatal cases—had been reported in mainland China—in 10 provinces and two municipalities. Although the animal reservoir of A(H7N9) infection involved in this outbreak has yet to be confirmed, it is probably poultry and most transmission to humans probably occurs in markets selling live poultry. The Chinese Ministry of Agriculture has already tested more than 1.2 million birds and other animals—from more than 69,000 different sites—for A(H7N9). By 9 December 2013, only 68 non-human samples had been found positive for the virus. (Vong et al., 2014, p. 304)

Information acquired by the collection and processing of population health data becomes the basis for knowledge in the field of **public health**. There is an ever-increasing need for timely information about the health of communities, states, and countries. Knowledge about disease trends and other threats to community health can improve program planning, decision making, and care delivery. Patients seen from the perspective of major health threats within their communities can benefit from opportunities for early intervention.

This chapter focuses on the application of informatics methods to public health surveillance. The availability of clinical information for public health has been fundamentally changed by the introduction of the electronic health record (EHR) and health information technology (IT), which now give public health "an unprecedented opportunity to leverage the information, technologies and standards to support critical public health functions such as alerting and surveillance" (Garrett, 2010).

Core Public Health Functions

The core public health functions are "The assessment and monitoring of the health of communities and populations at risk to identify health problems and priorities; The formulation of public policies designed to solve identified local and national health problems and priorities; To assure that all populations have access to appropriate and cost-effective care, including health promotion and disease prevention services, and evaluation of the effectiveness of that care" (Medterms Medical Dictionary, 2007). "Public health is a field that encompasses an amalgam of science, action, research, policy, advocacy and government" (Yasnoff, Overhage, Humphreys, & LaVenture, 2001, p. 536).

Historically, Dr. John Snow can be designated as the "father" of **public health informatics** (PHI). In 1854, he plotted information about cholera deaths and was able to determine that the deaths were clustered around the same water pump in London. He convinced authorities that the cholera deaths were associated with that water pump; when the pump handle was removed, the cholera outbreak ended. It was Dr. Snow's focus on the cholera-affected population as a whole rather than on a single patient that led to his discovery of the source of the cholera outbreak (Vachon, 2005).

Florence Nightingale should also be recognized as an early public health informaticist. Her recommendations about medical reform and the need for improved sanitary conditions were based on data about morbidity and mortality that she compiled from her experiences in the Crimea and England. Her efforts led to a total reorganization of how and which health care statistics were collected (Dossey, 2000).

Just as information has been recognized as an asset in the business world, so health care is now recognized as an information-intensive field requiring timely, accurate information from many different sources. Health information systems address the collection, storage, analysis, interpretation, and communication of health data and information. Many health disciplines, such as medicine and nursing, have developed their own concepts of informatics integrating computer, information, and cognitive science with the science of the professional domain. That trend has reached the field of public and community health. PHI represents "a systematic application of information and computer science and technology to public health (PH) practice, research and learning" (Yasnoff, O'Carroll, Koo, Linkings, & Kilbourne, 2000, p. 67). This area of informatics differs from others because it is focused on the promotion of health and disease prevention in populations and communities. PHI efficiently and effectively organizes and manages data, information, and knowledge generated and used by public health professionals to fulfill the core functions of public health: assessment, policy, and assurance (Agency for Toxic Substances and Disease Registry, 2003). Public health changes the social conditions and systems that affect everyone within a given community. It is because of public health initiatives that people understand the importance of clean water, the dangers of secondhand smoke, and the fact that seat belts really do save lives (Public Health Institute, 2007).

The scope of PHI practice includes knowledge from a variety of additional disciplines, including management, organization theory, psychology, political science, and law and fields related to public health, such as **epidemiology**, microbiology, toxicology, and statistics (O'Carroll, Yasnoff, Ward, Ripp, & Martin, 2003, p. 5). PHI focuses on applications of IT that "promote the health of populations rather than individuals, focus on disease prevention rather than treatment, focus on preventive intervention at all vulnerable points" (O'Carroll et al., 2003, pp. 3–4). PHI addresses the data, information, and knowledge that public health professionals generate and use to meet the core functions of public health (Public Health Data Standards Consortium [PHDSC], 2007b). Yasnoff et al. (2000) defined four principles that define and guide the activities of PHI: (1) applications promote the health of populations, (2) applications focus on disease and injury prevention, (3) applications explore prevention at "all vulnerable points in the causal changes," and (4) PHI reflects the "governmental context in which public health is practiced" (p. 69).

The Institute of Medicine defines the role of public health as "fulfilling society's interest in assuring conditions in which people can be healthy" (Khoury, 1997, p. 176). Functions of public health include prevention of epidemics and the spread of disease, protection against environmental hazards, promotion of health, disaster response and recovery, and providing access to health care (PHDSC, 2007a).

The initiative of integrating the health care enterprise to ensure that health care information can be shared more easily and used more effectively has inspired the creation of the domain known as quality, research, and public health (QRPH). Participants in this domain address the repurposing of clinical, demographic, and financial data collected in the process of providing clinical care to the monitoring of disease patterns; incidence, prevalence, and situational awareness of such patterns; and the identification of new patterns of disease not previously known or anticipated. Such data can be incorporated within existing public health population analyses and programs for direct outreach and condition management through registries and locally determined appropriate treatment programs or protocols (QRPH, 2010).

Community Health Risk Assessment: Tools for Acquiring Knowledge

As the public has become more aware of harmful elements in the environment, **risk assessment** tools have been developed. Such tools allow assessment of pesticide use, exposure to harmful chemicals, contaminants in food and water, and toxic pollutants in the air to determine if potential hazards need to be addressed. A risk assessment may also be called a "threat and risk assessment." A "**threat**" is a harmful act, such as the deployment of a virus or illegal network penetration. A "**risk**" is the expectation that a threat may succeed and the potential damage that can occur (PCMag.com Encyclopedia, 2007). "**Risk factor** assessments complement vital statistics data systems and morbidity data systems by providing information on factors earlier in the causal chain leading to illness, injury or death" (O'Carroll, Powell-Griner, Holtzman, & Williamson, 2003, p. 316).

"Health risk assessments are used to estimate whether current or future exposures will pose health risks to broad populations" (California Environmental Protection Agency [CEPA], 1998, p. 4) and are used to weigh the benefits and costs of various program alternatives for reducing exposure to potential hazards. They may also influence public policy and regulatory decisions. Health risk assessment is a constantly developing process based in sound science and professional judgments. There are usually four basic steps ascribed to risk assessment:

1. *Hazard identification* seeks to determine the types of health problems that could be caused by exposure to a potentially hazardous material. All research studies related to the potentially hazardous material are reviewed to identify potential health problems.
2. *Exposure assessment* is done to determine the length, amount, and pattern of exposure to the potentially hazardous material.
3. *Dose–response assessment* is an estimation of how much exposure to the potential hazard would cause varying degrees of health effects.
4. *Risk characterization* is an assessment of the risk of the hazardous material causing illness in the population (CEPA, 1998).

The overall question the risk assessment has to answer is, "How much risk is acceptable?" Risk factor systems are used throughout the United States and may be local, regional, or national in scope. Specific risk assessment tools exist for specific health issues, such as the **Suicide Prevention Community Assessment Tool**, which addresses general community information, prevention networks, and the demographics of the target population and community assets and risk factors. Other risk assessment tools include the **Youth Risk Behavior Surveillance System**, the **Behavioral Risk Factor Surveillance System**, and the **National Health and Nutrition Examination Survey**.

Determining the presence of risk factors in community is a key part of a **community risk assessment** (CRA). Communities may be concerned about which elements in the environment affect or may affect the community's health, the level of environmental risk, and other factors that should be included in public health planning. Ball (2003) defines value as "a function of cost, service, and outcome" (p. 41). The value of a CRA derives from its ability to provide information crucial to planning, build consensus regarding how to mobilize community resources, and allow for comparison of risks with those of other communities. The goal of a CRA is risk reduction and improved health. A CRA may identify unmet needs and opportunities for action that may help set new priorities for local public health units. It may also be used to monitor the impact of prevention programs.

Processing Knowledge and Information to Support Epidemiology and Monitoring Disease Outbreaks

There is a need to define the role of federal, state, and local public health agencies in the development of PHI and IT applications. The availability of IT today challenges all stakeholders in the health of the public to adopt new systems that can provide adequate disease surveillance; it also challenges people to improve outmoded processes.

Preparedness in public health requires more timely detection of potential health threats, situational awareness, surveillance, outbreak management, countermeasures, response, and communications. Surveillance uses health-related data that signal a sufficient probability of a case or an outbreak that warrants further public health response.

Although historically syndromic surveillance has been used to target investigations of potential infectious cases, its use to detect possible outbreaks associated with **bioterrorism** is increasingly being explored by public health officials (CDC, 2007). Early detection of possible outbreaks can be achieved through timely and complete receipt, review, and investigation of disease case reports; by improving the ability to recognize patterns in data that may be indicative of a possible outbreak early in its course; and through receipt of new types of data that can signify an outbreak earlier in its course. Such new types of data might include identification of absences from work or school; increased purchases of health care products, including specific types of over-the-counter medications; presenting symptoms to health care providers; and laboratory test orders (CDC, 2007). The University of Pittsburgh Realtime Outbreak and Disease Surveillance Laboratory (RODS), for example, developed the National Retail Data Monitor (NRDM) system. The NRDM collects data on over-the-counter medications and other health care products from 28,000 stores and uses computer algorithms to detect unusual purchase patterns that might potentially signal a disease outbreak (RODS Laboratory, 2013). A comprehensive surveillance effort supports timely investigation and identifies data needs for managing the public health response to an outbreak or terrorist event. Informatics tools are becoming increasingly important in these public health efforts.

To appropriately process public health data, PHI has a need for a standardized vocabulary and coding structure. This is especially important as national public health data are collected and data mining performed so that data variables can be understood across systems and between agencies. Health information organizations (HIOs) have been established to support data sharing via health information exchanges (HIE) promoted by the meaningful use criteria of the electronic health record (EHR). Central to these initiatives is the need for standardized codes and terminologies that may be used by the HIOs to map data from disparate sources (Shapiro, Mostashari, Hripcsak, Soulakis, & Kuperman, 2011).

In the early 1990s, the CDC launched a plan for an integrated surveillance system that moved from stand-alone systems to networked data exchange built with specific standards. Early initiatives were the National Electronic Telecommunications System for Surveillance and the Wide-Ranging Online Data for Epidemiologic Research. Six current initiatives reflect this early vision:

1. PulseNet USA: A surveillance network for food-borne infections.
2. National Electronic Disease Surveillance System: Facilitates reporting on approximately 100 diseases, with data feeding directly from clinical laboratories, which allows for early detection.
3. Epidemic Information Exchange: A secure communication system for practitioners to access and share preliminary health surveillance information.
4. Health Alert Network: A state and nationwide alert system.
5. Biosense: Provides improved real-time biosurveillance and situational awareness in support of early detection.
6. Public Health Information Network: Promotes standards and software solutions for the rapid flow of public health information.

Certainly, the events of September 11, 2001, which indicated the need for the United States to increase its efforts directed toward prevention of terrorism, accelerated the need for informatics in public health practice. Today, response requirements include fast detection, science, communication, integration, and action (Kukafka, 2006). In 2005, the CDC created the **National Center for Public Health Informatics** to provide leadership in the field. This center aims to protect and improve health through PHI (McNabb, Koo, Pinner, & Seligman, 2006).

Information is vital to public health programming. The data processed into public health information can be obtained from administrative, financial, and facility sources. Included in this data stream may be encounter, screening, registry, clinical, and laboratory and surveillance data. It has been recommended that the functions of population health beyond surveillance be integrated into the EHR and the personal health record. Such an initiative might allow for population-level alerts to be sent to clinicians through these electronic record systems. Systems now being developed allow for automated syndromic surveillance of emergency department records and media surveillance, which in turn supports early detection of potential pandemic occurrences. Such systems were tested during the 2009 H1N1 flu outbreak. The public health–enhanced electronic medical record can provide immediate detection and reporting of notifiable conditions. The incorporation of geographic information systems allows public health data to be mapped to specific locations that may indicate an immediate need for intervention (Grannis & Vreeman, 2010).

Vital statistics from state and local governments are also used for public health purposes. It should be noted that databases created with public funds are public databases that are available for authorized public representatives for public purposes (Freedman & Weed, 2003).

Widespread implementation of EHRs is likely to facilitate the concept of a public health–enabled record, which can automatically send patient information alerts from the point of care to public health departments when reportable symptoms, conditions, or diseases are encountered. A public health–enabled EHR can be bidirectional, allowing public health information and recommendations for treatment to be accessible at the point of care. One public health EHR prototype addresses the information flow related to newborn screenings (Orlova et al., 2005).

Potential applications of HIE to public health have been described by Shapiro et al. (2011). They include syndromic surveillance using data generated from mandated and nonmandated laboratory results, physician diagnoses, and emergency or clinic chief complaints; strategies to locate loved ones in mass-casualty events; and public health alerts at the individual and population levels.

Applying Knowledge to Health Disaster Planning and Preparation

The availability of data and the speed of data exchange can have a significant impact on critical public health functions, such as disease monitoring and syndromic surveillance. Currently, surveillance data are limited and historical in nature, although this situation is rapidly changing. Nevertheless, special data collections are needed to address specific public health issues, and investigations and emergencies are still frequently addressed and managed with paper. In the future, PHI will make real-time surveillance data available electronically, and investigations and emergences will be managed with the tools of informatics (Yasnoff et al., 2004). "**Surveillance data systems** such as infectious disease trackers that collect data on adverse health effects are invaluable tools for public health officials to tap for planning, evaluation, or implementation of **public health interventions**" (Agency for Toxic Substances and Disease Registry, 2003). "Syndromic surveillance for early outbreak detection is an investigational approach where health department staff, assisted by automated data acquisition and generation of statistical signals, monitor disease indicators continually (real-time) or at least daily (near real-time) to detect outbreaks of diseases earlier and more completely than might otherwise be possible with traditional public health methods" (Buehler, Hopkins, Overhage, Sosin, & Tong, 2004, para. 7). Traditionally, there has been no common infrastructure to respond to pandemics, but the development of health IT is creating opportunities that go far beyond national boundaries to impact global public health initiatives.

In New York City, a primary care information project funded by the CDC has developed a multifaceted initiative, the Center for Excellence in Public Health Informatics, to address issues of measurement of meaningful use, disease and outbreak surveillance, and decision support alerts at the point of care (Buck, Wu, Souliakis, & Kukalka, 2010).

Informatics Tools to Support Communication and Dissemination

The revolution in IT has made the capture and analysis of health data and the distribution of health care information more achievable and less costly. Since the early 1960s, the CDC has used IT in its practice; PHI emerged as a specialty in the 1990s. PHI has become more important with improvements in IT, changes in the care delivery system, and the challenges related to emerging infections, resistance to antibiotics, and the threat of chemical and biologic terrorism. Two-way communication between public health agencies, community, and clinical laboratories can identify clusters of reportable and unusual diseases. In turn, health departments can consult on case diagnosis and management, alerts, surveillance summaries, and clinical and public health recommendations. Ongoing health care provider outreach, education, and 24-hour access to public health professionals may lead to the discovery of urgent health threats. The automated transfer of specified data from a laboratory database to a public health data repository improves the timeliness and completeness of reporting notifiable conditions.

Public health information systems represent a partnership of federal, state, and local public health professionals. Such systems facilitate the capture of large amounts of data, rapid exchange of information, and strengthened links among these three system levels. Dissemination of prevention guidelines and communication among public health officials, clinicians, and patients has emerged as a major benefit of PHI. IT solutions can be used to provide accurate and timely information that guides public health actions. In addition, the Internet has become a universal communications pathway and allows individuals and population groups to be more involved and take greater responsibility for management of their own health status.

Few public health professionals have received formal informatics training, and many may not be aware of the potential impact of IT on their practice. A working group formed at the University of Washington Center for PHI has published a draft of PHI competencies needed (Karras, 2007). These competencies include the following (Center for Public Health Informatics, 2007):

- Supporting development of strategic direction for PHI within the enterprise
- Participating in development of knowledge management tools for the enterprise
- Using standards
- Ensuring that the knowledge, information, and data needs of project or program users and stakeholders are met
- Managing information system development, procurement, and implementation
- Managing IT operations related to a project or program (for public health agencies with internal IT operations)
- Monitoring IT operations managed by external organizations
- Communicating with cross-disciplinary leaders and team members
- Participating in applied public health informatics research
- Developing public health information systems that are interoperable with other relevant information systems
- Supporting use of informatics to integrate clinical health, environmental risk, and population health
- Implementing solutions that ensure confidentiality, security, and integrity while maximizing availability of information for public health
- Conducting education and training in PHI

Using Feedback to Improve Responses and Promote Readiness

Improvement of community health status and population health depends on effective public and health care infrastructures. In addition to information from public health agencies, there is now interest in the capture of information from hospitals, pharmacies, poison control centers, laboratories, and environmental agencies. Timely collection of such data allows early detection and analysis, which can increase the rapidity of response with more effective interventions. Yasnoff et al. (2000) identified the "grand challenges" still facing PHI as the development of national public health information systems, a closer integration of clinical care with public health, and concerns of confidentiality and privacy.

Population health data must be considered an important part of the infrastructure of all **regional health information exchanges**, which are the building blocks for a **national health information network**. Organizations and agencies interested in promoting and protecting the public's health must commit to collaboration and seamless data sharing (PHDSC, 2007b). Public health data include data related to surveillance, environmental health, and preparedness systems as well as client information, such as data from immunization registries and laboratory results reporting and analysis. These types of data can provide information about outbreaks, patterns of drug-resistant organisms, and other trends that can help improve the accuracy of diagnostic and treatment decisions (LaVenture, 2005). A regional health information exchange and national health information network can also support public health goals through broader opportunities for participation in surveillance and prevention activities, improved case management and care coordination, and increased accuracy and timeliness of information for disease reporting (LaVenture, 2005).

Much of the information presented here is focused on reaction to issues and timely intervention rather than harnessing information technology for disease prevention. Fuller (2011) has advocated for a shift to prevention informatics by harnessing real-time social data and aggregating and representing these data in a meaningful way so that an appropriate prevention response can be mounted. For example, Internet searches related to flu symptoms might prompt a public health prevention response, such as a school closure to minimize spread. Newer software tools to support mapping and real-time data visualization include Riff and Ushahidi, each of which supported "gathering of distributed data from the web and other data streams" (Fuller, 2001, p. 40). "Prevention informatics offers a useful paradigm for re-imagining health information systems and for harnessing the vast array of data, tools, technologies and systems to respond proactively to health challenges across the globe" (p. 41).

The emergence of the **one health** approach is a solid one that should be implemented: interprofessional teams working together to improve the health of animals and humans alike to enhance the collective health of a community or population. Vong et al. (2014) summarized as follows:

> *China's prompt response to the emergence of the A(H7N9) virus as a human pathogen—which spanned multiple governmental departments and ministries at national, provincial and municipal level—was mainly the result of strong leadership in a critical situation. We believe that strong and well integrated coordination between veterinary and public health services can be best sustained by joint preparedness planning and the creation of joint response systems. (p. 306)*

This one health approach is continuing to evolve internationally.

Harnessing data from **social media** such as Twitter and Facebook provides yet another example of using citizen-generated information (**crowdsourcing**) in community health. Merchant, Elmer, and Lurie (2011) have described how mining data generated in social media can improve response to mass disasters by helping responders locate people who need help and identify areas where to send resources, build social capital, and promote community resilience post-disaster. "Tweets and photographs linked to timelines and interactive maps can tell a cohesive story about a recovering community's capabilities and vulnerabilities in real time" (Merchant et al., 2011, p. 291). These authors caution, however, that social media should be used to augment—not replace—current disaster response and communication systems, as not all communications in social media are entirely trustworthy.

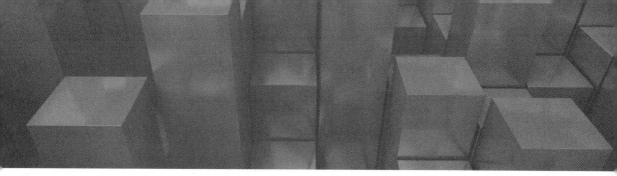

Summary

Public health informatics strives to ensure that evolving health data systems will meet the data needs of all organizations interested in population health as national and international standards are developed for health care data collection. This includes standardization of environmental, sociocultural, economic, and other data that are relevant to public health (PHDSC, 2007b). **Table 14-1** provides the names, addresses, and URLs for important organizations dedicated to public health data and informatics. **Table 14-2** lists abbreviations commonly used in PHI.

TABLE 14-1	IMPORTANT PHI SITES	
Name	Address	Website
American Public Health Association	APHA 800 I Street, NW Washington, DC 20001	www.apha.org
Center for Public Health Informatics	CPHI University of Washington 1100 NE 45th Street, Ste 405 Seattle, WA 98105	www.cphi.washington.edu
Centers for Disease Control and Prevention	Centers for Disease Control and Prevention 1600 Clifton Road Atlanta, GA 30333	www.cdc.gov
National Center for Public Health Informatics	The National Center for Public Health Informatics (NCPHI) 1600 Clifton Road, NE Mailstop E-78 Atlanta, GA 30333	https://web.archive.org/web/20110123075557/http://www.cdc.gov/ncphi/
Public Health Data Standards Consortium	Public Health Data Standards Consortium c/o Johns Hopkins Bloomberg School of Public Health 624 N Broadway, Room 325 Baltimore, MD 21205	www.phdsc.org
Public Health Institute	Public Health Institute 555 12th Street, 10th Floor Oakland, CA 94607	www.phi.org

TABLE 14-2	ABBREVIATIONS USED IN PHI
BRFSS	Behavioral Risk Factor Surveillance System
CDC	Centers for Disease Control and Prevention
CEPA	California Environmental Protection Agency
CPHI	Center for Public Health Informatics
CRA	Community Risk Assessment
EPI-X	Epidemic Information Exchange
HAN	Health Alert Network
IOM	Institute of Medicine
IT	Information Technology
NCPHI	National Center for Public Health Informatics
NEDSS	National Electronic Disease Surveillance System
NETSS	National Electronic Technology System for Surveillance
NHANES	National Health and Nutrition Examination Survey
NHIN	National Health Information Network
PH	Public Health
PHDSC	Public Health Data Standards Consortium
PHI	Public Health Informatics
PHIN	Public Health Information Network
PHRAP	Pennsylvania's Health Risk Assessment Process
QRPH	Quality, Research, Public Health
RHIO	Regional Health Information Exchanges
SPRC	Suicide Prevention Community Assessment Tool
WONDER	Wide-ranging Online Data for Epidemiologic Research
YRBSS	Youth Risk Behavior Surveillance System

The future of practice in public health depends on how efficiently and effectively public health data are captured, analyzed, and disseminated for regional, national, and global health planning and management. In an ideal world, we would see seamless data collection and sharing and a commitment to global health planning.

Thought-Provoking Questions

1. Imagine that you are a public health informatics specialist and that you and your colleagues are concerned about a new strain of influenza. Which public health data are used to determine the need for a mass inoculation? Which data will be collected to determine the success of such a program?
2. What are the advantages and disadvantages of using crowd sourced social media data during a disaster response?

Apply Your Knowledge

All health care professionals, regardless of discipline, may be called to serve in the case of a community disaster. Disasters may include such things as tornados, hurricanes, massive snowstorms, chemical spills, terrorist attacks, and so on. Search for information about the disaster preparedness (readiness) plans for your community.

1. How accessible was the plan? Is it easily understood by community members?
2. How is information managed in this plan?
3. Are there informatics tools that could be incorporated to improve disaster response and management?
4. What are the advantages and disadvantages of using crowdsourced social media data during disaster response?

References

Agency for Toxic Substances and Disease Registry. (2003). ATSDR glossary of terms. http://www.atsdr.cdc.gov/glossary.html

Ball, M. (2003). Better health through informatics: Managing information to deliver value. In P. O'Carroll, W. L. Yasnoff, M. E. Ward, L. Ripp, & E. Martin (Eds.), *Public health informatics and information systems* (pp. 39–51). New York: Springer-Verlag.

Buck, M., Wu, W., Souliakis, N., & Kukalka, R. (2010). *Achieving excellence in public health informatics: The New York City experience.* Washington, DC: AMIA.

Buehler, J. W., Hopkins, R. S., Overhage, J. M., Sosin, D. M., & Tong, V. (2004). Framework for evaluating public health surveillance systems for early detection of outbreaks. http://www.cdc.gov/mmwr/preview/mmwrhtml/rr5305a1.htm

California Environmental Protection Agency. (1998). A guide to health risk assessment. http://www.oehha.ca.gov

Center for Public Health Informatics. (2007). *Draft competencies V7 for the public health informatician.* Seattle: University of Washington.

Centers for Disease Control and Prevention. (2007). http://www.cdc.gov

Dossey, B. M. (2000). *Florence Nightingale: Mystic, visionary, healer.* Springhouse, PA: Springhouse.

Freedman, M. A., & Weed, J. A. (2003). National vital statistics system. In P. O'Carroll, W. Yasnoff, M. Ward, L. Ripp, & E. Martin (Eds.), *Public health informatics and information systems* (pp. 269–285). New York: Springer-Verlag.

Fuller, S. (2011). From intervention informatics to prevention informatics. *Bulletin of the American Society for Information Science & Technology, 38*(8), 36–41.

Garrett, N. (2010). Leveraging the EHR for public health alerting. CDC Clinician Outreach & Communication Activity conference call, June 22, 2010.

Grannis, S., & Vreeman, D. (2010). *A vision of the journey ahead: Using public health notifiable condition mapping to illustrate the need to maintain value sets.* Washington, DC: AMIA.

Karras, B. (2007). *Competencies for the public health informatician.* Seattle: University of Washington.

Khoury, M. J. (1997). Genetic epidemiology and the future of disease prevention and public health. *Epidemiology Reviews, 19*(1), 175–180.

Kukafka, R. (2006). *Public health informatics.* Medical Informatics Course for Health Professionals. Woods Hole, MA.

LaVenture, M. (2005, May). *Role of population/public health in regional health information exchanges.* PHDSC/eHealth Initiative Annual Conference, Washington, DC.

McNabb, S., Koo, D., Pinner, R., & Seligman, J. (2006). Informatics and public health at CDC. http://www.cdc.gov/mmwr/preview/mmwrhtml/su5502a10.htm

Medterms Medical Dictionary. (2007). http://www.medterms.com

Merchant, R., Elmer, S., & Lurie, N. (2011). Integrating social media into emergency-preparedness efforts. *New England Journal of Medicine, 365*(4), 289–291. doi: 10.1056/NEJMp1103591

O'Carroll, P. L., Powell-Griner, E., Holtzman, D., & Williamson, G. D. (2003). Risk factor information systems. In P. O'Carroll, W. Yasnoff, M. Ward, L. Ripp, & E. Martin (Eds.), *Public health informatics and information systems* (pp. 316–334). New York: Springer-Verlag.

O'Carroll, P., Yasnoff, W., Ward, M., Ripp, L., & Martin, E. (Eds.). (2003). *Public health informatics and information systems.* New York: Springer-Verlag.

Orlova, A., Dunnagan, M., Finitzo, T., Higgins, M., Watkings, T., Tien, A., et al. (2005). *An electronic health record–public health (EHR-PH) system prototype for interoperability in 21st century healthcare systems* (pp. 575–579). AMIA, Annual Symposium Proceedings.

PCMag.com Encyclopedia. (2007). http://www.pcmag.com/encyclopedia

Public Health Data Standards Consortium. (2007a). Tutorial module 1: What is public health. http://www.phdsc.org/knowresources/Tutorials/module1

Public Health Data Standards Consortium. (2007b). Tutorial module 8: Viewing public health data and data standards in a larger context. http://www.phdsc.org/knowresources/tutorials/module1

Public Health Institute. (2007). http://www.phi.org

QRPH. (2010). http://www.interoperabilityshowcase.org/.../HIMSS09_interop_QRPH

RODS Laboratory. (2013). About the National Retail Data Monitor. http://www.rods.pitt.edu/site/content/blogsection/4/42/

Shapiro, J. S., Mostashari, F., Hripcsak, G., Soulakis, N., & Kuperman, G. (2011). Using health information exchange to improve public health. *American Journal of Public Health, 101*(4), 616–623. doi: 10.2105/AJPH.2008.158980

Vachon, D. (2005). Dr John Snow blames water pollution for cholera epidemic. *Old News, 16*(8), 8–10. http://www.ph.ucla.edu/epi/snow/fatherofepidemiology.html

Vong, S., O'Leary, M., & Feng, Z. (2014). Early response to the emergence of influenza A(H7N9) virus in humans in China: The central role of prompt information sharing and public communication. *Bulletin World Health Organization, 92*, 303–308.

Yasnoff, W., Humphreys, B., Overhage, J., Detmer, D., Brennan, P., Morris, R., et al. (2004). A consensus action agenda for achieving the national health information infrastructure. *Journal of the American Medical Informatics Association, 11*(4), 332–338.

Yasnoff, W., O'Carroll, P., Koo, D., Linkings, R., & Kilbourne, E. (2000). Public health informatics: Improving and transforming public health in the information age. *Journal of Public Health Management Practice, 6*(6), 67–75.

Yasnoff, W., Overhage, M., Humphreys, B., & LaVenture M. (2001). A national agenda for public health informatics. *Journal of the American Medical Informatics Association, 8*(6), 535–545.

Section IV

Advanced Concepts in Health Informatics

Health informatics (HI) provides more tools and capabilities than can at times be imagined. Just as HI has changed the ways that professionals practice, so too has it dramatically affected the ways that professionals are educated.

Health care professional education is evolving with the increased integration of technology tools to promote learning. The tools that are available must be used prudently by reflecting on and applying knowledge on teaching styles, learning styles, and other pedagogic concerns. As informatics capabilities continue to expand, a phenomenal amount of potential for virtual reality–embedded education looms on the horizon. Once the purview of gamers and geeks, virtual reality has exploded onto the academic scene. The use of virtual reality has the potential for cross-pollination between fields of inquiry across the curriculum, the university, and even learning systems. Many university departments will experiment with virtual reality in hopes of staying current and appealing to their young and demanding "Generation Next" constituency. However, much of society loves the feel of books too much to dismiss them as archaic. There is room for both books and technology in education. Students, educators, and administrators will ultimately return to a modified form of face-to-face classroom teaching, even with the availability of newer and more adventuresome teaching technologies. Furthermore, after fast, high-burn technologies stop flooding the marketplace and big business provides opportunities for proprietary online universities, modified traditions will take their place, creating new spaces for nontraditional students and members of the Net generation, with both being anxious for technology use in the classroom for very different reasons.

Informatics has also dramatically altered research practices. Health care research has evolved with technology. In the era of evidence-based practice, clinicians must continue to think critically about their actions. What is the science behind interventions? Things must no longer be done a certain way just because they have always been done that way. Instead, one should research the problem, use evidence-based resources, critically select electronic and non-electronic references, consolidate the research findings and combine and compare the conclusions, present the findings, and propose a solution. The health care professional may be the first to ask *why*, thereby becoming a key player in making change happen.

HI enhances and facilitates collaboration; improves access to online libraries; provides research tool transparency for collection, analysis, and dissemination of research knowledge; and facilitates the development of a common data language. It provides organizational and informational support to advance translational research, helping to fill the gap between research findings and practice implementation. Repeat studies are needed to provide meaningful meta-analyses and systematic reviews of evidence to advance disciplinary practice. Technology advancement in the area of incorporating evidence into clinical tools must continue. Removing the barriers to knowledge-seeking behavior and providing access to evidential resources promotes knowledge use and, in the end, improves patient outcomes. In addition, HI provides support for powerful research techniques such as data mining and research involving biological processes and genomics that hold the promise of discovering new knowledge to improve clinical practices.

The material in this book is placed within the context of the Foundation of Knowledge model (**Figure IV-1**) to meet the needs of health care delivery systems, organizations, patients, and professionals. Health care professional education promotes scholarship and evidence-based teaching and learning. Through the sound integration of information management and technology tools, teaching and learning strategies promote the social and intellectual growth of the learner. As teachers and learners quest for knowledge, the need for pursuit of lifelong learning is instilled. Teachers and learners involved in the process of education are also involved with all levels of the model. Typically, they acquire and process data and information and generate and disseminate knowledge within the frame of reference of their educational institution. Their

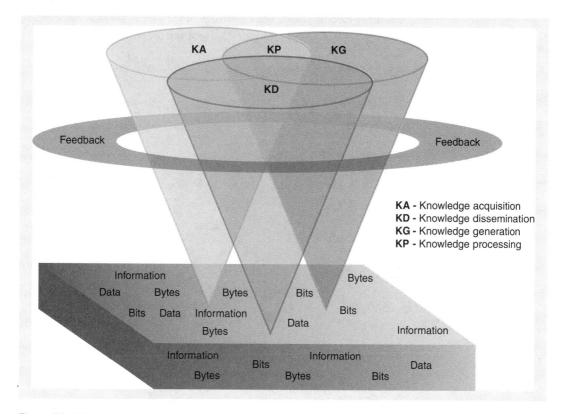

Figure IV-1 Foundation of Knowledge Model
Source: Designed by Alicia Mastrian.

knowledge generation remains on a limited, individual/course/school basis unless they become involved with developing publications and educational research that informs others in the health care professions.

Research is conducted to generate knowledge that is used to meet the needs of health care delivery systems, organizations, patients, and health care professionals. In relation to the model, researchers are involved with every aspect—from acquiring (collecting) and processing (analyzing) data and information to generating knowledge to disseminating the results or findings (knowledge). Through this work, the researcher generates knowledge for the health care professions. Knowledge generation is extremely important in the advancement of the disciplinary sciences.

The reader of this section is challenged to ask the following questions: (1) How can I apply the knowledge I gain from my education to benefit my patients and enhance my practice? (2) How can I help my colleagues, patients, and fellow students understand and use the current technologies to promote learning? (3) How can I use my wisdom to help create the theories, tools, and knowledge of the future? (4) How can I utilize research as evidence to enhance my knowledge base and my practice?

15

Informatics Tools to Support Health Care Professional Education and Continuing Education

Heather E. McKinney, Sylvia DeSantis, Kathleen Mastrian, and Dee McGonigle

OBJECTIVES

1. Describe health professional education in relation to the Foundation of Knowledge model.
2. Explore knowledge acquisition and sharing.
3. Assess technology tools and delivery modalities used in health care professional education and in continuing education.

Introduction: Professional Education and the Foundation of Knowledge Model

Health informatics facilitates the integration of information, data, and knowledge to support health care professionals, patients, and other providers in their various settings and decision-making roles. The **Foundation of Knowledge model** specifically prompts health care professionals to extend their theoretical and metaphorical knowledge into practical, holistic determinations based on a variety of factors and contexts. Because competencies in informatics include but are not limited to **information literacy**, computer literacy, and the ability to use strategies

Key Terms
Asynchronous
Audiopod
Avatars
Blended hybrid
Blog
Collaboration
Compact disk read-only memory
Computer-assisted instruction
Computer based
Continuing education
Copyright
Digital versatile disk or digital video disk
(continues)

and system applications to manage data, knowledge, and information, the ability of students to use technology-mediated communication skills is essential to their success in the profession and as a means to improve patient safety.

The rise of telecommunications, computer-mediated communications, and virtual technologies has opened up opportunities for improving communication and extending care within the health care industry (Barnes & Rudge, 2005). Proponents of instructional applications of computer technology view it as a way to erase geographic boundaries for students, enhance the presentation of content, improve learning outcomes, and even tailor instruction to individual learning needs. When carefully matched with curricular objectives, technology becomes an efficient and affordable avenue through which faculty may provide useful knowledge to their students, thereby facilitating the learning process (Hebda & Czar, 2013). Now going far beyond the simple applications of word processing software or spreadsheets, technology applications have evolved greatly, taking advantage of modern capabilities to provide health care students with simulations, complex multimedia, virtual reality–assisted clinical scenarios, and a host of information and literature-gathering Internet tools.

Knowledge Acquisition and Sharing

The shift from computer literacy to information literacy and management has drawn attention to interactivity and design as the most important components of interactive **Web-enhanced** and **Web-based** courses in providing effective learning environments. Thurmond and Wambach (2002) discussed the four types of interactions related to Web-enhanced courses based on their literature review: (1) learner–learner, (2) learner–content, (3) learner–instructor, and (4) learner–interface interactions (para. 1). In traditional learner–learner exchanges, students interact with one another to troubleshoot, work out challenges, and exchange solutions generated from different perspectives. Traditional and familiar, both learner–content and learner–instructor interactions expect students to work directly with course content or the faculty member and then participate in relevant course activities, such as tests and reviews. Learner–interface interaction includes the ways students access their course work and their ultimate success or failure in finding, retrieving, and using what they need (Thurmond, 2003; Thurmond & Wambach, 2002). When Web enhanced, these interactions include **online chats**, forum discussions, participation in electronic mailing list groups, instant messaging, blogging, and use of e-mail, all of which ask the student to engage, digest, use, and disseminate information in new ways.

Hardware and Software Considerations

In the 21st century, health informatics has begun to rely heavily on technology usability, functionality, and accessibility. **Computer-assisted instruction** (CAI) has had an enormous impact on health informatics, with many CAI programs offering individualized instruction in the form of customizable scenarios, frameworks, and programs for study. Additionally, CAI contributes to better understanding of material by supporting all learning styles, types, and paces. Consequently, clinical skills have presented endless potential for software development, making the effective use of software and hardware by educators and students a prime necessity (Riley, 1996).

Recall that software comprises the instructions that direct a computer's hardware to work, whereas hardware consists of physical computer components, such as a mouse, keyboard, and monitor. Software essentially translates commands into computer language, allowing the hardware to perform its functions. Without hardware and software, computer technologies are moot; moreover, without software, hardware does not function (McHugh, 2006). Applications software refers to the various programs individuals use to communicate with others, do work, play games, or watch multimedia on a computer. The most common software package sold with computers is an office package, which generally includes a word processing program, spreadsheet capability, a presentation graphics program (e.g., PowerPoint), and some kind of database management system. Software packages are available on **compact disk–read-only memory** (CD-ROM), on **digital versatile disk or digital video disk** (DVD), or through the Internet, allowing the user to download the software directly from a vendor's website (McHugh, 2006).

Hardware decisions depend on the way a computer system will be used in addition to considerations related to cost, ease of use, and durability (Clochesy, 2004). Systems purchased for personal use may differ dramatically from those purchased for online learning laboratories or smart classrooms. Some factors to consider include where the system will be stationed (e.g., at home for personal use or in a learning laboratory for use by many students), how many desktops there will be (e.g., one or a few dozen), if it will be networked to a school's internal system, if printing will be available, and which level of security is needed (Hebda & Czar, 2013).

Delivery Modalities

Learning is a multispatial function, and in the age of technology innovation, instructional delivery can inhabit many forms in both physical and virtual spaces. Spaces in academia are no longer defined by a class or its content but instead by the learning the class is trying to promote. To this end, learning spaces should support multiple modes of learning and delivery, including reflection, discussion, and experience, and should facilitate face-to-face and online interaction within and beyond classrooms. Truly innovative delivery, whether face-to-face classroom interaction, online engagement, or a blended hybrid of technology and traditional classroom teaching, supports learning activities rather than standing independently of them (Oblinger & Oblinger, 2005).

Face-to-Face Delivery versus Collaborative Learning

Ridley (2007) suggests that although it is the most widely used teaching method among educators, traditional face-to-face lecture yields only a 5% information retention rate over a 24-hour period, a rate that compares unfavorably with demonstration (30%), discussion groups (50%), practice activities (75%), and peer teaching (90%) (as cited in Sousa, 1995). Additionally, the inability of physical space to keep pace with evolution of learning models inhibits the benefits gained from face-to-face interaction between teacher and student. For example, collaborative learning grinds to a halt when class is held in a room with chairs bolted to the floor, facing a lectern (Oblinger & Oblinger, 2005); this kind of spatial arrangement prohibits a sense of classroom community by inhibiting easy peer interaction, reducing students' ability to see one another, and concentrating all attention on the professor.

Conversely, in a collaborative learning environment, the professor guides conversation and sets up discussion, acting less as classroom authority and more as facilitator, helping students maintain focus, gently guiding discussion, and ultimately empowering students to push knowledge boundaries in a safe and secure atmosphere of peer support. This inductive, epistemological approach promotes active, critical thinking skills and assists students in not only learning facts but also how to learn. As future health care professionals determined to rely on quantification and rationale, students will benefit from face-to-face classroom interaction that hones their ability to manufacture new personal truths through interaction with people and ideas in ways that cannot always be measured and counted.

Ridley (2007) suggests that such interactive, cooperative learning strategies might include gaming, **role playing**, and problem-based learning. Because games are non-threatening and fun, they promote critical thinking and teamwork by pushing students to work together in groups to find answers and achieve success. Role playing is similar in that it allows students to try on real-life scenarios by filling either prescripted or ad-libbed roles (occupational or physical therapy assistant, dietician, patient, and so on) without the fear or pressure of putting another's life at risk while trying to determine the best course of action or find a solution for a fictitious patient's health issue.

Problem-based learning, a well-accepted form of interactive learning, takes assignments out of a contextual vacuum and applies real-life scenarios to problems or challenges. Students work in groups to solve the dilemma presented by real patient cases and build on prior knowledge, using higher-level thinking skills and progressive inquiry to resolve the problem (Ridley, 2007). This enhances the student's critical skills for acquiring and maintaining knowledge in practice.

Online Delivery

E-learning, online learning, and Web-based education have caused a significant shift in student–teacher relationships in health care professional education. According to Oblinger and Oblinger (2005), not only are learning spaces no longer physical or formal, especially on campuses with wireless capabilities, but students also expect to make use of wide ranges of cutting-edge technology during their academic tenure, exchanging the traditional "sage on the stage" for a technologically savvy "guide on the side" (Leasure, Davis, & Thievon, 2000) who gives up the role of gatekeeper and instead promotes and facilitates dialogue as central to teaching–learning (Aquino-Russell, Maillard Strüby, & Reviczky, 2007).

Student centered and no longer limited to the domain of the classroom, laboratory, or even a patient's bedside, online learning allows educators to translate theory into practice, creating a virtual classroom space that promotes **collaboration**, engagement, discussion, and analysis. Detractors of online learning initiatives suggest, however, that sharing an online space undermines the student–teacher relationship, makes building peer relationships difficult, and generally disrupts the normal classroom dynamic, thereby creating an unfamiliar, uncomfortable atmosphere. Despite these concerns, studies show that Web-based courses not only continue to gain in popularity but also enhance learning in ways that encourage students to share personal experiences and support. Researchers cite many factors that make online learning laudable, with accessibility and convenience being two of the most frequently cited issues (Aquino-Russell et al., 2007).

The **asynchronous** and time-independent elements of Web-based courses respond to the huge need for flexible class times among today's growing population of nontraditional learners. Additionally, Web-based and place-independent learning allows participation by anyone, anywhere in the world, with access. Exposure to online learning during health care professional education programs will facilitate continuing professional education during the practice tenure.

It is important to use tools that facilitate learning, such as the introduction of social media, into health care professional education. Twitter (http://www.twitter.com) can be used to focus and hone student perspectives. Each posting, or tweet, cannot exceed 140 characters. As they critically think about what they want to add to the discussion, students must act as wordsmiths to express their views succinctly given the character limitation; that is, they must present their viewpoints concisely. Other social media that can be used in education include the following sites:

- Diigo (https://www.diigo.com), a social bookmarking tool to collect, tag, and share online sources (Meyer, 2015)
- Feedly (https://feedly.com/i/welcome), an online feed aggregator to notify the subscriber of new content on blogs and websites of interest (Meyer, 2015)
- Flickr (http://www.flickr.com), for photo sharing
- Glogster (http://www.glogster.com), a graphical blog
- Instagram (http://instagram.com), for customizing and sharing photos and videos (Meyer, 2015)
- Pinterest (https://www.pinterest.com), a social bookmarking tool used to prime discussions (Meyer, 2015)
- Pixton (http://www.pixton.com), to create comics or cartoons
- Prezi (http://www.prezi.com), to create zooming presentations
- Scoop.it (http://www.scoop.it), an online content curation tool used to collect Web resources, comment on them, and publish the source and commentary (Meyer, 2015)
- Slideshare (http://www.slideshare.net), a community for sharing presentations
- VoiceThread (http://voicethread.com), for sharing images, videos, documents, and commentary (Meyer, 2015)

- Wordle (http://www.wordle.net), to create word clouds from text
- YouTube (http://www.youtube.com), to watch and share videos

These sites can be used by students to facilitate their presentations and team collaboration. The use of social media not only exposes the students to their use but also promotes the development of skills that will support professional collaboration as students enter the practice arena. Meyer (2015) reported that using social media in education helps students put concepts into context and maintain currency in course content and fosters a sense of community.

Hybrid or Blended Delivery

Traditional courses are more frequently being offered as online, virtual classes (i.e., **distance education**)—learning that occurs elsewhere than in the traditional classroom and consequently requires special course design, planning, techniques, and communication. A **hybrid** of this delivery mode includes learning in which traditional classroom time is enhanced or broken up with online components, thereby creating a class in which **blended hybrid** learning occurs. Forms of hybrid learning include Web-enhanced learning, such as asking students to **blog** responses to a reading or class discussion, and learning that takes place in and makes use of smart classrooms (e.g., teaching in a wired room equipped with classroom learning technologies, such as the Blackboard Learning System).

Smart classrooms, also known as digital and multimedia classrooms, integrate computer and audiovisual technologies by providing a ceiling-mounted projector with an access point at the front of the room, an instructor podium or workstation, sound, and network access. An enhanced smart classroom also provides networked student workstations instead of traditional desks, allowing students to follow along online and perform network or Web searches, chat, blog, or myriad other activities as dictated by the professor. For example, at Penn State University, users can access announcements, course materials, faculty information, websites, and other tools through the electronic course management system, enabling the faculty to extend learning beyond the physical classroom walls.

Technology Tools Supporting Education

Certain social trends emerging from the morass of both traditional and innovative technology tools include the use of technologies attempting to meet the needs of members of the **Net generation** or Millennial generation. These are students who have grown up inside a wired world of instant access and online everything and who are connected, digital, experiential, and social learners. Through the use of software, hardware, drivers, dedicated servers, plug-ins, and an Internet connection, students can chat, collaborate, play games, or interact electronically with a peer in some way, all with little to no learning curve or effort. Because visual media are now the vernacular of this highly digital culture, students and faculty are also embracing technology tools that allow for the creation and interpretation of visual images (Oblinger & Oblinger, 2005). Such tools might take the shape of interactive tutorials, a created city within a virtual reality land-scape, high-fidelity simulations, serious games, or even a multimedia action maze that prompts users to choose different outcomes within a scenario.

Tutorials

Modern **tutorials** mimic lectures by guiding users through a series of objectives or tasks, usually allowing the user to do the work at his or her own pace (Edwards & Drury, 2000). Tutorials generally stand alone as autonomous multimedia that may use anima-tion, text, graphics, sound, questions, and different kinds of interactivity to engage and intrigue the user. They tend to promote active learning by prompting the user to answer sets of questions, follow clickable **hypertext**, or complete quizzes. For example, users might be asked to fill in worksheets after reviewing anatomy concepts, take a quiz, post an answer to a question, or even click through a scenario by choosing the best course of action in a mock clinical situation.

Because most students benefit from being able to contextualize a lesson's framework and purpose, the most effective tutorials provide users with understandable navigation, such as a table of contents at its beginning, or additional navigational aids, such as icons, buttons, or text that indicate where and how they need to progress (Dewald, 1999).

Although most tutorials are created to stand alone, some may also benefit and supplement face-to-face instruction, such as the interactive information skills tuto-rial developed at the Institute for Health and Social Care Research in Salford, United Kingdom. This tutorial divides a traditional lecture series into chunks, incorporating questions that would normally arise during the session into the text and providing hyperlinks. This organization allows users to browse to different parts of the tutorial, open a database in a new window to perform a practice search, and access other fea-tures (Grant & Brettle, 2006). Tutorials in all their iterations urge students to hone and develop effective critical thinking skills. Short tutorials may also be created on an organization's intranet for continuing education of practicing professionals introducing a new policy or procedure. Since the tutorial is electronic, access and time spent on the tutorial can be easily tracked.

Case Scenarios

Professional organizations are increasingly recommending performance-based assess-ments of students in professional degree programs, and enacting case scenarios pro-vides an opportunity for students to practice procedural responses and improve patient safety. Case **scenarios**, a form of problem-based learning, are now available through simulation software and virtual reality programming as well. This kind of testing, in which students must respond within context to a perceived situation rather than a theoretical or fact-based question, allows educators to gauge procedural knowledge; it allows them to determine well how a student executes a skill or applies concepts and principles to specific situations (Garavalia, 2002). For example, in a clinical con-text, a student could explain a specific procedure, but such knowledge is declarative rather than procedural and, therefore, for some evaluators, not as valuable. Conditional knowledge is often also reflected in procedural knowledge, demonstrating a student's ability to know when and why action is or is not taken and how.

Portfolios

Viewed in the 1980s as realistic evaluative tools of student accomplishment and learning, portfolios in health care professional education are growing in popularity as useful tools for documenting students' exposure to educational experiences. A **portfolio** allows a student to document a variety of sometimes unquantifiable skills, such as creativity, communication, and critical thinking. Further, portfolios can reflect achievement of goals, self-evaluation, and professional development, also providing a way for returning students to log and document past work or life experiences in a creative but structured way without taking a standardized test. The usefulness of a portfolio for an undergraduate depends on a structured system of organization: an identification page with résumé, a table of contents, separate and clearly marked sections, and so forth. In this way, portfolios can monitor program outcomes, positively influence employment and graduate school admission, and provide a clear snapshot of a student's strengths and abilities. See **Box 15-1** for an overview of electronic portfolios and specific information on developing a professional portfolio.

Simulations *(with Contributions by Nickolaus Miehl)*

Used within health care circles for more than 15 years, the use of **simulations** in health care professional education have experienced a recent upsurge in popularity, in part due to the more widespread availability of high-quality simulation equipment and a reduction in price for this technology. Ranked by fidelity, or the level of realism the equipment resembles, simulation may take various forms: from computer-based simulation, in which software is used to simulate a subject or situation (e.g., an interactive tutorial featuring a nurse–patient situation), to full-scale simulation, in which all the elements of a health care situation are re-created using real physiology, people, and interaction to resemble an environment as closely as possible to immerse students in the experience (Seropian, Brown, Gavilanes, & Driggers, 2004). A simulator in essence is any device that is used to create a realistic learning experience for the learner but that removes the risk associated with learning during hands-on patient care. A simulator offers the unique ability to create a realistic learning environment that is safe, structured, and supportive for the learner (Bligh & Bleakley, 2006). Task and skill training rank as the most popular forms of simulation. Simulators encompass a broad range of devices, such as partial task trainers (e.g., an IV insertion arm); screen-based simulations, including simulated electronic health records, simulated documentation, and simulated environments replicating a realistic patient care area; and complex computer-driven human patient simulation mannequins. Although each of these simulation modalities can be used alone, collectively they can be powerful learning tools when used together to create a realistic patient care scenario. The goal of simulation, according to Gaba (2004), is a seamless immersion into the simulated practice environment during which learners are drawn into the reality of the environment or task at hand. Hertel and Millis (2002)

BOX 15-1   WHAT IS AN ELECTRONIC PORTFOLIO?

Glenn Johnson and Jeff Swain

Today's information technology infrastructure allows users to easily build Web-based collections that include evidence of their knowledge and skills. Users can upload artifacts that represent evidence of their learning experiences both inside and outside of the classroom. Electronic portfolios (e-portfolios) may also contain a blog element where students reflect on their total experience and demonstrate growth in their areas of study.

E-portfolios can be built using a range of different technologies. Some individuals use PowerPoint presentations to capture and present evidence. Web-based e-portfolios are built using common **Web publishing** tools to create webpages, such as Web 2.0 or open-source tools; the webpages are then published on the Internet (Barrett, 2012). In addition, an increasing number of institutional e-portfolio systems have emerged through which users can log in and then upload, enter, and share information or evidence related to their experiences. Examples of such systems include the following:

- Association for Authentic, Experiential and Evidence-Based Learning: http://www.aaeebl.org
- Digication: http://www.digication.com
- Epsilen: http://www.epsilen.com/Epsilen/Public/Home.aspx
- Facebook: http://www.facebook.com
- iWebfolio: http://www.iwebfolio.com
- LiveText: http://www.livetext.com
- MySpace: http://www.myspace.com
- PebblePAD: http://www.pebblepad.com
- TaskStream: https://www.taskstream.com/pub
- TypePad: http://www.typepad.com

WHY CREATE AN E-PORTFOLIO?

Although academic institutions may use e-portfolios for assessment of student learning, for the individual, e-portfolios are all about opportunity. Such opportunities might include supporting a working relationship with a mentor, networking with other professionals, or representing certain qualities and characteristics to prospective employers. In all of these cases, having gone through the process of developing an e-portfolio requires critical examination of which qualities make individuals who they are and why these qualities are important to them and their profession. It is important for all professionals to have a foundational understanding of where they are in their career trajectory and how this fits their long-term professional goals.

Practically speaking, e-portfolios are efficient. When introducing oneself in an e-mail message, a self-starting individual who has taken the initiative to develop and publish an e-portfolio can add this line to the message: "Here is a link to my e-portfolio." The recipient can click on this link, which automatically opens that individual's e-portfolio in a Web browser. Metaphorically, the senders of such messages have just walked into the recipient's office with information that illustrates who they are, what they know, what they can do, and what they value as important; they have just walked in with what could be a multimedia showcase of their qualities. The Internet is a very powerful communication medium, and individuals with professional e-portfolios are simply taking advantage of this fact.

E-PORTFOLIOS IN HIGHER EDUCATION

As an instructional strategy, portfolios have been around for a long time. Instructionally, portfolios, whether electronic or paper based, require students to demonstrate or provide evidence that they have attained specific learning outcomes. For example, in the arts, portfolios have been used to demonstrate the depth and breadth

(*continues*)

BOX 15-1   WHAT IS AN ELECTRONIC PORTFOLIO? (continued)

of the work of an artist. Although performance-based programs of study are more likely to be familiar with the concept of the portfolio as a demonstration of what a student knows and can do, other areas of study have also begun to adopt this method of assessment.

Portfolios can be particularly helpful in areas where higher-level thinking and analysis are essential. For example, being a good health care professional encompasses much more than simply being able to get high scores on examinations. Professionals need to be able to collect information, analyze the information presented, relate it to past experience, apply related knowledge, and evaluate various options and from this present a diagnosis and a plan of action. In short, health care professionals need to be able to think critically and make informed decisions. In learning to become a health care professional, portfolios can be used to capture, support, and improve this type of thinking as it develops.

Like the artist, the health care professional student can connect, share, and present cases and findings and include with this evidence the reflective commentary that serves to unveil how he or she arrived at a decision, which information or experiences were vital, and how his or her action plan evolved. However, given the vast variety of evidence that individuals might potentially use to represent themselves, what should one select and how should this be shared?

E-PORTFOLIOS FOR PROFESSIONAL DEVELOPMENT
Using an e-portfolio to support professional networking involves a predetermined and focused purpose. This purpose may be to foster better communication between oneself and a mentor, or it may be to establish how what a professional is doing fits with the goals of the institution or perhaps an institution for which the individual would like to work. A professional e-portfolio is evidence based and uses this evidence to make a case that highlights the individual's capacity not only to perform but also to grow and develop professionally within his or her chosen field.

THE E-PORTFOLIO PROCESS
The four steps involved in developing an e-portfolio are recursive in nature, meaning that during the process one can backtrack to fill in missing pieces or reevaluate earlier decisions that were made. The four steps are (1) collect, (2) select, (3) reflect, and (4) connect.

Collect
Evidence should demonstrate what a person knows, what he or she can do, or the values that the person holds as being important. When it comes to developing e-portfolios, it is important to think of evidence in very broad terms. This evidence might include the results of what someone has learned in courses taken as a student, especially in terms of demonstrating a new skill or increased knowledge of a subject. More importantly, evidence can come from experiences that take place outside of the classroom. For example, someone may have been involved in an internship or clinical observation where he or she had the opportunity to connect what was learned in the classroom with how this information is applied in a real-world setting. Not only is such an experience valuable, but it also represents the individual's understanding of how this knowledge can be applied; thus, it enhances others' perception of the depth of what the person knows.

Résumés are evidence documents. They are very important, and every professional should have an updated copy available. However, résumés simply list an individual's experiences or accomplishments. E-portfolios, by comparison, go beyond the résumé to emphasize personal attributes that are very important in the specific profession. These attributes include but are not limited to interpersonal skills, leadership skills, appreciation of diversity, ability to work in a team, and self-sufficiency. These attributes are difficult, if not impossible, to demonstrate in a résumé.

BOX 15-1   WHAT IS AN ELECTRONIC PORTFOLIO? (continued)

When reflective commentary accompanies evidence of an individual's involvement, these attributes and values can become the highlights of an e-portfolio.

Select

Everyone has his or her own unique pool of evidence from which to pull, and over time this evidence pool can become quite large. What will someone choose to feature and why? Putting together a professional e-portfolio requires that two intertwining questions related to purpose and audience be addressed.

What is the purpose? What is it that someone is attempting to gain by putting an e-portfolio together? Is the purpose related to personal development (i.e., feedback and advice about the professional direction that is being taken)? Is the purpose to connect with colleagues? An individual may, for example, be interested in using his or her e-portfolio to find a job or to gain admission into a graduate program.

Although an e-portfolio can link to everything that a person has accomplished, this may not be the best strategy. Instead, it is essential that an individual consider the audience and establish a plan that enables the person to select the most appropriate pieces of evidence for his or her particular purpose and audience. A helpful way to start is to select the top five pieces of evidence that support the plan. Next, the individual should consider why he or she selected these pieces of evidence. What it is about each piece of evidence that makes it representative of who the individual is, what he or she knows, what he or she can do, and what he or she values as important.

Reflect

Reflection and reflective commentary take an e-portfolio to the next level. This component may take the form of a single reflective statement, or it may be attached to the evidence throughout the e-portfolio. Reflective comments should open up a window into why an individual thinks this evidence is important, the ways in which the individual values what he or she learned, or why the person thinks it is important for the larger profession. For example, the individual may present an experience where he or she was challenged to provide assistance. Describing this experience would be important; however, the reflective comments can extend this description, enabling the person to talk about the alternatives considered as the basis for how he or she made a decision to provide the specific type of assistance and the manner in which it was provided. By itself, a description of this experience is good. With reflective comments, readers have a much more thorough perception of and insight into an individual's professional thinking. This is where having a blog element as part of an e-portfolio becomes extremely powerful.

Unlike static webpages, a blog page is a space designed to be interactive. The blog owner posts commentary, thoughts, and experiences for others to read and respond. Regular entries on a blog give others a reason to return to one's e-portfolio site over and over again. It is an opportunity to share one's perspective on topics of interest and critical to the chosen field. A blog is a place where conversation happens. It provides a nice counterbalance to the static webpages, such as a résumé and project pieces.

Most blogging platforms allow users to select from a range of templates that include a blogging element along with static webpages. Such platforms as WordPress, MoveableType, and Google are free for at least the basic service, enabling the user to create a dynamic e-portfolio without having to build webpages. Most platforms allow entries to be in both text and multimedia format, so the blog becomes the perfect place for personal expression. A blog is quickly becoming a standard part of an e-portfolio.

Connect (Connections) and Feedback

The connection and feedback step is important to validate the assertions someone makes about what it is he or she knows, understands, or values. Individuals may choose to receive feedback from those who are close to them and

(continues)

BOX 15-1   WHAT IS AN ELECTRONIC PORTFOLIO? (continued)

from here reach out to others who may provide different perspectives. For example, if a health care professional was thinking about using his e-portfolio to apply for a position, he might want to start by first getting feedback from friends and family. He might also share his e-portfolio with a mentor or faculty member, raising the bar by getting professionally grounded feedback before sharing the e-portfolio with a prospective employer.

CHALLENGES AND ISSUES: PRIVACY AND SECURITY
The ease and popularity of both Web-based social networking and professional e-portfolio tools also raises several challenges and issues for users. Never before has information for individuals been so accessible, and never before has such personal information been so readily made public. For this reason, issues related to **privacy** and security need to be addressed. What might be appropriate socially can be deadly in a professional context.

E-PORTFOLIO PROCESS: SUMMARY COMMENTS
In summary, one might think about the process of developing a professional e-portfolio as boiling down to the telling of a rather simple story albeit a story that has three parts: looking back, looking around, and looking ahead. Readers should think of their own evidence pool as they answer these questions:

1. Looking back: What have you done? In which activities and with which organizations have you been involved? Where have you been? With whom have you worked? How did this help get you where you are today?
2. Looking around: In what are you currently involved? Why are you doing this? What are you getting out of it?
3. Looking ahead: Where would you like to be in 2 years? Where would you like to be in 5 years? Why do you feel this way? What makes you think your goals are realistic?

REFERENCE
Barrett, H. (2012). ePortfolios. http://electronicportfolios.org/eportfolios/index.html

---

note that this is a cooperative process whereby learners come together in an authentic setting and begin to learn from one another.

Considering the realistic nature of simulation and its hands-on active approach to learning, it seems that the use of simulation modalities can be a powerful tool in moving health care professionals toward achieving the informatics competencies.

The most useful teaching simulations combine **high-fidelity** equipment with **real-time** demonstrations of simulated medical emergencies, such as those enacted by the patient simulator laboratory at the Patient Safety Institute, a training subcenter of the North Shore–Long Island Jewish Health System. Home to programmable human simulator mannequins (including an infant) that can exhibit a variety of symptoms resembling various patient scenarios, the patient simulator laboratory tests and trains staff in responding to simulated medical emergencies using real-time demonstrations and gives immediate feedback on their video-recorded activities. Intended to help improve both clinical and decision-making skills, the mannequins mimic human responses, such as breathing, coughing, and speaking, and are anatomically accessible in their ability to be intubated, catheterized, and auscultated (Spillane, 2006). Simulated experiences in health care professional education (and continuing education) provide important opportunities for students and professionals to hone critical thinking and clinical skills in a safe and supportive environment. Simulation scenarios may also provide a better variety of clinical experiences than those available in a real setting and also provide faculty the opportunity to track student progress and development against specific learning objectives.

Virtual Reality

In traditional **virtual reality**, the user receives multiple sensory inputs, either mediated or generated by a computer, through visual stimulation (glasses, goggles, and screens), audio input (earphones, microphones, and synthesizers), and touch (smells, gloves, and bodysuits). A form of simulation training that was once considered a science fiction technology of the future, virtual reality health care training has been widely used by medical students and surgeons in training in recent years, as it allows individuals to practice an operation before working on a real patient (Turley, 2000). The current spotlight in virtual reality systems focuses on **Second Life**, an online virtual world created by San Francisco–based Linden Lab in 2003 that has multiple teaching applications.

Virtual worlds are online environments in which the residents are **avatars** who, in turn, represent individuals participating online. Virtual world participants have an opportunity to design nearly every aspect of their environment, from their avatars' clothing, gender, and appearance (EDUCAUSE Learning Initiative, 2006) to more complex elements that openly lend themselves to teaching approaches supported by the Foundation of Knowledge model, such as how the avatars communicate, move, interact, and create. Because virtual worlds are so versatile in their setup and preselected environments are highly customizable, health care instructors have the opportunity to create learner-led scenarios rather than relying on outcome-based models of knowledge development (EDUCAUSE Learning Initiative, 2006), thereby creating opportunities for "mediated immersion" (Dede, 2005), a "neomillennial learning style" (Skiba, 2007b, p. 156) that promotes the ability to negotiate multiple media and simulation-based virtual settings and communal learning, providing an important and valuable balance among experiential learning and guided mentoring (Dede, 2005).

No longer limited to the purview of computer geeks, virtual worlds like Second Life have drawn the attention of large organizations, such as the American Cancer Society and the Centers for Disease Control and Prevention (Skiba, 2007b). Educational institutions have also recognized the benefits of educating students in a virtual world that not only resembles the real world but can also be modified to enhance learning. At Chamberlain College of Nursing, Dr. Dee McGonigle directs the use of Second Life with graduate nursing students in their practicum experiences across the education, executive, informatics, and health care policy tracks. Because this environment lends itself to collaboration, nursing and other health care professionals, engineering, and business students are able to participate in cooperative interdisciplinary learning episodes.

Because virtual worlds foster unintentional learning through gamer-like technology in which students discover and create knowledge to accomplish something, rather than experiencing traditional outcome-based learning, their experiences result in greater comprehension and deeper knowledge. In a virtual clinical scenario, for example, a simulated, immersive environment presents invaluable learning opportunities for the student who is assuming the role of health care provider. Faculty can monitor the interaction and interrupt as necessary to provide advice or suggestions, while students negotiate the real and virtual world components of the scenario and their avatar patients, thereby becoming aware of how, why, and when to apply specific skills within a clinical setting (EDUCAUSE Learning Initiative, 2006).

Because so much of the data health care professionals rely on are complex and so many patient cues are lacking in concrete language or responses, virtual worlds' animated, immersive, three-dimensional environment allows students to practice skills, try new ideas, and learn from their mistakes while receiving feedback from educators within a globally networked classroom environment. Some students may struggle to participate in virtual communities for various reasons. Increasing comfort with multidisciplinary learning among students and educators improves patient safety and encourages the refinement of best practices for effective integration of these tools into mainstream education (EDUCAUSE Learning Initiative, 2006).

Serious Games *(Contributed by Brett Bixler)*

An educational game—one designed for learning—is a subset of both play and fun and is sometimes referred to as a "serious game" (Zyda, 2005). Many different types of games exist, and each type has a different potential for educational use. To learn to respond quickly and hone reflexes, action games may be used. Adventure games may be used to discover the unknown, such as diagnosing a patient illness. Construction and building games could be used for building complex mental constructs that can be understood only through knowledge of their constituent parts and the ways in which they interrelate. Strategy games are great for health care professional education teaching moments where careful, up-front planning is critical and on-the-fly adjustments to one's plan may be needed to ensure its success. In role-playing games, the player takes on the role of one or more characters and improves them while progressing through a story line. Role-playing games are an excellent way for educators to guide students through any situation where a sequenced step-by-step introduction to the parts of the job or skill is required. Fairly new are casual games, also known as mini-games. These games are designed to be played in a short time span or for a few minutes a day over several days, weeks, or even months. Many online browser-based games fit this category. Casual games may be useful for continuous reinforcement of basic concepts, for emulating a slowly changing environment, and for modifying the player's attitudes on a given topic over a period of time. To date, these games remain largely untapped as educational tools.

Two important websites to watch for emerging games are the Serious Games Initiative (http://www.seriousgames.net) and Games for Health (http://www.gamesforhealth.org).

The use of educational games, simulations, and virtual worlds for education continues to grow, with a great deal of research effort and funds directed toward the discoveries of their best uses. Educational games, simulations, and virtual worlds all share some characteristics, and it is difficult to find a pure experience in any of the genres. Simulations may have game-like qualities, and virtual worlds may be used to present a simulation.

Internet-Based Tools

The general consensus in health care professional education suggests that any technology that allows users to interact and engage both materials and one another is useful. More specifically, the Foundation of Knowledge model qualifies this observation with the caveat that technology must display user-friendly capabilities to provide benefits to its users, thereby allowing students not just to find information and one another online, but also to engage, challenge, and institute their discoveries. Providing students with easy-to-use, free Internet tools for reaching the first step in this process (gaining access to materials and peers) has been addressed by the proliferation of communication technologies available to any user with an Internet connection. Beyond the gadgetry, with the development of new strategies, practices, applications, and resources in technology comes the need for instructional strategies that not only appeal to this newer generation of students but also enhance learning. Such strategies, when coupled with easily accessible and highly functional tools, encourage students to see beyond the right answer and to seek out information that encourages them in developing approaches to issues and resolutions for problems (Bassendowski, 2005).

Webcasts and Webinars

Webcasts are broadcasts that are typically live presentations delivered by way of the Web. Webcasts offer great potential for helping students and faculty to engage both information and one another globally, by tapping into students' multiple intelligences to enable them to access what they need. Because of the growing ease of producing streaming video and subsequently delivering it via larger bandwidth, Webcasts have grown in popularity and are especially favored by programs that feature distance education components. Although some institutions create their own Webcast delivery system, most users rely on a few standard providers that, in turn, present the Webcast online. Although these presentations are often delivered live, allowing audience members to participate in the broadcast, many instructors use Webcasts as an access point for prerecorded archives of lectures and presentations by experts whom their students would not otherwise have the opportunity to see or hear. Studies show that students enthusiastically embrace Webcast technology, accessing archived presentations more repeatedly than traditionally filmed sessions of guest lecturers; this dynamic level of engagement aids students in better grasping the subject manner. Like much dynamic technology, Webcasts are an innovative component that keeps students engaged but tends to work best when learners are provided with learning outcomes before viewing them (Bell, 2003).

Webinars are Web-based seminars that use Web conferencing software that allows educators to share their computer screen and files and interact with their students. According to Moreau (2013), "Depending on what type of webinar service you decide to use, there are interactive sections that the audience can use to ask questions" (para. 5). Webinars are typically delivered live but can be recorded. Moreau equates this presentation form to Skype. In our geographically dispersed, online world of learners, webinars provide another avenue for sharing and collaborating.

There is a key difference between Webcasts and webinars. Webcasts present material to the audience with limited or no interactivity. By comparison, webinars are generally live, interactive, educational sessions. Both of these venues provide access to the educator and, depending on the level of interactivity, sometimes to other learners.

Searching

One of the most common and proliferate search tools in technology today is the **wiki**. Wikis are websites or hypertext document collections that allow users to edit and add content in an open-ended forum. The appeal of (and objection to) wikis resides in their ability to let anyone with an interest and an Internet connection participate in a once-exclusive community of knowledge creators and seekers. As an environment that encourages practice and learning, wikis support learning communities where students collaborate online (Skiba, 2007a). Higher education has evolved from a place of straightforward knowledge transmission to a place where one strives to become a member of an expert community, and wikis promise to create opportunities for individuals to participate in this community in heretofore untapped ways.

The most objectionable aspects of wikis are their lack of organizing principle (many are organized alphabetically) and the ability for anyone to edit entries, the latter of which creates new intellectual property right challenges. Wikipedia, for example, is the best-known wiki project on the Web; it is an online encyclopedia of sorts whose open-access policy regarding its content keeps educators and professionals wary of inaccurate information to be found there (Skiba, 2007a). For more information on the appropriate use of Wikipedia, see the online tutorial: http://www.libraries.psu.edu/psul/tutorials/wikipedia.html.

Instant Messaging

Instant messaging, one of many collaborative Web chat tools available to any user with a computer and Internet access, continues to establish itself as a working, useful tool for informatics learning, providing instant access to and communication among people, information, and technology. Although some **instant message** services provide voice and video messages, all instant messaging clients provide real-time text, allowing users to interact in the form of an on-screen conversation through a technology that is free, is already quite popular with users, is Web based, does not require additional hardware or software, and has a very low learning curve for those few to whom it is unfamiliar. Beyond having a real-time conversation, instant messaging an individual allows the user to share links, pictures, and files. This kind of easy accessibility allows students, when logged on, to collaborate; seek real-time help from professors or librarians; and engage others working on questions, studying for clinical examinations, or reviewing information or notes (Chase, 2007).

Chats and Online Discussions (Blogs)

Real-time chats occur all over the Internet, at each hour of every day. The best-known chat tools are instant messenger clients, but chatting also refers to real-time discussion venues in which users meet in virtual chat rooms to engage in conversations by posting messages; this provides a comfortable, recognizable way of communicating for Net generation students used to surfing the Web and interacting online. In a chat, students can meet, discuss, and engage one another over any given topic. Chats take various forms, the most complex of which involve highly evolved virtual communities in which users step into various rooms where they interact with other individuals who are in the room at the same time. Initially the exclusive purview of gamers or hard-core programmers creating private online communities, chat rooms now exist for a wide variety of topics and interests.

Web logs, also known as "blogs," have emerged as low-investment and easy-to-use writing tools that, through their very setup and appearance, enhance health professionals' communication, writing, reading, information-gathering, and collaboration skills (Maag, 2005). Blogs are a kind of online journal created by individuals who then invite comments from visitors to that Web space. Compared to technically complex online projects, such as tutorials and various multimedia, blogs are immediate, free to set up and access with an Internet connection, and easily negotiable by even the technically ambivalent. By their very nature, blogs present a built-in discussion area to the user, so they are especially useful for study groups interested in reflecting on material and evaluating ideas in a collective, collaborative way (Shaffer, Lackey, & Bolling, 2006).

Electronic Mailing Lists

One low-investment information-gathering tool for use by nursing professionals is membership in an **electronic mailing list**. These electronic discussion groups use **e-mail** to communicate and promote communication and collaboration with others interested in a particular field of study (Hebda & Czar, 2013). Electronic mailing lists have very few requirements to participate—usually just a free subscription and e-mail capability. Such lists are available on any subject, but most share common features, such as the need to subscribe and then log in to participate. The moderators of an electronic mailing list have specific instructions on how to post messages and how to set subscription controls. Posting information means that when a user replies to a topic thread, he or she generally has sent information to every member of the list. Like other technologies, the capabilities of electronic mailing lists continue to change and expand, providing ongoing viability for use in health care professional education.

Portals

Similar to electronic mailing lists in the way they deliver specific information to one's e-mail, a **portal** allows the personalization of a specific website. Portals organize information from webpages into simple menus so that users may choose what they want to view and how they want to view it (Hebda & Czar, 2013). For example, WebMD is one of the most popular and best-known portals, allowing users to create accounts, bookmark their favorite information, and sign up for e-mail notifications. Portals, like most Web technologies, require an Internet connection and a free subscription that allows the user to log in. Portals need users to register in order to collect information from them to personalize features for each individual user as they use the portal (Hebda & Czar, 2013).

Podcasts: Audiopods and Videopods

Podcasts are audio recordings linked to the Web that are then downloaded to an MP3 player (Gordon, 2007), a **smartphone**, or a computer where the listener accesses the recording or video. An outgrowth of the Apple iPod market, podcasts are developed and delivered by way of the Internet and require minimal investment—namely, a microphone, an Internet connection, and (often free) editing software.

Beyond possibilities for global accessibility to whatever information the user may record, podcasts allow for automatic updates in the form of a **really simple syndication** (RSS) (also known as a **resource description framework** [RDF] site summary) feed that lets subscribers receive automatic notification whenever a podcast is updated (Gordon, 2007). Refer to **Box 15-2** for more information.

Audiopods

Audiopod is a term used to describe a traditional or audio-based podcast. Participating in podcasting can exercise not just basic technology skills but also writing, editing, and speaking skills. Writing scripts for a podcast can be an excellent exercise in critical thinking and information delivery, whereas the technology itself allows global access to information by faculty, teachers, and students anywhere at any time (Gordon, 2007). Both faculty and students can create audiopods with little difficulty, and most use podcasts to share additional class materials, updates, and even entire lectures (Oblinger & Oblinger, 2005).

Videopods

Similar to an audiopod in setup and accessibility, a **videopod** is a podcast that provides video in addition to audio functionality. Faculty might use videopodcasts to demonstrate concepts, interview experts in the field, and even assess student progress (Gordon, 2007). Libraries and other institutions have even begun using the videopod as a learning alternative to the ubiquitous and often-mocked information video, finding that highly mobile students are more readily embracing this technology (Oblinger & Oblinger, 2005).

Multimedia

As technologically savvy students continue to demand accessible, interactive learning tools to keep them engaged, an increasing number of instructors are experimenting

BOX 15-2 PODCASTS

Jackie Ritzko

A basic Web search using the search term *free health care professional podcasts* returned nearly 5 million hits on one search engine. But what does this mean in the context of health informatics? The implication is that there are many resources on the Internet that somehow involve podcasts with a health care focus. How these sites might be of use to a professional in the health care field is the focus of this feature. Before any discussion of the educational uses of a technology tool can take place, however, there needs to be an understanding of the hardware, software, training, and support that are required to use the tool as well as the history of the development of the tool.

Podcast is a term coined from the words *iPod* and *broadcast*. **iPod** is the name given to a family of portable MP3 players from Apple Computer. MP3 is a common file format for electronic audio files. Audio files—in particular, MP3 files—can contain verbal speech, music, or a combination of both. MP3 files can be played or listened to using an MP3 player. MP3 players can be portable devices, such as the iPod, or an MP3 player can simply be software that is installed and used on a computer, a tablet, or a smartphone. Thus, a podcast is simply an MP3 file that can be played on an MP3 player. *Broadcast*, in its simplest usage, refers to the ability to send out. In terms of podcasts, broadcasting is the ability to share MP3 files in such a way that the files are delivered to the user whenever new versions are available through a subscription. This ability to share resources and access the most up-to-date resources is a great advantage, especially for the educational community.

We will now discuss podcasts in terms of function, ranging from the more basic to the more advanced functions: finding podcasts, listening to podcasts, creating podcasts, and sharing podcasts. Finding podcasts at a minimal level requires only an Internet connection and a web browser. As noted earlier, a basic Web search for the term *health care professional podcast* found many sites. Performing a basic Web search, however, may provide a user with only limited search capabilities. An **MP3 aggregator** is a program that can facilitate the process of finding, subscribing to, and downloading podcasts. One popular aggregator is Apple Computer's iTunes, which is a free program available as a download from Apple.com. Although iTunes is widely used, it is not the only program of this type. A program such as iTunes gives the user the ability to search for podcasts based on many criteria, including category, author, or title. The iTunes program provides access to audio downloads that may be either songs or podcasts. In both cases, users may find downloads that are free and those that require payment.

Because podcasts are largely MP3 audio files (Advanced Audio Coding [AAC] is a newer format but is not as widely used), an MP3 player is needed to listen to a podcast. As noted, this can be done on a smartphone, a computer with an MP3 player, or a portable MP3 player. Podcasts can be downloaded in two ways: manually or by subscribing to a podcast. In the case of a subscription, once a new track is added to the podcast, iTunes automatically delivers it to a computer. Continuing to use iTunes as an example, once a podcast is found, it can also be manually downloaded from iTunes to a computer. Once on the computer, it can be listened to or transferred to a portable device or accessed via a tablet or smartphone.

Users may also choose to produce or record podcasts. As with most technology solutions, hardware and software requirements typically must be met to create podcasts. The hardware for recording a podcast can vary. In a stationary setup, a microphone can be connected to a desktop or laptop computer. Stand-alone audio recorders can also record podcasts, and some MP3 players contain built-in recorders. Free recording software is available for most computer platforms.

Sometimes a podcast is created for the sole use of the creator. More often, however, a podcast is created with the intention of its being shared with and listened to by others. Podcasts can be stored on Web servers for distribution and can also be shared via tools, such as iTunes. Within iTunes, for example, educational institutions are able to host podcasts in the area known as iTunesU.

(continues)

BOX 15-2 PODCASTS (continued)

Podcasts have many uses in education in general and in health care education in particular. Informal learning can take place when a student listens to podcasts. Listening to or creating podcasts may be a formal class assignment, providing new ways to interact with course material.

Short discussions of what is new in the field may appear as podcasts on the Internet, in particular on news and research sites. Learners may rely on the portability of MP3 players to take learning with them on the road. Commuters and walkers and joggers are often seen listening to MP3 players. Because creating podcasts is relatively easy and inexpensive, such presentations can be produced by students as review files for common terms or used as ways for students to self-assess their ability to discuss topics. The uses of podcasts from an educational perspective are limitless.

Bringing the discussion of podcasts back to the Foundation of Knowledge model, for each task or process in the model, one can see how podcasts fit with that concept. Podcasts can be used to acquire new knowledge from sources on the Web. Listening to podcasts provides learners with another tool for learning in addition to readings and lectures, thereby addressing a wider audience whose members have varying learning styles. Because podcast creation is simple and inexpensive, podcasts are an ideal way to generate and disseminate knowledge.

---

with and incorporating multimedia into their courses. Generally, **multimedia** refers to a **computer-based** technology that incorporates traditional forms of communication to create a seamless and interactive learning environment, such as interactive tutorials, streaming video, and problem-solving programs. Health care educators have long relied on traditional multimedia, such as slide presentations, overhead projections, and training videos, for **continuing education** (CE) of staff, classroom learning, and patient education (Edwards & Drury, 2000). Now, however, new advances in multimedia allow faculty to add such innovations as simulations and virtual reality to their health care training, providing a way for students to learn procedural skills, such as range-of-motion exercises and physical assessment, without any risks to an actual patient.

Research suggests that the seeing, hearing, doing, and interacting afforded by multimedia facilitate learning retention, with multimedia being at least as effective as traditional instruction but offering the benefit of greater learner satisfaction. Authoring software—that is, programs that allow users of varied technical skill to design and create webpages and movies—has greatly facilitated the use of multimedia by faculty (Hebda & Czar, 2013). Nevertheless, the most effective multimedia relies on the careful and pedagogically appropriate combination of textual material, graphics, video, animation, and sound (Edwards & Drury, 2000)—a distinctly separate skill set from teaching and instructing. Some schools have instructional designers on staff to assist faculty with the development of multimedia to support learning.

Beyond providing a flexible method of delivery for instructional information, multimedia promises to motivate students by requiring them to analyze evidence in ways that require higher-order thinking and problem-solving skills. Similarly, faculty can begin to think about their classes in new ways and accommodate different student learning styles (Oblinger & Oblinger, 2005). **Box 15-3** looks at the capabilities of smartphones.

BOX 15-3   SMARTPHONES AND OTHER SMART DEVICES IN HEALTH CARE EDUCATION

Dee McGonigle and Kathleen Mastrian

Smartphones are another tool for the educational arena. As Yu (2012) stated, "Smart phone technology, with its pervasive acceptance and powerful functionality, is inevitably changing peoples' behaviors" (para. 6).

Our educational uses of a technology such as smartphones not only affect the learning episode but also influence how we prepare students to embrace and use technologies appropriately. As educators, we want our students to remain competitive in a highly technologically dependent world. Health care is a data- and information-driven profession, and health care professionals must rely on technologies to provide the data and information necessary to provide safe, high-quality care to our patients.

If students have smartphones, we can share text, graphics such as PowerPoint presentations, podcasts, and other audio/video media with them prior to the learning episode. When all students have access to the same information, it enhances the dialogue and topical discussion centered on that information. Educators can use smartphones to distribute announcements, reminders, and even pertinent notes that the students need. Students can also be polled using these devices. Smartphones can even replace huge textbooks with electronic files. Smart devices and their calendars and messaging features help both educators and students organize their lives and keep their hectic schedules straight. The use of smart technologies can facilitate interactions around the world. Students can consult with other students and experts from anywhere on the globe. As this brief list of applications suggests, we have only just begun to think of ways in which to incorporate smartphones into our learning episodes.

In conclusion, we would like to leave you thinking about a money-saving alternative for many schools. Instead of requiring a laptop computer, what if your school required every student to have a smartphone? Could we replace the expensive computer labs on our campuses while better connecting our online and blended students to their educational milieu?

REFERENCE

Yu, F. (2012). Mobile/smart phone use in higher education. http://www.swdsi.org/swdsi2012/proceedings_2012/papers/Papers/PA144.pdf

Promoting Active and Collaborative Learning

A collaborative, student-centered approach uses the best tenets of inductive teaching by imposing more responsibility on students for their own learning than is assumed in the traditional lecture-based deductive approach. These constructivist methods are built on the widely accepted principle that students are constantly constructing their own realities rather than simply absorbing versions presented by their teachers. Collaborative methods often involve students' discussion of questions and in-class problem solving, with much of the work (in and out of class) done by students in groups rather than individually (Felder & Prince, 2007).

Johnson and Johnson (2009) have identified significant elements for successful collaborative and cooperative learning that are still pertinent today:

1. Face-to-face interaction between students, allowing them to build on one another's strengths
2. Mutual learning goals that, in turn, prompt students to exhibit positive interdependence rather than individualized competition

3. Equal participation in the work process and personal accountability for the work one contributes
4. Regular debriefing sessions as a group after meetings or presentations during which time feedback is shared and observations analyzed
5. Use of cooperative group process skills learned in the classroom

Especially useful for students is the collaborative fieldwork model in which two or more students share a clinical setting and the same fieldwork educator. In this model, learning happens in a reciprocal fashion, with students constructing knowledge by watching each other and exchanging ideas. The most effective fieldwork experiences are highly structured with clear outlines of responsibilities, duties, and expectations, ensuring that the experience matches the learner's expectations. All activities performed by students, such as conducting evaluations, are done jointly so that peers provide each other with objective feedback, leading to eventual increased self-confidence (Costa, 2007). In this way, suggests Costa, individuals with different viewpoints and experiences create a space where new knowledge emerges and existing knowledge can be restructured (as cited in Cockrell, Caplow, & Donaldson, 2000).

Libraries have also begun to recognize their role in students' success with and predisposition toward collaborative learning by creating redesigned spaces that reflect students' need to huddle in small groups, sit closely together without barriers, chat about their work, and view digital information without physical hindrances, such as carrels or work stalls. A leader in this movement has been Indiana State University, whose new information commons features completely overhauled furniture, software, monitors, processing power, and wireless access to the university's network. Students can now collect as a group at kidney-shaped tables; better see the information loaded on the flat-screen monitors; make use of brainstorming, design, and planning software; and discuss their work in a chat-friendly zone. Some faculty members have even scheduled classes at the learning stations, and students have responded enthusiastically to the evolved space (Gabbard, Kaiser, & Kaunelis, 2007).

In addition to adaptable physical spaces that encourage discussion and group work, students require a supportive infrastructure that provides essential elements necessary to successful research and scholarship. These include professional development support in the form of workshops that help students acquire or refresh skill sets, presentation opportunities, and hardware, software, and resource support. One such example involves the participation by nursing students at the University of Texas Medical Branch School of Nursing in the Scholarly Talk About Research Series, in which students and faculty give presentations of their work before presenting those materials at professional conferences (Froman, Hall, Shah, Bernstein, & Galloway, 2003), thereby eliciting collegial feedback, collaborative troubleshooting, and shared research ideas. Imagine how powerful such a process would be in a cross-discipline health care education school.

Preceptors and mentors help students learn by acting as clinical practitioner role models from whom the students can copy appropriate skills and behaviors. Preceptors enhance clinical competence through direct role modeling, which is especially valuable in a field where competence and clinical ability are paramount (Armitage & Burnard, 1991). Mentors, similar to preceptors, provide equally valuable assistance to students in the form of a facilitator. Mentors are most often used in health care education to support new professionals who are trying to fulfill the rigors of a new position while negotiating the stress inherent to a new environment (Gagen & Bowie, 2005). Mentors tend to address student needs through open conversation, student advocacy, feedback on student progress, facilitation, teaching, and general support (Neary, 2000).

Generally, these and other forms of institutional support promote students' adoption of a meaning-oriented approach to learning as opposed to a surface or memorization-intensive approach. Collaborative, inductive learning promotes intellectual development that challenges the dualistic thinking that characterizes many entering college students, which holds that "all knowledge is certain, professors have it, and the task of students is to absorb and repeat it" (Felder & Prince, 2007, p. 55). Further, this kind of learning helps students acquire the self-directed learning and critical thinking skills that characterize the best scientists and engineers (Felder & Prince, 2007). The active, engaging elements of collaborative learning increase self-confidence, promote autonomy in students, and foster a commitment to lifelong learning (Costa, 2007)—all necessities for the success of a new millennial information-literate student.

Knowledge Dissemination and Sharing

Sharing stories and experience from a clinical point of view accomplishes much more than simply promoting camaraderie or empathy (although this kind of engagement is infinitely valuable in its own way); sharing experiences of clinical learning can help convey lifesaving information to other clinicians in a way that is more memorable and palatable and less imposing than warnings delivered outside a social context. Clinical and caring knowledge, often rooted in everyday exchanges, become socially embedded such that those with experience in particular clinical settings share common knowledge and understanding. The social embeddedness of caring and clinical knowledge is a result of shared and shaped collective understanding of practice and sometimes provides an alternative view. The power of pooled knowledge, in combination with knowledge produced in dialogue with others, helps to limit tunnel vision and is a powerful strategy for maximizing the clinical knowledge of a group.

Networking

Considered crucial to career development because of opportunities for collaboration and information exchange, networking encourages professional support by making successful professionals accessible to their colleagues.

Because health care professionals tend to gather their information from personal networks, such as colleagues or professional meetings, the increased availability of technology to assist in networking has greatly facilitated information exchange. Blogs, e-mail, websites, electronic mailing lists, and other communicative technologies have opened up an endless stream of collaboration and networking possibilities, allowing professionals to more easily access and learn from colleagues' experiences.

Membership and participation in professional associations also provide ways to network and advance one's profession. Professional associations represent venues through which members may set standards for professional practice, establish codes of ethics, become involved in advocacy, engage in continuing education opportunities, access job banks, subscribe to professional journals, and act as a common voice for the profession. Barriers to joining and participating in professional organizations include cost, distance to meetings, lack of activities in their geographic area, and inability to attend meetings. Recognizing that networking creates fertile areas for the development of new ideas, partnership, jobs, and strategies, both national and state associations are increasingly creating opportunities for health care practitioners to earn continuing education credit and network with others in their field using technology.

Presenting and Publishing

Much in the way that accrediting agencies maintain standards for education, professional journals also hold their contributors to similarly rigorous standards and provide a valuable venue in which professionals might share ideology and innovations in the field. With the proliferation of online journals and the availability of health care information via multiple media, publishing remains an excellent way to participate in the dissemination of professional information. Both magazines and journals reach considerable audiences; journal distinctions lie in their authorship and audience. Although journal articles are written by and for scholars, with refereed or peer-reviewed journals requiring a blind review by a group of reviewers to eliminate bias, magazine articles may be written by a professional in the field, an editor, a freelancer, or another author. Publishing provides excellent opportunities to extend knowledge and share research.

Similar to publishing, making presentations at contemporary professional conferences allows educators and students to gain experience and share scholarship with colleagues. Presentations must meet certain standards for an audience to find them credible and effective.

Conferences often host poster presentations that enable contributors to share research findings, innovations, and exemplar programs in a low-investment but visually captivating way. Because posters are primarily visual, with little or no verbal supplementation, most important for consideration are room elements, such as size, space limitations, and lighting. A high-tech alternative to a paper poster is an electronic poster—that is, a continuously running PowerPoint presentation either projected for larger audiences or left to run from a laptop or desktop for smaller audiences (Bergren, 2000). Both publishing and presenting provide opportunities for the health care professionals to disseminate new knowledge and stay abreast of information in the field. Some educational institutions provide opportunities for undergraduates to showcase projects and research at undergraduate research conferences. These conferences are excellent ways for developing professionals to hone knowledge dissemination skills that will serve them well in their professional practice.

Continuing Education and Recertification

Nationally, health care employers and institutions have, because of budgetary constraints, begun to eliminate continuing education programs traditionally reliant on classes, conferences, and workshops; consequently, reliance on outside agencies and technology has increased to meet this need. The traditional approach to obtaining continuing education credits has included home study offered by professional journals and organizations in which the client reads articles, answers related questions, and sends in the test form and fee. Although fairly straightforward, this technique provides little in the way of peer interaction (Hebda & Czar, 2013).

With the ubiquitous technology influx and the accessibility it affords, obtaining continuing education credits through e-learning is considered a beneficial delivery method for mandatory educational programs and other programs that provide employees with opportunities to maintain or improve skills. Benefits of e-learning for continuing education training include the ability to access information at any time (thus creating a flexible schedule) and experience instant feedback and individualized instruction by seeking out specific, additional information as needed.

E-learning can also benefit administrative support of continuing education credits by providing instantly accessible computerized records and other tracking features, such as records of success and completion, associated costs of program development, and staff productivity. Allowing professionals to complete mandatory training on demand represents a huge benefit of e-learning, with the best programs allowing for customization to accommodate program revisions and regulation changes (Hebda & Czar, 2013).

In some cases, acquiring continuing education credits may also help the professional achieve recertification. Available through myriad professional organizations, recertification ensures that professionals are staying current in their field. As an added benefit, some employers may provide higher salaries to professionals who seek and maintain certification.

Fair Use and Copyright Restrictions

Fair use refers to a legal concept that permits the use of copyrighted works for specific purposes without obtaining permission from the author or without paying for the use of the work. Originally, fair use evolved for written work and allowed for uses that include journalists reporting the news, teaching, or scholarly research. As digital technology and the Web burst on the scene, fair use expanded to apply to the copying and redistribution of digital media, including photographs, graphics, music, videos, audio, and software or computer programs.

Four factors must be considered in determining whether a particular use is fair. These factors are derived directly from the fair use provision (http://www.copyright.gov/fls/fl102.html) of Section 107 of the U.S. Copyright Law (U.S. Copyright Office, n.d.):

1. The purpose and character of the use, including whether such use is of commercial nature or is for nonprofit educational purposes
2. The nature of the copyrighted work

3. The amount and substantiality of the portion used in relation to the copyrighted work as a whole

4. The effect of the use upon the potential market for or value of the copyrighted work

The first factor tends to favor educational institutions and nonprofit entities. The second factor relates to the nature of the work: Courts have consistently protected creative works and those that have not yet been published. The third factor that must be considered relates to the amount of use. Typically, you should determine how much of the overall work you are using; if it represents the core or essence of the work, you should not replicate or use it. The fourth and final factor relates to the effect on the creator's market share. If you are using a substantial portion of a text or software work that is offered for sale, you can adversely affect its owner's earning potential. The term itself should make you reflect on all of these factors and decide whether your proposed use is fair.

Copyright refers to the exclusive right of the creator of a work to distribute, sell, publish, copy, lease, or display that work in whatever manner he or she so chooses. Copyright laws are not only misinterpreted but are constantly being challenged by our advancing technological capabilities. Even though you use American Psychological Association (APA) formatting, for example, and cite the authors, you might be overstepping your rights and infringing on the author's copyright; you might not be accused of plagiarism, but you should always cite where you obtained your information or digital media.

All users of others' work, in whatever medium, must fully understand, be well aware of, and comply with copyright and fair use principles. Typically, you should try to think of what is reasonable use and always make sure that you cite the authors. Reflect on all four fair use factors before making your decision to use another's work for educational purposes.

The Future

Virtual reality–embedded education holds phenomenal promise for the future. Once the purview of gamers and geeks, virtual reality has exploded onto the academic scene and offers the potential for cross-pollination between fields of inquiry across the curriculum, university, and even learning systems. All kinds of university departments will undoubtedly experiment with virtual reality in hopes of staying current and pleasing their young and demanding constituency; however, much in the way society loves the feel of a book too much to make it archaic, so too will students, educators, and administrators ultimately return to some form of face-to-face classroom teaching, even as newer and more adventuresome teaching technologies emerge. Further, once fast, high-burn technologies stop flooding the marketplace and making education an even bigger business for proprietary online universities, modified traditions will take their place, creating new spaces for nontraditional students and the Internet generation—both groups that are anxious for technology use in the classroom for very different reasons.

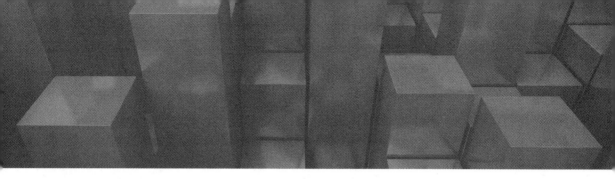

Summary

In an ideal world, health care professionals will work against the assumption that technology runs itself and take proactive roles in helping to design the education necessary best to prepare them for real-world scenarios. Consider that flash is not substance and that drama is not depth; technology performs only as well as the pedagogy that undergirds and sustains it. Use technology with care so that its best features consequently enrich your role as a learner.

Thought-Provoking Questions

1. What are some of the forces behind the push toward a more wired learning experience in health care education?
2. Which of the technologies discussed here most appeals to you? Why?
3. Explore one of the newer learning technologies in more depth. How would the use of this technology benefit you in your practice or education setting? Why do you find this tool useful? From your perspective, how could you enhance this tool?
4. Jean, a physical therapist assistant, recently read an article in an online journal that she accessed through her health agency's database subscription. The article provided a comprehensive checklist for preventing falls in older adults that Jean prints out and distributes to her patients as she visits them in their homes. Does this constitute fair use, or is it a copyright violation? Explain your answer.
5. Reflect on virtual learning opportunities. Develop a detailed list of pros and cons from your perspective. Provide rationale for each pro and con you delineate.

Apply Your Knowledge

Several informatics tools support education, but, even better, they support continuing education of professionals. Most professionals will need continuing education credits to maintain licensure, but all professionals should commit to lifelong learning and keep up with advances in their respective professions.

1. Choose an informatics tool that supports education and explore the advantages and disadvantages of engaging in this type of continuing education.

If your discipline requires a license and continuing education, obtain a copy of the law governing your practice and the acceptable continuing education activities.

Additional Resources

Association for Authentic, Experiential and Evidence-Based Learning
http://www.aaeebl.org

Digication
http://www.digication.com
Diigo
https://www.diigo.com
Epsilen
http://www.epsilen.com/Epsilen/Public/Home.aspx
Facebook
http://www.facebook.com
Feedly
https://feedly.com/i/welcome
Flickr
http://www.flickr.com
Games for Health
http://www.gamesforhealth.org
Glogster
http://www.glogster.com
Instagram
http://instagram.com
iWebfolio
http://www.iwebfolio.com
LiveText
http://www.livetext.com
MySpace
http://www.myspace.com
PebblePAD
http://www.pebblepad.com
Pinterest
https://www.pinterest.com
Pixton
http://www.pixton.com
Prezi
http://www.prezi.com
Scoop.it
http://www.scoop.it
Serious Games Initiative
http://www.seriousgames.net
Slideshare
http://www.slideshare.net
TaskStream
https://www.taskstream.com/pub
Twitter
http://www.twitter.com
TypePad
http://www.typepad.com
U.S. Copyright Office
http://www.copyright.gov/fls/fl102.html
VoiceThread
http://voicethread.com
Wikipedia Online Tutorial
http://www.libraries.psu.edu/psul/tutorials/wikipedia.html
Wordle

http://www.wordle.net
YouTube
http://www.youtube.com

References

Aquino-Russell, C., Maillard Strüby, F. V., & Reviczky, K. (2007). Living attentive presence and changing perspectives with a Web-based nursing theory course. *Nursing Science Quarterly*, *20*(2), 128–134.

Armitage, P., & Burnard, P. (1991). Mentors or preceptors? Narrowing the theory–practice gap. *Nurse Education Today*, *11*, 225–229.

Barnes, L., & Rudge, T. (2005). Virtual reality or real virtuality: The space of flows and nursing practice. *Nursing Inquiry*, *12*(4), 306–315.

Bassendowski, S. L. (2005). NursingQuest: Supporting an analysis of nursing issues. *Journal of Nursing Education*, *46*(2), 92–95.

Bell, S. (2003). Cyber-guest lecturers: Using webcasts as a teaching tool. *TechTrends*, *47*(4), 10–14.

Bergren, M. D. (2000). Power up your presentation with PowerPoint. *Journal of School Nursing*, *16*(4), 44–47.

Bligh, J., & Bleakley, A. (2006). Distributing menus to hungry learners: Can learning by simulation become simulation of learning? *Medical Teacher*, *28*(7), 606–613.

Chase, D. (2007). Transformative sharing with instant messaging, wikis, interactive maps, and Flickr. *Computers in Libraries*, *27*(1), 7–56.

Clochesy, J. M. (2004). Hardware and software options. In J. Fitzpatrick & S. Montgomery (Eds.), *Internet for nursing research* (pp. 120–128). New York: Springer.

Cockrell, K., Caplow, J., & Donaldson, J. (2000). A context for learning: Collaborative groups in the problem-based learning environment. *Review of Higher Education*, *23*(3), 347–363.

Costa, D. M. (2007). The collaborative fieldwork model. *OT Practice*, *12*(1), 25–26.

Dede, C. (2005). Planning for neomillennial learning styles. *EDUCAUSE Quarterly*, *28*(1).

Dewald, N. H. (1999). Transporting good library instruction practices into the Web environment: An analysis of online tutorials. *Journal of Academic Librarianship*, *25*(1), 26–32.

EDUCAUSE Learning Initiative. (2006, June). 7 things you should know about . . . virtual worlds. http://www.educause.edu/library/resources/7-things-you-should-know-about-virtual -worlds

Edwards, M. J. A., & Drury, R. M. (2000). Using computers in basic nursing education, continuing education, and patient education. In M. J. Ball, K. J. Hannah, S. K. Newbold, & J. V. Douglas (Eds.), *Nursing informatics: Where caring and technology meet* (pp. 49–68). New York: Springer.

Felder, R., & Prince, M. (2007). The case for inductive teaching. *Prism*, *17*(2), 55.

Froman, R. D., Hall, A. W., Shah, A., Bernstein, J. M., & Galloway, R. Y. (2003). A methodology for supporting research and scholarship. *Nursing Outlook*, *51*(2), 84–89.

Gaba, D. (2004). The future vision of simulation in health care. *Quality and Safety in Healthcare*, *13*, 2–10.

Gabbard, R. B., Kaiser, A., & Kaunelis, D. (2007). Redesigning a library space for collaborative learning. *Computers in Libraries*, *27*(5), 6–12.

Gagen, L., & Bowie, S. (2005). Effective mentoring: A case for training mentors for novice teachers. *Journal of Physical Education, Recreation and Dance*, *76*(7), 40–45.

Garavalia, L. S. (2002). Selecting appropriate assessment methods: Asking the right questions. *American Journal of Pharmaceutical Education*, *66*, 108–112.

Gordon, A. M. (2007). Sound off! The possibilities of podcasting. *Book Links*, 16–18.

Grant, M. J., & Brettle, A. J. (2006). Developing and evaluating an interactive information skills tutorial. *Health Information and Libraries Journal*, *23*(2), 79–88.

Hebda, T., & Czar, P. (2013). *Handbook of informatics for nurses and health care professionals* (5th ed.). Upper Saddle River, NJ: Prentice Hall.

Hertel, J. P., & Millis, B. J. (2002). *Using simulations to promote learning in higher education: An introduction*. Sterling, VA: Stylus.

Johnson, R., & Johnson, D. (2009). An Overview of Cooperative Learning. http://clearspecs.com/joomla15/downloads/ClearSpecs69V01_Overview%20of%20Cooperative%20Learning.pdf

Leasure, A., Davis, L., & Thievon, S. (2000). Comparison of student outcomes and preferences in a traditional vs. World Wide Web–based baccalaureate nursing research course. *Journal of Nursing Education, 39*, 149–154.

Maag, M. (2005). The potential use of "blogs" in nursing education. *CIN: Computers, Informatics, Nursing, 23*(1), 16–26.

McHugh, M. L. (2006). Computer hardware. In V. K. Saba & K. McCormick (Eds.), *Essentials of nursing informatics* (4th ed., pp. 517–532). New York: McGraw-Hill.

Meyer, L. (2015). 6 alternative social media tools for teaching and learning. http://campustechnology.com/Articles/2015/01/07/6-Alternative-Social-Media-Tools-for-Teaching-and-Learning.aspx?Page=1

Moreau, E. (2013). What is a webinar? http://webtrends.about.com/od/office20/a/What-Is-AWebinar.htm

Neary, M. (2000). Supporting students' learning and professional development through the process of continuous assessment and mentorship. *Nurse Education Today, 20*, 463–474.

Oblinger, D., & Oblinger, J. (2005). Educating the Net Generation. http://net.educause.edu/ir/library/pdf/PUB7101.pdf

Ridley, R. T. (2007). Interactive teaching: A concept analysis. *Journal of Nursing Education, 46*(5), 206–209.

Riley, J. B. (1996). Educational applications. In V. K. Saba & K. A. McCormick (Eds.), *Essentials of computers for nurses* (2nd ed., pp. 527–573). New York: McGraw-Hill.

Seropian, M. A., Brown, K., Gavilanes, J. S., & Driggers, B. (2004). Simulation: Not just a manikin. *Journal of Nursing Education, 43*(4), 164–170.

Shaffer, S. C., Lackey, S. P., & Bolling, G. W. (2006). Blogging as venue for nurse faculty development. *Nursing Education Perspectives, 27*(3), 126–128.

Skiba, D. J. (2007a). Do your students wiki? *Nursing Education Perspectives, 26*(2), 120–121.

Skiba, D. J. (2007b). Nursing education 2.0: Second Life. *Nursing Education Perspectives, 28*(3), 156–157.

Sousa, D. A. (1995). *How the brain learns*. Reston, VA: National Association of Secondary School Principals.

Spillane, J. (2006). Virtual reality takes on patient safety. *Nursing Spectrum (New York/New Jersey Metro Edition), 18A*(7), 13.

Thurmond, V. (2003). Defining interaction and strategies to enhance interactions in Web-based courses. *Nurse Educator, 28*(5), 237–241.

Thurmond, V., & Wambach, K. (2002). Understanding interactions in distance education: A review of the literature. http://www.itdl.org/journal/jan_04/article02.htm

Turley, J. P. (2000). Nursing's future: Ubiquitous computing, virtual reality, and augmented reality. In M. J. Ball, K. J. Hannah, S. K. Newbold, & J. V. Douglas (Eds.), *Nursing informatics: Where caring and technology meet* (pp. 49–68). New York: Springer.

U.S. Copyright Office. (n.d.). Copyright law of the United States of America and related laws contained in Title 17 of the United States code. http://www.copyright.gov/title17/92chap1.html#107

Zyda, M. (2005). From visual simulation to virtual reality to games. *Computer, 39*(9), 25–32.

Data Mining as a Research Tool

*Dee McGonigle, Kathleen Mastrian,
and Craig McGonigle*

OBJECTIVES

1. Describe big data.
2. Assess knowledge discovery in data.
3. Explore data mining.
4. Compare data mining models.

Introduction: Big Data, Data Mining, and Knowledge Discovery

Data mining methods have been developed over time using research. As data mining evolves, we have not only become able to navigate our data in real time but also progressed beyond mere access to retrospective data with navigational improvements. Using data warehousing and decision support, we could, for example, answer the question "What was the most commonly diagnosed disease in our nine-site practice last April?" We could then drill down to one practice site. As we have developed big data collection capabilities, data capture, data transmission, storage capabilities, powerful computers, statistics, artificial intelligence, high-functioning relational database engines with data integration, and advanced algorithms, we have realized the ability to data mine our big data to predict and deliver prospective and proactive information. We can begin to predict by answering a question such as "What is likely to be the most commonly diagnosed disease next month and why?" Data mining includes tools for visualizing relationships in the data and mechanizes the process of discovering predictive information in massive databases.

Key Terms
Algorithms
Bagging
Big data
Boosting
Brushing
Classification
Classification and regression trees
Data mining
Data set
Decision trees
DMAIC (define, measure, analyze, improve, control)
Drill-down
Exploratory data analysis
Knowledge discovery and data mining
Knowledge discovery in data
Knowledge discovery in databases
(continues)

Pattern discovery entails much more than simply retrieving data to answer an end user's query. Data mining tools scan databases and identify previously hidden patterns. The predictive, proactive information resulting from data mining analytics then assists with development of business intelligence, especially in relation to how we can improve. Much of our big data is **unstructured data**; unstructured big data reside in text files, which represent more than 75% of an organization's data. Such data are not contained in databases and can be easily overlooked; moreover, it is difficult to discern trends and patterns in such data. Data mining is an iterative process that explores and models big data to identify patterns and provide meaningful insights.

As we evolve the tools with which we can collect, access, and process data and information, it is necessary to concomitantly evolve how we analyze and interpret the data and information. IBM (2013) describes **big data** in a way that is easy to understand:

Every day, we create 2.5 quintillion bytes of data—so much that 90% of the data in the world today has been created in the last two years alone. This data comes from everywhere: sensors used to gather climate information, posts to social media sites, digital pictures and videos, purchase transaction records, and cell phone GPS signals to name a few. This data is big data. (p. 1)

According to Tishgart (2012), "More data means more knowledge, greater insights, smarter ideas and expanded opportunities for organizations to harness and learn from their data" (para. 2).

Data mining is the process of using software to sort through data to discover patterns and ascertain or establish relationships. This process may help to discover or uncover previously unidentified relationships among the data in a database with a focus on applications. This information can then be used to increase profits or decrease costs, or a combination of the two. In health care, it is being used to improve efficiency and quality, resulting in better health care practices and improved patient outcomes. As we hone our analytical skills, we will be able to clarify and explain patterns existing in our big data related to improved patient responses to select treatments in order to strive for optimal patient outcomes (Liebeskind, 2015). We can then drill down for each treatment to examine the conditions the patient presented with and the number of visits they made. The data can then be explored to refine the output. For example, it would be very important to know more about all patients such as if they had other conditions or diseases, comorbidities that could affect their outcomes as well as their age, gender, educational level, and so on. See **Box 16-1** for health care practice quotes.

Data mining projects help organizations discover interesting knowledge. These projects can be predictive, exploratory, or focused on data reduction. Data mining focuses on producing a solution that generates useful forecasting through a four-phase process: (1) problem identification, (2) exploration of the data, (3) pattern discovery, and (4) knowledge deployment, or application of knowledge to new data to forecast or

BOX 16-1 HEALTH CARE PRACTICE QUOTES

Moskowitz, McSparron, and Celi (2015) stated,

> *Beyond simple user principles, trainees do not learn the skills and concepts necessary for the optimal use of EMRs, including knowledge creation and personalized clinical decision making through analysis of large data sets. To date, this is largely because such systems have not been designed or implemented with these goals in mind. In the coming era of "Big Data," our community of medical educators and researchers must leverage digital systems for this purpose and find a way to prepare trainees for this critical role. (para. 9)*

Their next steps concluded that "the time has come to leverage the data we generate during routine patient care to formulate a more complete lexicon of evidence-based recommendations and support shared decision making with our patients" (para. 19).

PHYSICAL THERAPY
According to Stout and Mack (2014),

> *Data mining is not a new concept and can be considered the harbinger of big data. Many [physical therapy] practices currently data-mine their own information to look for patterns of referrals, payer types, recruiting issues, clinical outcomes, productivity, profitability and other areas of interest in practice management. (para. 8)*

Hayhurst (2015) viewed data mining as the ability "to make predictions, which in turn might be used to direct clinical decision-making and boost outcomes even more, or to demonstrate efficiency, or to improve practice management" (para. 12). As stated in the title of the article, Hayhurst said, "while the use of predictive analytics in physical therapy is still in its infancy, early adopters see great potential for it to transform the profession and society."

OCCUPATIONAL THERAPY
Braveman (2014) stated,

> *Occupational therapy practitioners . . . as professionals with a specific knowledge base we can contribute to understanding the needs of individuals, communities and populations and to help design interventions at all levels and interpret big data to translate it to meeting the needs of individuals. (para. 1)*

DIETITIAN
Frederico (2015) stated that "RDNs interpret & follow sensor data with clients. . . . RDNs are nutrition informatics experts!" (slide 46). FitBit data can be evaluated by dieticians who focus on wellness while understanding disease management.

RADIOGRAPHERS
Fratt (2013) concluded that "big data applications in radiology include automated alerts, computer-aided diagnosis and real-time issues reporting for quality monitoring" (para. 8).

(continues)

BOX 16-1   HEALTH CARE PRACTICE QUOTES (continued)

Siegel (2014) described two challenges in imaging informatics as communication of information and how to better handle imaging's big data. He stated,

The second major challenge for imaging informatics is figuring out how to tag and index the incredible amount of data that we routinely acquire in diagnostic imaging. Our counterparts in astronomy, chemistry, and other disciplines have created means of structuring, tagging, and indexing their information in a logical and machine-readable fashion. Our colleagues in cardiology and other disciplines in medicine have found ways to make their results available in a highly structured fashion, which allows them to be discovered and utilized by the algorithms that represent clinical pathways and decision-support systems. In the near future, computers will assist much more than today in ensuring patient safety, minimizing disparity of treatment by different physicians in different areas, and in day-to-day clinical decision support. (para. 11)

Steere (2014) concluded that

big data is particularly important to radiology, a specialty in the business of big information and a key specialty in individualized decision making. Given the changing healthcare climate, radiology departments have to watch their spending due to heightened competition, declining reimbursement and pressure from payers to eradicate unnecessary imaging. It will become increasingly difficult for radiologists to obtain reimbursement and funding if people can't see the data, and thereby value, in scans and reports. This is where big data comes into play. (para. 6)

Vasko (2013) described the issue with saving and tagging imaging information when he stated, "Variability isn't limited to image acquisition. Different vendors' workstations also use proprietary methods of saving and tagging information, and even DICOM structured reporting fails to specify a standardized mechanism across different users and systems" (para. 7).

RESPIRATORY THERAPIST
Mussa (n.d.) concluded that

the information systems used by respiratory therapists appear to have marginal utility and have problems with data storage and retrieval. This is due to the prevalence of information systems that do not employ computerized databases and computerized databases that are not equipped with a full-scale database management system (DBMS). This is a significant finding since accepted computer science database theory asserts that an inadequate data storage and retrieval system compromises data integrity and consistency of data. Furthermore, inadequate data storage and retrieval results in data redundancy and ultimately, inaccurate information. Development of data models specific to the respiratory care profession may also be necessary to build databases with conceptual schemas that accurately reflect the professional activities of respiratory therapists. (para. 5) generate predictions. Data mining is an analytic, logical process with the ultimate goal of forecasting or prediction. It mines or unearths concealed predictive information, constructing a picture or view of the data that lends insight into future trends, actions, or behaviors. This data exploration and resulting knowledge discovery foster proactive, knowledge-driven decision making.

Problem identification is the initial phase of data mining. The problem must be defined, and everyone involved must understand the objectives and requirements of the data mining process they are initiating.

Exploration begins with exploring and preparing the data for the data mining process. This phase might include data access, cleansing, sampling, and transformation; based on the problem you are trying to solve, data might need to be transformed into another format. To ensure meaningful data mining outcomes, you must comprehend and truly understand your data. The goal of this phase is to identify the relevant or important variables and determine their nature.

Sometimes known as model building or pattern identification, *pattern discovery* is a complex phase of data mining. In this phase, different models are applied to the same data to choose the best model for the data set being analyzed. It is imperative that the model chosen should identify the patterns in the data that will support the best predictions. The model must be tested, evaluated, and interpreted. Therefore, this phase ends with a highly predictive, consistent pattern-identifying model.

The final phase, *knowledge deployment*, takes the pattern and model identified in the pattern discovery phase and applies them to new data to test whether they can achieve the desired outcome. In this phase, the model achieves insight by following the rules of a decision tree to generate predictions or estimates of the expected outcome. This deployment provides the organization with the actionable information and knowledge necessary to make strategic decisions in uncertain situations.

Data mining develops a model that uses an algorithm to act on a **data set** for one situation where the organization knows the outcome and then applies this same model to another situation where the outcome is not known—an extension known as **scoring**. Data mining is concerned with extracting what is needed, and it applies statistics so that organizations can gain an advantage by manipulating information for practical applications. In our information-overloaded health care world, all too often we find ourselves grasping for knowledge that is currently nonexistent or fleeting. Data mining is a dynamic, iterative process that is adjusted as new information surfaces. It is a robust, predictive, proactive information and knowledge tool that, when used correctly, empowers organizations to predict and react to specific characteristics of and behaviors within their systems.

Data mining is also known as **knowledge discovery and data mining** (KDD), **knowledge discovery in data**, and **knowledge discovery in databases**. The term *knowledge discovery* is key, as data mining looks at data from different vantage points, aspects, and perspectives and brings new insights to the data set. This analysis then sorts and categorizes the data and finally summarizes the relationships identified. In essence, then, data mining is the process of finding correlations or patterns among the data.

Health care, as noted earlier, generates big data. Data mining tools, in turn, are able to analyze enormous databases to determine patterns and establish applications to new data. Health care organizations clearly need to invest more in big data and data mining analysis: The "big data market [reached an estimated] $2.2 billion in 2011, [but] only 6% of that investment came from health care" (Tishgart, 2012, para. 2).

The health care sector has discovered data mining through the realization that knowledge discovery can help to improve health care policymaking, health care practices, disease prevention, detection of disease outbreaks, prevention of sequelae, and prevention of in-hospital deaths. On the business side, health care organizations use data mining for the detection of falsified or fraudulent insurance claims. According to Manyika et al. (2011),

> If US healthcare were to use big data creatively and effectively to drive efficiency and quality, the sector could create more than $300 billion in value every year. Two-thirds of that would be in the form of reducing US healthcare expenditure by about 8 percent. (para. 2)

If they are to develop a successful data mining process, organizations must have the data needed to create meaningful information. In health care, we are honing our ability to analyze our data by making sure that those data are comprehensive and complete, meet our needs, and are cleansed and prepared for the data mining process. Many facilities are using data warehouses to store data and facilitate this pre-data mining process. We are learning to ask the right questions during the data mining process to gain a thorough understanding of our data. The following pages introduce the concepts, techniques, and models used in data mining.

KDD and Research

According to IBM (2013), big data does not just refer to size but rather "is an opportunity to find insights in new and emerging types of data and content, to make your business more agile, and to answer questions that were previously considered beyond your reach" (p. 6). We now have advanced analytical software designed to facilitate data mining. The knowledge discovery capabilities continue to evolve. Goodwin et al. (1997), for example, reported on their collaborative data mining research, which explored the relationship between clinical data and adult respiratory distress syndrome in critically ill patients. DeGruy (2000) indicated that big data in health care needed to be analyzed using KDD tools and applications to determine trends and relationships with the ultimate goal of decreasing health care costs while improving quality. Madigan and Curet (2006) described the **classification and regression trees** (CART) data mining method for analyzing the outcomes and service use in home health care for three conditions: chronic obstructive pulmonary disease, heart failure, and hip replacement. They

CASE STUDY

In a large teaching hospital, there is a high rate of readmission for patients with community-acquired pneumonia who are being treated at the facility. The chief information officer wants to know the cause of the readmissions, as the rate at this facility is almost twice that of competing health care entities in the area. The chief information officer works with the respiratory therapy department to research the cases and address this situation.

The researchers begin to scour the electronic health records (EHRs) of more than 10,000 community-acquired pneumonia hospitalizations in the past 5 years to determine the cause of the situation. As they begin to understand this data set, they are able to build a data mining model using algorithms to discover patterns and relationships in the data. Based on the old data, they determine that the key factor for readmission was the length of time it took to follow up at home with discharged patients.

In response to this new knowledge, a program in which nurses contact patients with community-acquired pneumonia the day after their discharge by phone was developed, and a home visit is scheduled for the second day post-discharge to ensure a smooth transition to home or an assisted living facility. This follow-up within the first 4 days of discharge has reduced readmissions by 40%. The model that was used with the old data is being applied to the new data.

found that four factors—patient age, type of agency, type of payment, and ethnicity—influenced discharge destination and length of stay.

Over the last several decades, the KDD capability has improved as the analytical power of data mining tools has increased, thereby facilitating the recognition of patterns and relationships in big data. Trangenstein, Weiner, Gordon, and McNew (2007) described how their faculty used data mining to analyze their students' clinical logs, which enabled them to make programmatic decisions and revisions and rethink certain clinical placements. Zupan and Demsar (2008) described the open-source tools developed by data mining researchers that they felt were ready to be used in biomedical research. Fernández-Llatas et al. (2011) described work flow mining technology as a means to facilitate relearning in dementia processes. Lee et al. (2011) discussed the application of data mining to identify critical factors. As we intervene with patients, we must be able to evaluate our interventions related to our practice area and patient context. Lee, Lin, Mills, and Kuo (2012) used data mining to determine risk factors related to each stage of pressure ulcers and identified five predictive factors: hemoglobin level, weight, sex, height, and use of a repositioning sheet. Based on the results of this data mining analysis, the interprofessional health care team can better target their interventions to prevent pressure ulcers. Green et al. (2013) identified differences in limb volume patterns in breast cancer survivors; their results have the potential to influence clinical guidelines for the assessment of latent and early-onset lymphedema.

As this example suggests, we must collaborate with the interprofessional health care team to continue to employ data mining to reduce inefficiencies, improve quality, and support transformations using data-driven models of care.

Data Mining Concepts

Bagging is a term for the use of voting and averaging in predictive data mining to synthesize the predictions from many models or methods or the use of the same type of a model on different data. This term can also refer to the unpredictability of results when complex models are used to mine small data sets.

Boosting is what the term infers—a means of increasing the power of the models generated by weighting the combinations of predictions from those models into a predicted classification. This iterative process uses voting or averaging to combine the different classifiers.

Data reduction shrinks large data sets into manageable, smaller data sets. One way to accomplish this is via aggregation of the data or clustering.

Drill-down analysis typically begins by identifying variables of interest to drill down into the data. You could identify a diagnosis and drill down, for example, to determine the ages of those diagnosed or the number of males. You could then continue to drill down and expose even more of the data.

Exploratory data analysis (EDA) is an approach or philosophy that uses mainly graphical techniques to gain insight into a data set. Its goal varies based on the purpose of the analysis, but it can be applied to the data set to extract variables, detect outliers, or identify patterns.

Feature selection reduces inputs to a manageable size for processing and analysis, as the model either chooses or rejects an attribute based on its usefulness for analysis.

Machine learning is a subset of artificial intelligence that permits computers to learn either inductively or deductively. Inductive machine learning is the process of reasoning and making generalizations or extracting patterns and rules from huge data sets—that is, reasoning from a large number of examples to a general rule. Deductive machine learning moves from premises that are assumed true to conclusions that must be true if the premises are true.

Meta-learning combines the predictions from several models. It is helpful when several different models are used in the same project. The predictions from the different classifiers or models can be included as input into the meta-learning. The goal is to synthesize these predicted classifications to generate a final best predicted classification—a process also referred to as stacking.

Predictive data mining identifies the data mining project as one with the goal of identifying a model that can predict classifications.

Stacking or stacked generalization synthesizes the predictions from several models.

Data Mining Techniques

It is important to understand your data before you begin the data mining process so that you can choose the best technique and get the most from the data mining. The commonly used techniques in data mining are neural networks, decision trees, rule induction, algorithms, and the nearest neighbor method.

Neural networks represent nonlinear predictive models. These models learn through training and resemble the structure of biological neural networks; that is, they model the neural behavior of the human brain. Computers are fast and can respond to instructions or programs over and over again. Humans use their experience to generalize the world around them. Neural networks are a way to bridge the gap between computers and humans. Neural networks go through a learning process or training on existing data so that they can predict, recognize patterns, associate data, or classify data.

Decision trees are so named because the sets of decisions form a tree-shaped structure. The decisions generate rules for classifying a data set. CART and chi-square automatic interaction detection are two commonly used types of decision tree methodologies. See **Box 16-2** and **Figure 16-1** for an overview of decision tree analysis.

BOX 16-2   DECISION TREE ANALYSIS

Steven L. Brewer Jr.

Decision trees are a statistical technique based on numerous algorithms to predict a dependent variable. These predictions are determined by the influence of independent variables. Decision trees help researchers understand the complex interactions between variables generated from research data. The entire data set is split into child nodes based on the impact of the independent predictors. The most influential variable is situated at the top of the tree; the subsequent nodes are ranked by the significance of the remaining independent predictors.

Graphically, decision trees produce a tree (as illustrated in **Figure 16-1**) that consists of a root node and child nodes. The tree is an inverted, connected graphic. The graphic representation of the decision tree helps general users, such as practitioners, understand the complex interrelationships between the independent and dependent variables in a large data set.

Within the graphical display, there are three major components: the root node, the child node, and the terminal node. The root node represents the dependent variable, and the child nodes represent the independent variables. The root node is essentially the base of the tree or the top node. It contains the entire sample, while each child node contains a subset of the sample within the node directly above it. In Figure 16-1, the root node represents a sample of women who were either reassaulted or not reassaulted in a domestic violence database. Data in the root node are then partitioned and passed down the tree.

The number of child nodes will vary depending on the classification procedure that is used to determine how the data are split. In Figure 16-1, the first child node is "women's perception of safety." This node suggests that the most influential predictor in domestic violence reassault for this sample is the women's perception of safety. The tree produces additional child nodes based on the responses to that variable. Node 1 represents the women who responded "no" when asked whether they felt safe in the relationship. For this node, women had a 90% chance of being reassaulted. In contrast, node 2 represents the women who responded "yes" when asked whether they felt safe in the relationship. These women had only a 72% chance of being reassaulted.

The decision tree in Figure 16-1 splits the entire sample into subsamples, which in turn allows for different predictions for different groups within the sample. For example, women who felt safe in their relationship (node 2) and experienced controlling behaviors (node 6) had an 80% chance of being reassaulted. In contrast, women who did not feel safe (node 1) and were in a relationship characterized by controlling behaviors (node 6) had a 97.3% chance of being reassaulted. The splitting of the data continues until the data are no longer sufficient to predict the remaining variables or there are no additional cases to be split.

(continues)

BOX 16-2   DECISION TREE ANALYSIS (continued)

Classification trees share commonalities with nonlinear traditional methods, such as discriminant analysis, cluster analysis, nonparametric statistics, and nonlinear estimation; however, the technique differs significantly from linear analyses. In general, the decision tree technique does not rely on "multiplicative" or "additive" assumptions, such as regression, to predict the outcome of y. The flexibility of classification trees is one characteristic that makes them attractive to researchers. The trees are not bound or limited to examining all predictor variables simultaneously. Therefore, each predictor variable can be examined as a singularity to produce univariate splits in the tree. Additionally, classification trees can handle a mixture of categorical and continuous variables when univariate splits are used. While this flexibility offers advantages over traditional methods, classification trees are not limited to univariate splits.

Decision trees have become a popular alternative to methods such as regression and discriminate analysis for data mining big data. Such trees use algorithms from one of the numerous classification procedures to separate the data into different branches or child nodes that predict y. The dependent variable (y) is represented by the root node.

These algorithms have three main functions: (1) They explain how to separate or partition the data at each split, (2) they decree when to stop or end the splitting of data, and (3) they determine how to predict the value of y for each x in a split. The child nodes are separated into homogeneous groups by the algorithms from different classification procedures. This process of partitioning is the main purpose of classification procedures. First, the procedure clusters and creates child nodes. Second, it ranks them based on their predictive values of y. Hence, the most influential variable(s) will be located at the base of the tree. From this point, the classification procedures further expand the child nodes by finding the next best factor. The tree is expanded until the algorithm is unable to find a clearly distinguishable split within the data.

Based on the results of the sample decision tree analysis presented in Figure 16-1, practitioners would conclude that women should be attuned to their perception of safety in a relationship, as those who feel unsafe have a much higher chance of another assault.

Decision trees are a powerful tool that can be used to mine large data sets and discover previously unknown relationships among the data. The predictive relationships uncovered by the decision tree analysis may be useful in directing approaches to future care interventions.

Rule induction is based on statistical significance. Rules are extracted from the data using *if-then* statements, which become the rules.

Algorithms are typically computer-based recipes or methods with which data mining models are developed. To create the model, the data set is first analyzed by the algorithm, looking for specific patterns and trends. Based on the results of this analysis, the algorithm defines the parameters of the data mining model. The identified parameters are then applied to the entire data set to mine it for patterns and statistics.

Nearest neighbor analysis classifies each record in a data set based on a select number of its nearest neighbors. This technique is sometimes known as the *k*-nearest neighbor.

Text mining for text is equivalent to data mining for numerical data. Because text is not always consistent in health care because of the lack of a generally accepted terminology structure, it is more difficult to analyze. Text documents are analyzed by extracting key words or phrases.

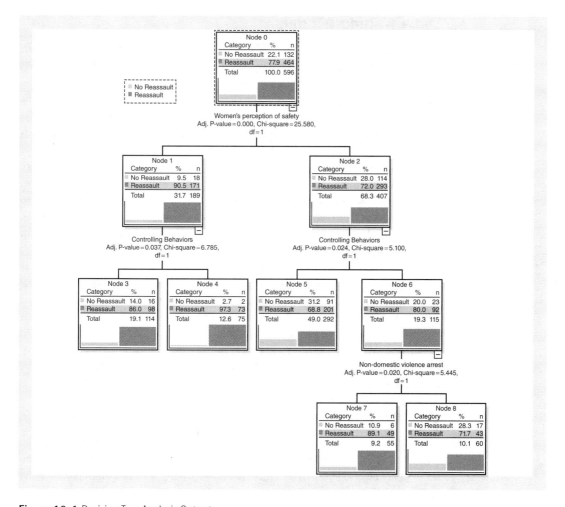

Figure 16-1 Decision Tree Analysis Output

Online analytic processing (OLAP) (also known as fast analysis of shared data) generates different views of the data in **multidimensional databases**. These perspectives range from simplistic views, such as descriptive statistics, frequency tables, or comparative summaries, to more complicated analyses requiring various forms of cleansing the data, such as removing outliers.

Brushing is a technique in which the user manually chooses specific data points or observations or subsets of data on an interactive data display. These selected data can be visualized in two-dimensional or three-dimensional surfaces as scatter plots. Brushing is also known as graphical exploratory data analysis.

Data Mining Models

To generate predictions and infer relationships, the data set, statistics, and patterns identified in existing data must be applied to new data. A data mining model is developed by exercising more than algorithms on data. Specifically, the data mining model consists of a mining structure plus an algorithm. The data mining model remains empty until it applies the algorithm or processes and analyzes the data provided by the mining structure. This model stores the information obtained from a statistical analysis of the data, identifying patterns and gaining insights. It then contains metadata that specify the name and definition of the model, the server location or other place where it is stored, definitions of any filters applied when processing the model, columns from the mining structure that were used to build the model, and the algorithm used to analyze the data. The columns, their data types, any filters, and the algorithm used are all choices that are made in the data mining process, and each of these decisions can greatly influence the data mining results. The same data can be used to create many models; one type of model could organize the data into trees, for example, whereas another type of model might cluster the data in groups based on the rules applied. Different results can be achieved from the same mining structure, even though it is used in many models, based on the filtering method or analysis conducted. Therefore, each decision made along the way is very important.

There are many models. We will review the following models here: Cross-Industry Standard Process for Data Mining (CRISP-DM), Six Sigma, and SEMMA (sample, explore, modify, model, access).

CRISP-DM

The CRISP-DM model follows a path or series of steps to develop a business understanding by gaining an understanding of the business data collected and analyzed. The six steps are business understanding, data understanding, data preparation, modeling, evaluation, and deployment.

The CRISP-DM model begins with an understanding of the business. The situation must be assessed to establish the data mining goals and produce the project plan. You must be able to answer the following questions: What are the business objectives? What are the requirements? Have we specifically defined the problem? The answers to these questions help transform the business perspective knowledge into a data mining problem definition and initial plan to meet the objectives.

Data understanding begins with the preliminary data collection and assimilation of the data. It is during this step that the data will be described and explored to facilitate the user's comprehension of the data. As the user gains familiarity with the data, data quality issues are identified and the quality of the data is verified.

The data are cleansed and transformed during the data preparation step. First, one must select the data, attributes, and records to be used. These data are then cleansed, constructed, integrated, and properly formatted. At this point, the final data set is constructed from the data; this data set will be processed by the model.

Modeling involves selection of the modeling methods and their application to the prepared data set. Parameters are calibrated, a test design is generated, and the model is built and assessed. This step might require you to revisit data preparation if the format of the data does not meet the specific requirements of the methods.

During the evaluation step, the degree to which the objectives were met is assessed from a business perspective. A key question is, Were any important business issues not considered? The model was built for high-quality data analysis. To see whether this goal has been met, the process is reviewed, results are evaluated, and the model is interpreted. This is where you determine whether the model should be implemented or whether more iterations must occur before its deployment. The project may not be completed, or a new data mining project might be initiated. If the project is deployed, this step is when you must decide how the results from the data analysis will be used.

Deployment is the final step, in which the model is finally implemented. The plan must be monitored and maintained and the project reviewed. The six-step process should yield a reliable, repeatable data mining process. The knowledgeable insights gained from the implementation of the model must be organized and presented in such a way that they can be used. The final project report is generated to document the process and share this enhanced knowledge of the data.

The CRISP-DM model employs a process that has been proven to make data mining projects both more rapid and more effectual. Using this model helps to avoid typical mistakes while assessing business problems and detailing data mining techniques.

Six Sigma

Six Sigma is a data-driven method to eliminate defects, avoid waste, or assess quality control issues. It aims to decrease discrepancies in business and manufacturing processes through dedicated improvements. Six Sigma uses the **DMAIC** steps: define, measure, analyze, improve, and control.

The first step defines the goals of the project or the goals for improvement. During this step, you can use data mining techniques to discover prospective ideas for implementing the project.

In the measure step, exploratory and descriptive data analyses are used on the existing system to enhance the understanding of the data. Reliable, valid, and accurate metrics with which to measure goal achievement in each of the steps are identified.

The analysis step should assess the system to identify discrepancies between the current big data and the goal. Statistical methods guide this analysis.

Improvements must be made to the current system to attain the organizational goals. The use of project management skills facilitates the application of the new methodology and processes. Statistical methods assess the improvements and any deficiencies that exist.

The final step of the model is control. Controlling the system is important so that discrepancies are remedied before they cause a disruption.

The Six Sigma model applies a different mentality to the same old business model or way of thinking. The DMAIC steps that are implemented typically result in success.

SEMMA

According to SAS (n.d.), "The acronym SEMMA—sample, explore, modify, model, assess—refers to the core process of conducting data mining" (para. 1). This model is similar to Six Sigma but concentrates more on the technical activities characteristically involved in data mining.

The first step is to sample the data. Sampling is optional but creates a more robust data mining effort. Using a "statistically representative sample of your data, SEMMA makes it easy to apply exploratory statistical and visualization techniques, select and transform the most significant predictive variables, model the variables to predict outcomes, and confirm a model's accuracy" (SAS, n.d., para. 1). Creating a target data set shrinks the data to a manageable size yet maintains the important information necessary to mine.

The exploration of the data seeks to discover discrepancies, trends, and relationships in the data. It is at this point that ideas about the data should emerge to help the organization understand the data and its implications for the organization's business. In health care, for example, it would be important to determine how many people use the emergency department each year and how many of those people are admitted, released, and return and to identify any disparities in care and diagnoses. What did you discover? What are the trends and relationships that emerge from the data mining?

After exploring, you should modify your data based on the information discovered. It might be important to modify the data based on groupings such as "all people who are diagnosed with congestive heart failure who present with shortness of breath" if the trending and relationships indicate that this subgroup is significant. Other variables can also be introduced at this time to help gain a further understanding of the data.

The data are modeled to predict outcomes based on analytically searching the data. Combinations of data must be identified to predict desired outcomes.

During the assessment phase, the data as well as the models are assessed for not only the reliability of the discoveries but also the usefulness of the data mining process. Assessment is key to determine the success of the data mining approach.

SEMMA focuses on the tasks of modeling. This approach has been praised for its ability to guide the implementation of data mining. Conversely, it has been criticized for omitting the critical features of the organization's business. SEMMA is logical and can be robust from sampling through assessment.

Based on the needs of the organization, a variety of models can be used in combination. A coordinated, cooperative environment is necessary for complicated data mining projects because they require organizational commitment to ensure their success. As described in this section, models such as CRISP-DM, Six Sigma, and SEEMA have been designed as blueprints to deal with the dilemma of how to integrate data mining techniques into an organization. They facilitate the gathering of data, the analysis of those data, the conversion of the data into information, and the dissemination of this information in a format that is easy to digest and understand so as to inform organizational decision making. It is imperative that the results of the data mining process be implemented and any resultant improvements monitored and evaluated.

Benefits of KDD

KDD can enhance the business aspects of health care delivery and help to improve patient care. Some examples of how KDD can be applied effectively follow:

- A durable medical equipment company analyzed its recent sales and enhanced its targeting of hospitals and clinics that yielded the highest **return on investment** (ROI).
- Several plastic surgery suites were bought by the same group of surgeons. They wanted to know how those organizations were the same and how they were different. They ran analytics for disparities while looking for patterns and trends that led them to develop standardized policies and modify treatment plans.
- Analytic techniques were used in the clinical trials of a new oral contraceptive to aid in monitoring trends and disparities.
- Hidden patterns and relationships between death and disease in selected populations can be uncovered.
- Government spending on certain aspects of health care or specific disease conditions can be analyzed to discover patterns and relationships and to distinguish between the real versus desired outcomes from the investment.
- Patient data can be analyzed to identify effective treatments and discover patterns or relationships in the data to predict inpatient **length of stay** (LOS).
- Data can be analyzed to help detect medical insurance fraud.

Even though KDD can be complex, this process tends to yield a potent knowledge representation. As analytics evolve, KDD will almost certainly become easier to use, more efficient, and more effective in facilitating data mining in health care.

Ethics of Data Mining

Data mining in health care is dependent on the use of private health information. Practitioners engaging in data mining must ensure that such data are de-identified and that confidentiality is maintained. Because most data mining depends on the aggregation of data, maintaining individual patient confidentiality should be relatively straightforward. You can follow changes and specific requirements for compliance with the Health Insurance Portability and Accountability Act (HIPAA) at this website: http://www.hhs.gov/ocr/privacy/hipaa/understanding/special/research/index.html.

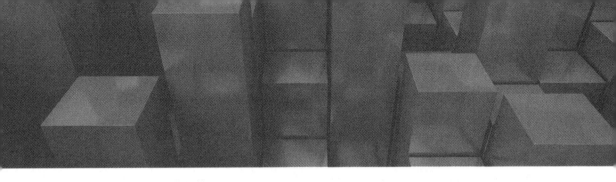

Summary

Big data is everywhere—we collect and store data every second of every day. The data in big clinical data sets can get lost, however, diminishing its value. Therefore, in health care, it is imperative that we use KDD to analyze these data sets and discover meaningful information that will influence our practice. Our existing data repositories are ripe for the picking; they contain hidden patterns, trends, and undiscovered nuggets that we must mine to continue to hone our understanding and improve health care.

Data management is essential so that this process can begin with clean, good data. The decisions that are made when conducting the analysis and when developing the model and algorithms enable us to predict and discover patterns and trends in the data, thereby making them meaningful. We must be able not only to extract meaningful information and knowledge but also to share and disseminate what we are learning and the new knowledge we are generating.

Thought-Provoking Questions

1. Reflect on these terms: database, data warehouse, and data mining. What do they have in common? How do they differ?
2. Describe an issue associated with health care data that impedes the construction of meaningful databases and inhibits the data mining process. Which strategies would you use to remedy this situation? Thoroughly describe one strategy and its potential outcomes.
3. Suggest a data mining project for your practice. Which information would you like to have about your practice area that could be extracted using data mining strategies?
4. Data mining is associated with numerous techniques and algorithms. How can you make sure that you select and develop those that best fit your data?

Apply Your Knowledge

Data mining projects help organizations and professionals discover interesting knowledge. These projects can be predictive, exploratory, or focused on data reduction. Data mining focuses on producing a solution that generates useful forecasting through a four-phase process: (1) problem identification, (2) exploration of the data, (3) pattern discovery, and (4) knowledge deployment, or application of knowledge to new data to forecast or generate predictions. Data mining is an analytic, logical process with the ultimate goal of forecasting or prediction. It mines or unearths concealed predictive information, constructing a picture or view of the data that lends insight into future trends, actions, or behaviors. This data exploration and resulting knowledge discovery foster proactive, knowledge-driven decision making.

1. List and describe some of the issues associated with health care data that impede the construction of meaningful databases. You might need to revisit Chapter 2 for some of these insights.
2. List and describe some of the specific applications of data mining in health care.
3. Suggest a data mining project for your practice other than those mentioned in the reading. What information would you like to have about your practice area that could be extracted using data mining strategies?

Additional Resources

Health Insurance Portability and Accountability Act
http://www.hhs.gov/ocr/privacy/hipaa/understanding/special/research/index.html

References

Braveman, B. (2014). More about big data. http://otconnections.aota.org/community_blogs/b /brentbraveman/archive/2014/12/28/more-about-big-data.aspx

DeGruy, K. B. (2000). Healthcare applications of knowledge discovery in databases. *Journal of Healthcare Information Management, 14*(2), 59–69.

Fernández-Llatas, C., Garcia-Gomez, J. M., Vicente, J., Naranjo, J. C., Robles, M., Benedi, J. M., & Traver, V. (2011). Behaviour patterns detection for persuasive design in nursing homes to help dementia patients. *Conference Proceedings IEEE Engineering in Medicine & Biology Society,* 6413–6417.

Fratt, L. (2013). Big data & radiology. http://www.healthimaging.com/topics/health-it/big -data-radiology

Frederico, C. (2015). Riding the wave of EHRs for nutrition practice. http://files.himss .org/2015Conference/handouts/183.pdf

Goodwin, L., Saville, J., Jasion, B., Turner, B., Prather, J., Dobousek, T., & Egger, S. (1997). A collaborative international nursing informatics research project: Predicting ARDS risk in critically ill patients. *Studies in Health Technology Informatics, 46,* 247–249.

Green, J., Paladugu, S., Shuyu, X., Stewart, B., Shyu, C., & Armer, J. (2013). Using temporal mining to examine the development of lymphedema in breast cancer survivors. *Nursing Research, 62*(2), 122–129.

Hayhurst, C. (2015). The power of prediction. While the use of predictive analytics in physical therapy is still in its infancy, early adopters see great potential for it to transform the profession and society. http://www.apta.org/PTinMotion/2015/6/Feature/PowerofPredictionIBM. (2013). Big data at the speed of business. http://www-01.ibm.com/software/data/bigdata

Lee, T., Lin K., Mills, M., & Kuo, Y. (2012). Factors related to the prevention and management of pressure ulcers. *Computers Informatics Nursing, 30*(9), 489–495.

Lee, T., Liu, C., Kuo, Y., Mills, M., Fong, J., & Hung, C. (2011). Application of data mining to the identification of critical factors in patient falls using a Web-based reporting system. *International Journal of Medical Informatics, 80*(2), 141–150.

Liebeskind, D. (2015). Big and bigger data in endovascular stroke therapy. http://informahealthcare .com/doi/pdf/10.1586/14737175.2015.1018893

Madigan, E., & Curet, O. (2006). A data mining approach in home healthcare: Outcomes and service use. *BMC Health Services Research, 6,* 18.

Manyika, J., Chu, M., Brown, B., Bughin, J., Dobbs, R., Roxburgh, C., & Byers, A. (2011). McKinsey Global Institute: Big data: The next frontier for innovation, competition, and productivity. http://www.mckinsey.com/insights/business_technology/big_data_the_next_frontier_for_innovation

Moskowitz, A., McSparron, J., & Celi, L. (2015). Preparing a new generation of clinicians for the era of big data. http://www.hmsreview.org/?article=preparing-new-generation-clinicians-era-big-data

Mussa, C. (n.d.). Is respiratory care informatics a legitimate area of study within the science of respiratory care? http://extww02a.cardinal.com/mps/focus/respiratory/abstracts/abstracts/ab2004/OF-04-241%20Mussa.aspSAS. (n.d.). SAS enterprise miner. http://www.sas.com/offices/europe/uk/technologies/analytics/datamining/miner/semma.html

Siegel, E. (2014). Radiology's future in big data [*Radiology Today* interview with Eliot Siegel, MD]. *Radiology Today, 15*(2), 22. http://www.radiologytoday.net/archive/rt0214p22.shtml

Steere, A. (2014). Diving into the business of big data in radiology. http://www.healthimaging.com/topics/imaging-informatics/diving-business-big-data-radiology?nopaging=1

Stout, C., & Mack, B. (2014). "Big data" and physical therapy. http://physical-therapy.advanceweb.com/Business-and-Practice-Management/Archives/Article-Archives/Big-Data-and-Physical-Therapy.aspx

Tishgart, D. (2012). Why security matters for big data and health care: Data integrity requires good data security. http://soa.sys-con.com/node/2389698

Trangenstein, P., Weiner, E., Gordon, J., & McNew, R. (2007). Data mining results from an electronic clinical log for nurse practitioner students. *Studies in Health Technology Informatics, 129*, 1387–1391.

Vasko, C. (2013). Five challenges facing radiology in the era of big data. http://www.imagingbiz.com/portals/medical-imaging-review/five-challenges-facing-radiology-era-big-data?nopaging=1

Zupan, B., & Demsar, J. (2008). Open-source tools for data mining. *Clinics in Laboratory Medicine, 28*(1), 37–54.

Finding, Understanding, and Applying Research Evidence in Practice

Jennifer Bredemeyer, Ida Androwich, Heather E. McKinney, Kathleen Mastrian, and Dee McGonigle

OBJECTIVES

1. Explore the acquisition of previous knowledge through Internet and library holdings.
2. Examine information fair use and copyright restrictions.
3. Assess informatics tools for collecting data and storing information.
4. Evaluate evidence-based practice and translational research.
5. Describe models for introducing research findings into practice.
6. Identify barriers to research utilization in practice.

Introduction

During rounds, Charles encounters a rare pulmonary condition he has never personally seen and only vaguely remembers hearing about in respiratory therapy school. He takes a few moments to prepare himself by searching the Internet. That evening, he does even more research so that he can assess and treat the patient safely. He searches clinical databases online and his own school textbooks. Most of the information seems consistent, yet some factors vary. Charles wants to provide the safest and highest quality of patient care. He wonders which resources are best, which are the most trusted, and which are the most accurate.

The **Foundation of Knowledge model** suggests that the most important aspect of information discovery, retrieval, and delivery is the ability to acquire, process, generate, and disseminate knowledge in ways that help those managing the knowledge reevaluate and rethink the way they understand and use what

Key Terms
Agency for Healthcare Research and Quality
American Library Association
Context of care
Copyright
Cumulative Index to Nursing and Allied Health Literature
Educational Resources Information Center
Evidence
Evidence-based practice
Fair use
Foundation of Knowledge model
Information literacy
Iowa model
MEDLINE
Meta-analysis

(continues)

they know and have learned. These goals closely reflect the Information Literacy Competency Standards for Higher Education, published by the **American Library Association** (ALA) in 2003 in response to changing perceptions of how information is created, evaluated, and used.

According to the ALA (2000), an information-literate individual is able to do the following:

- Determine the extent of information needed
- Access the needed information effectively and efficiently
- Evaluate information and its sources critically
- Incorporate selected information into one's knowledge base
- Use information effectively to accomplish a specific purpose
- Understand the economic, legal, and social issues surrounding the use of information and access and use information ethically and legally (para. 8)

In addition, new challenges arise for individuals seeking to understand and evaluate information because information is available through multiple media (graphical, aural, and textual). The sheer quantity of information does not by itself create a more informed citizenry without complementary abilities to use this information effectively. Most significantly, information literacy forms the basis for lifelong learning, serving as a commonality among all learning environments, disciplines, and levels of education (Association of College and Research Libraries [ACRL], 2000).

This chapter introduces the concepts of information literacy, fair use of information, translational research concepts, and their role in promoting evidence-based practice. Information management technologies are an integral part of evidence-based practice, and it is important for all health care disciplines to appreciate the contribution of this aspect of health informatics to patient care.

Information Literacy

Information literacy is an intellectual framework for finding, understanding, evaluating, and using information. These activities are accomplished in part through fluency with information technology and sound investigative methods but most importantly through critical reasoning and discernment. The ACRL (2000) has suggested that "information literacy initiates, sustains, and extends lifelong learning through abilities that may use technologies but are ultimately independent of them" (p. 5).

The ability to recognize the need for a specific kind of information and then locate, evaluate, and effectively use that information (ALA, 1989) within the health informatics paradigm will catapult some health care professionals ahead of other health care professionals in providing evidence-based care. Traditional approaches to care that adhere to the "we have always done it this way" adage are no longer good enough. Our patients deserve care that utilizes the best available research and practice evidence.

Acquiring Knowledge Through Internet and Library Holdings

In an environment characterized by rapid technological change, coupled with an overwhelming proliferation of information sources, health care professionals face an enormous number of options when choosing how and from where to acquire information for their academic studies, clinical situations, and research. Because information is available through so many venues—libraries, special interest organizations, media, community resources, and the Internet—in increasingly unfiltered formats, health care practitioners must inevitably question the authenticity, validity, and reliability of information (ACRL, 2000).

Often, the retrieval of reliable research and information may seem to be a daunting task in light of the seemingly ubiquitous amount of information found on the Web. Focusing on specific information venues not only aids this search but also assists in negotiating the endless maze of resources, allowing a professional to find the best and most accurate information efficiently.

Professional Online Databases

Professional databases represent a source of online information that is generally invisible to all Internet users except those with professional or academic affiliations, such as faculty, staff, and students. These databases, which range from specific to general, act as collection points by aggregating information, such as abstracts and articles from many different journals; two such databases include the **Cumulative Index to Nursing and Allied Health Literature** (CINAHL) and MEDLINE. CINAHL, for example, specifically includes information from all aspects of allied health, nursing, alternative medicine, and community medicine. The MEDLINE database contains more than 10 million records and is maintained and produced by the National Library of Medicine. Other databases, such as **PsycInfo** from the American Psychological Association and the **Educational Resources Information Center** (ERIC) database, may also benefit health care professionals. Still others are more specific by discipline, such as OTseeker (specific to occupational therapy), PEDro (specific to physical therapy), and speechBITE (for speech therapists). Many databases also offer full-text capabilities, meaning that entire articles are available online. The articles and abstracts contained within these databases have already withstood the rigors of publication in professional journals and, therefore, are considered viable and authentic peer-reviewed sources.

Libraries with subscriptions to databases often employ library professionals who are able to help patrons sift through the vast amounts of available electronic information; using the expert research capabilities of a health science librarian at one's local university is the best way to learn how to conduct database searches that yield the most efficient and useful results. Also useful are websites that provide tutorials on best searching practices specifically for medically oriented databases, such as the tutorials provided by EBSCO support to search the CINAHL database (http://support.epnet.com/training/flash_videos/cinahl_basic/cinahl_basic .html and http://support.epnet.com/training/flash_videos/cinahl_advanced/cinahl _advanced.html).

Search Engines

Search engines allow users to surf the Web and find information on nearly anything, although many involved in conducting scholarly research steer clear of search engines because of the vast amounts of unsubstantiated information they are likely to uncover. Because no legitimacy needs to be provided for any information that appears on the Web, an author can make claims, substantiated or not, and still use the Web as a publishing venue. Despite the pitfalls associated with search engines in general, they can yield a bounty of useful information when used with discretion.

Different search engines will produce different results when used for the same research. For example, one popular search engine ranks its results by number of hits that a page or site has received. Whereas the most popular research results are likely to be relevant, the order in which results appear does not indicate quality or viability of the source.

Different Web address (domain) suffixes (.com, .edu, .org, .gov, and so forth) indicate who is responsible for creating the website. Although an .edu site is hosted by an educational institution and for that reason may seem legitimate, consider that it could also belong to a student stating personal opinion, gossip, or guesswork. In contrast, .gov sites are maintained by the government and nearly always have professional contact information. Web hosts develop new domain suffixes constantly, so although looking at the suffix can be useful, it should not be the sole deciding factor when choosing to trust information.

One should never blindly trust information found on a webpage. When possible, check the date of the most recent update (How old is the page?), contact information (Is a bibliography or list of sources provided?), links to external sources (Do they seem relevant?), and previous attained knowledge from other reputable sources (Is the information too unbelievable?).

Fees and information retrieval charges should be approached with skepticism. Private companies do offer information aggregation services for a fee. In these cases, users pay a flat monthly fee for access to collections of articles in a particular field. What users (especially those affiliated with an academic institution) may not realize is that they are likely to have free access to the same, if not more complete, information through their institution's library system.

Some legitimate databases and traditional newspapers that maintain a Web presence do provide access for a small fee, but just as many others simply ask users to register to see articles for free. Many students and professionals affiliated with a university may find that their university library has already purchased access for those affiliated with the university—students, faculty, and staff.

Electronic Library Catalogs

Nearly all higher education institutions have placed their library catalogs online. Although this is an obvious convenience for many students, some health care professionals unaccustomed to working completely online may be intimidated by an e-catalog. Library professionals at the tiniest university and the busiest community college are available to demonstrate how to navigate a basic search of their library's catalog. Asking for assistance in learning how to access the vast assortment of journals, books, databases, and other resources available at one's college library is an excellent idea. Students in health care programs at larger universities will likely find free classes that specifically teach users how to navigate and use the online catalog. If smaller colleges and universities do not offer these services, one should take advantage of the library's online tutorials, help pages, frequently-asked-questions pages, and online reference service (if available). Local public libraries often have subscriptions to popular databases and offer free classes on searching techniques to patrons, providing yet another free access point to the best information for one's research needs. Making full use of available library resources serves to strengthen information literacy skills, enabling learners to master content and extend their investigations, become more self-directed, and assume greater control over their own learning (ACRL, 2000).

Information Sharing and Fair Use

Copyright laws in the world of technology are notoriously misunderstood. The same copyright laws that cover physical books, artwork, and other creative material apply in the digital world. Have you ever given a friend a CD that contains a computer game or some other type of software that you paid for and registered? Have you ever downloaded a song from the Internet without paying for it? Have you ever copied a section of online content from a reference site and used that content as if it were your own? Have you ever copied a picture from the Internet without asking permission from the photographer who took the picture? Have you ever copied and pasted information about a disease or drug from a website and then printed out the information to give to a patient or family member? These are all examples of the type of copyright infringements enabled by technology that occur almost without thought.

The value of creative material—whether it is written content, a song, a painting, or some other type of creative work—lies not in the physical medium on which it is stored but rather in the intangibles of creativity, skills, and labor that went into creating that item. The person who created the material should be properly credited and possibly reimbursed for the use of the material. How would musicians be reimbursed for their music if everyone just downloaded their songs illegally from the Internet? Imagine that you created a game to teach patients with type 1 diabetes how to manage their diet and other dieticians copied and distributed that game without getting your permission to do so. How would you feel?

Almost all software, music CDs, and movie DVDs come with restrictions on how and why copies can be made. The license included with the software clarifies exactly which restrictions are applicable. The most common type of software license is a "shrink wrap" license, meaning that as soon as the user removes the shrink wrap from the CD or DVD case, he or she has agreed to the license restriction. Most computer software developers allow for a backup copy of the software to be made without restriction. If the hard drive fails on the user's computer, the software can usually be reinstalled through this backup copy. Some software companies even allow the purchaser of a software package to transfer it to a new user. In this case, the software typically must be uninstalled from the original owner's computer before the new owner is free to install the software on his or her computer. Most of these restrictions depend on the honesty of the user in reading and following the licensing agreement. As a result of widespread abuses, however, the music and film industries commonly include hardware security features in their products that block users from making a working copy of a music CD or movie DVD.

The bottom line: Copyright laws also apply to the digital world, and copyright violations can lead to prosecution. Advances in technology have made the sharing of information easy and extremely fast. A scanner can convert any document to digital form instantly, and that document can then be shared with people anywhere in the world. Nevertheless, the person who originally created that document has the right to approve of the sharing of their work. Carefully read the fine print of any software purchased and be sure to clarify any questions regarding how that software can be copied. Avoid downloading music illegally from the Internet, and do not use information from the Internet without permission to do so or without citing the reference appropriately. Health care organizations that allow access to the Internet from a network computer should ensure that users are well aware of and compliant with all copyright and **fair use** principles.

Clarification of Research Terms

Evidence-based practice, translational research, and *research utilization* are all terms that have been used to describe the application of evidential knowledge to clinical practice. The following paragraphs explore the definitions of each term. Although these terms are related, they have slightly different meanings and applications.

Evidence-based practice (EBP), developed originally for its application to medicine, is defined by Sackett, Rosenberg, Gray, Haynes, and Richardson (1996) as "the conscientious, explicit and judicious use of current best evidence in making decisions about the care of individual patients" (p. 71). The "best evidence" in this context refers to more than just research. Goode and Piedalue (1999) state that EBP should be combined with other knowledge sources and "involves the synthesis of knowledge from research, retrospective or concurrent chart review, quality improvement and risk data, international, national, and local standards, infection control data, pathophysiology, cost effectiveness analysis, benchmarking data, patient preferences, and clinical expertise" (p. 15). EBP starts with a clinical question to resolve a clinical problem. For example, published research studies are used in health care quality initiatives as the evidence behind the development of practice algorithms designed to decrease practice variability, increase patient safety, improve patient outcomes, and eliminate unnecessary costs. Use of EBP promotes the use of clinical judgment and knowledge, with procedures and protocols being linked to scientific evidence rather than based on what is customary practice or opinion (Stevens, 2004).

Research utilization is the use of findings from one or more research studies in a practical application unrelated to the original study (Polit & Beck, 2008, p. 29) resulting in the generation of new knowledge. Stetler (2001) defines research utilization as the "process of transforming research knowledge into practice" (p. 274). Research utilization can be self-limiting if research is inconsistent or not enough research is available to develop a consensus regarding the answer to the clinical question (Kirchhoff, 2004).

Translational research (science) describes the methods used in translating medical, biomedical, informatics, and health care research into clinical interventions. Woolf (2008) describes translational research in two ways:

- T1: the transfer of clinical research to its first testing on humans
- T2: the transfer of clinical research to an everyday clinical practice setting

Difficulties in translating research to the T2 setting exist when research applications do not fit well within the clinical context or practical considerations within the organization constrain the application in a clinical setting. Translational research is complicated by the follow-up analysis, practice, and policy changes that occur when adopting research into practice; consequently, available evidence-based health care practices are often not fully incorporated into daily care (Titler, 2004, 2010). Organizational culture influences the changes made to a clinical application and establishes the groundwork and the support for change-making activities (Titler, 2004). The study of ways to promote the adoption of evidence in the health care context is called "translation science" (Titler, 2010).

History of EBP

Research results are crucial to furthering EBP. The concept of using randomized controlled trials (RCTs) and systematic reviews as the gold standard against which one should evaluate the validity and effectiveness of a clinical intervention was introduced in 1972 by Archie Cochrane (1972), a scientist and a physician. Cochrane's experiences as a prisoner of war and medical officer while interning during World War II led to his belief that not all medical interventions were needed and that some caused more harm than good. Cochrane viewed the randomized clinical trial as a means of validating clinical interventions and limiting the interventions to those that were scientifically based, effective, and necessary (Dickersin & Manheimer, 1998).

Cochrane's colleague, Iain Chalmers, began compiling a comprehensive clinical trials registry of 3,500 clinical trial results in the field of perinatal medicine. In 1988, after being published in print 3 years earlier, the registry became available electronically. Chalmers's methods for compiling the trials databases became a model for future registry assembly. Eventually, the National Health Service in the United Kingdom, recognizing the value of and need for systemic reviews for all of health care, developed the Cochrane Center. The Cochrane Collaboration (2004) was initiated in 1993 and expanded internationally to maintain systematic reviews in all areas of health care

(Dickersin & Manheimer, 1998). Many universities subscribe to the Cochrane Collaboration database, making this information easily accessible to students, faculty, and health care professionals who work for university hospital systems.

Evidence

The RCT is considered the most reliable source of evidence. Yet RCTs are not always possible or available; consequently, health care professionals must use critical analysis to base their clinical decision making on the best available evidence (Baumann, 2010). The updated Stetler model of research utilization (Stetler, 2001) identifies internal and external forms of evidence. External evidence originates from research and national experts, whereas internal forms of evidence originate from nontraditional sources, such as clinical experience and quality improvement data.

Evidence includes standards of practice, codes of ethics, philosophies of practice, autobiographic stories, aesthetic criticism, works of art, qualitative studies, and patient and clinical knowledge (Melnyk, Fineout-Overholt, Stone, & Ackerman, 2000). French (2002) summarizes evidence as "truth, knowledge (including tacit, expert opinion and experiential), primary research findings, meta-analyses and systematic reviews" (p. 254). Health care professionals may additionally draw on evidence from the **context of care**, such as audit and performance data, the culture of the organization, social and professional networks, discussion with stakeholders, and local or national policy (Rycroft-Malone et al., 2004, p. 86).

To use evidence in practice, the weight of the research, also called **research validity**, must be determined. Evidence hierarchies have been defined to grade and assign value to the information source. For example, an evidential hierarchy developed by Stetler et al. (1998) prioritizes evidence into six categories:

1. Meta-analysis
2. Individual experimental studies
3. Quasi-experimental studies
4. Nonexperimental studies
5. Program evaluations, such as quality improvement projects
6. Opinions of experts

The hierarchy identifies **meta-analysis** as the best-quality evidence because it uses multiple individual research studies to reach a consensus. It is interesting to note that opinions of experts are considered the least significant in this hierarchy, yet health care professionals most often seek the opinion of a more experienced colleague or peer when seeking information regarding patient care (Pravikoff, Tanner, & Pierce, 2005).

Qualitative research allows one to understand the way in which the intervention is experienced by the researcher and the participant and the value of the interventions to both parties (O'Neill, Jinks, & Ong, 2007). Qualitative research is not always considered in EBP because methods for synthesizing the evidence do not currently exist. The Cochrane Qualitative Research Methods Group (CQRMG) is developing search, appraisal, and synthesis methodologies for qualitative research (Joanna Briggs Institute, n.d.).

Bridging the Gap Between Research and Practice

The time between research dissemination and clinical translation may be significant, and this delay may adversely affect patient outcomes. Bridging the gap between
research and practice requires an understanding of the key concepts and barriers,
access to research findings, access to clinical mentors for research understanding, a
reinforcing culture, and a desire on the part of the clinician to implement best practices (Melnyk, 2005; Melnyk, Fineout-Overholt, Stetler, & Allen, 2005). In the **Iowa
model** of EBP, research and other evidential sources are adopted directly in the practice
setting with the goal of developing a standard of care (Titler, 2007). Additionally, the
groundwork required to create a conceptual framework supportive of an EBP includes
workplace culture change and support of the change through leadership (Stetler et al.,
1998). Beliefs and attitudes, involvement in research activities, information seeking,
professional characteristics, education, and other socioeconomic factors are potential determinants of research utilization (Estabrooks, Floyd, Scott-Findlay, O'Leary, &
Gushta, 2003); however, meta-analysis points out that too much original research and
not enough repetition of previous studies fails to advance the knowledge base.

Developing countries are often constrained economically from accessing research
sources. Such organizations as the Cochrane Collaboration provide free reviews to fill
this void. Even so, knowledge dissemination strategies and education are required to
take advantage of these resources (Cochrane Collaboration, 2004).

Barriers to and Facilitators of EBP

Barriers to the application of EBP include lack of time, lack of access to libraries within
a facility, lack of technology confidence, lack of knowledge on how to search for information, lack of value assigned to using research in practice (Pravikoff et al., 2005),
inadequate EBP knowledge and skills, lack of mentors in EBP, inadequate support
and resources from administration, and insufficient time (Melnyk, Fineout-Overholt,
Stillwell, & Williamson, 2009). McKnight (2006) noted that nurses on one unit felt
constrained by time and ethically obligated to provide patient care rather than spend
time looking up evidence-based references. Nurses may also see the job of interpreting
research as too complex or see the organizational culture as a barrier to implementation of EBP (McCaughan, Thompson, Cullum, Sheldon, & Thompson, 2002). Some
of these same attitudes toward EBP may be echoed by other health care professionals.
Heiwe et al. (2011) surveyed occupational therapists, physical therapists, and dieticians
to uncover attitudes, beliefs, knowledge, and practice related to EBP. They found generally positive attitudes toward using evidence to support clinical practice and confidence
among these clinicians in their ability to interpret and apply evidence in practice. Results
also indicated concern by professionals that EBP guidelines may not adequately reflect
patient preferences and that time was the major barrier that interfered with EBP use.

Yet, Melnynk et al. (2009) noted that a number of factors also facilitate the use of
EBP. These driving forces include knowledge and skills in EBP, having a conviction that
there is a value to using evidence in practices, and practicing in a supportive culture

with tools available to sustain evidence-based care, including access to computers and databases, evidence-based content at the point of care, and the presence of EBP mentors. Similarly, a pre–post study of allied health professionals demonstrated that a structured journal club was an effective tool among some professionals for improving understanding of EBP and attitudes toward using evidence in clinical practice (Lizarondo, Grimmer-Somers, Kumar, & Crockett, 2012).

Informatics Tools to Support EBP

Computers are used in all areas of research: (1) literature search databases, such as CINAHL; (2) online literature reference lists, such as RefWorks; (3) data capture, collection, and coding; (4) data analysis; (5) data modeling; (6) meta-analysis; (7) qualitative analysis; and (8) dissemination of results (e.g., via e-mail or Internet website) (Saba & McCormick, 2006). The context for health informatics has expanded to support dramatic changes in the way science is accomplished. Information need and the collaborative component of interdisciplinary research rely heavily on technology and informatics. Technologies, such as social networking (Web 2.0), may also improve collaboration. The use of technology and informatics in facilitating interdisciplinary and translational research is a key architectural component of the National Institutes of Health's reengineering of the clinical research enterprise as part of its road map initiative for medical research (National Institutes of Health, 2009).

An informatics infrastructure is critical to EBP. Bakken, Stone, and Larson (2008) discuss expanding the context of informatics to genomic health care, shifting research paradigms, and social web technologies. Ensuring the global collaborative nature of health care research for 2010–2018 requires an expansion of the research agenda to user information needs, data management, information support for health care professionals and patients, practice-based knowledge generation, and design evaluation methodologies. Giuse et al. (2005) describe the evolving role of the clinical informationist as being a partner on the health care team who provides timely clinical evidence for the clinical work flow. The National Institutes of Health provides awards under its Clinical and Translational Science Award (CTSA) program to accelerate the transfer of research to the clinical setting (National Institutes of Health, 2009). With the goal of promoting the use of research findings and tool use based on these findings, the **Agency for Healthcare Research and Quality** (AHRQ) became an active participant in pushing evidence forward into practice. The AHRQ is a government-sponsored organization with the mission of reducing patients' risk of harm, decreasing health care costs, and improving patient outcomes through the promotion of research and technology applications focused on EBP. In 1999, AHRQ implemented its Translating Research into Practice Initiative (TRIP) to generate knowledge about evidence-based care (AHRQ, 2001). In the second Translating Research into Practice Initiative (TRIP-II), the focus shifted to improving health care for underserved populations and using information technology to shape translational research and health policy. AHRQ, in partnership with the American Medical Association and the American Association of Health Plans, developed the **National Guideline Clearinghouse** (NGC). NGC is a comprehensive database of evidentially based clinical practice guidelines and related documents that are regularly published through the NGC electronic mailing list and are available on the NGC website (NGC, 2015). The NGC website allows users to browse for the clinical guidelines, view abstracts and full-text links, download full-text clinical guidelines to **personal digital assistant** (PDA) devices and smartphones, obtain technical reports, and compare guidelines. For example, a search (August 22, 2015) using "dental hygiene" as the key words yielded links to 52 guidelines—one of which was titled "Guideline on oral health care for the pregnant adolescent, created in 2007 and revised in 2012 (NGC, 2015). PubMed4Hh (PubMed for handheld devices) is a powerful, free application for smartphones that provides access to the National Library of Medicine and supports PICO (Population, Intervention, Comparison, Outcome) searches, clinical queries, and multi-language searches with links to consensus abstracts. Several universities have developed comprehensive research guides to assist health care professionals in finding evidence to support practice. One of the more comprehensive guides for allied health professionals is provided by Eastern Michigan University (http://guides.emich.edu/c.php?g=217258&p=1435210). Check your own library system as well for EBP resources.

In addition, a growing number of printed and electronic resources are available to assist in creating guidelines and offering information about EBP. A selection of existing websites is shown in **Table 17-1**.

TABLE 17-1 THE ROLE OF INFORMATICS: ONLINE EVIDENCE-BASED RESOURCES

Website	Description
Academic Center for Evidence-Based Practice (ACE) http://www.acestar.uthscsa.edu	The School of Nursing at the University of Texas Health Science Center at San Antonio sponsors the Academic Center for Evidence-Based Practice. The center's ultimate goal is to bring research to practice to improve patient care, outcomes, and safety. The center is also home to the ACE star model of knowledge transformation.
The Agency for Healthcare Research and Quality http://www.ahrq.gov	The agency for Healthcare Research and Quality contains a wealth of information regarding healthcare quality. There is no charge for access to the site or its resources.
BMJ Publishing http://clinicalevidence.bmj.com/x/index.html	The BMJ publishing group provides clinical databases by prescription. The BMJ Clinical Evidence site allows the download of some clinical papers and some interesting risk tools without charge.
The Center for Evidence-Based Practices (CEBP) http://www.evidencebasedpractices.org	The Center for Evidence-Based Practices of the Orelena Hawks Puckett Institute focuses on research to practice initiatives related to early intervention, early childhood education, parent and family support, and family-centered practices.
Centre for Evidence Based Medicine http://www.cebm.net	The Center for Evidence Based Medicine, located in Oxford in the UK, is devoted to developing and promoting evidence-based resources for healthcare professionals. In addition to free articles, the site also provides free teaching resources and presentation.

(*continues*)

TABLE 17-1 THE ROLE OF INFORMATICS: ONLINE EVIDENCE-BASED RESOURCES (continued)

Website	Description
CINAHL http://cinahl.com	CINAHL information systems offers a multitude of online services, which include website link sources, CINAHL'S online nursing and allied health database, document delivery, and search services.
The Cochrane Collaboration http://www.cochrane.org	The Cochrane Collaboration provides reviews for free, but fulltext articles are by subscription.
Entrez PubMed http://www.ncbi.nlm.nih.gov /guide/all/#databases_	Entrez PubMed is a service provided by The National Library of Medicine (NLM). The NLM was developed by the National Center for Biotechnology Information (NCBI), which provides access to life science journals and MEDLINE citations. Some of the journal links are free, and some require a subscription.
PubMed Central http://www.pubmedcentral .nih.gov	PubMed Central (PMC) is a free digital archive of science-related articles managed by the NCBI. BioMed Central (an open-source online archive) may be accessed here.
The Joanna Briggs Institute http://www.joannabriggs .org/index.html	The Joanna Briggs Institute was established in 1996 as a resource for best care practices. Joanna Briggs was first matron of the Adelaide Hospital in Australia and is recognized for her financial and organizational support. The Joanna Briggs Institute is a leader in developing evidence-based practices.
Information & Resources for Nurses Worldwide http://www.nurses.info /specialty_evidenced _based_orgs.htm	This website provides searchable links to evidence-based practice organizations by specialty.
The Iowa Model of Evidence-Based Practice http://www.nnpnetwork.org /ebpresources/iowa-model	This website provides a brief overview of the Iowa Model for Evidence-Based Practice.
The Johns Hopkins Bloomberg School of Public Health http://www.jhsph.edu/epc	The Johns Hopkins Evidence-Based Practice Center was established in 1997 and is one of 14 such centers producing comprehensive, systematic reviews for the AHRQ.
Trip database http://www.tripdatabase .com	The Trip database is a clinical search tool to allow clinicians to identify the best evidence for clinical practice.
University of Iowa College of Nursing http://www.nursing .uiowa.edu/hartford	The John A. Hartford Foundation Center of Geriatric Nursing Excellence at the University of Iowa has evidence-based practice resources available at this site for a nominal fee.
World Views on Evidence-Based Nursing http:// blackwellpublishing.com /wvn	Through Blackwell Publishing, this magazine, sponsored by Sigma Theta Tau, is dedicated exclusively to evidence-based nursing articles. The magazine is also offered online by subscription.

Developing EBP Guidelines

Several models have been developed to guide organizations into translating research into practice. Brief descriptions of these models are provided in **Table 17-2**. As an example, Titler (2007) identifies the steps in the Iowa model for translating research into practice as (1) identifying the problem, issue, or topic in professional practice; (2) research and critique of related evidence; (3) adaptation of the evidence to practice; (4) implementation of the EBP; and (5) evaluation of patient outcomes and care practices. Careful analysis and discussion of the research or other forms of evidence in this scenario may reveal that given the context, implementation may not be practical. Following implementation, results must be monitored to determine whether the application works for the context. Thoughtful discussion of the findings will help the clinical team determine if further research is warranted or if further change is needed.

Information technology is important in synthesizing the research regardless of the model. Bakken (2001) recommends (1) standardized nomenclature required for the electronic health record (standardized terminologies and structures), (2) digital sources of evidence, (3) standards that facilitate healthcare data exchange among heterogeneous systems, (4) informatics processes that support the acquisition and application of evidence to a specific clinical situation, and (5) informatics competencies (p. 1999). Bakken's recommendations encourage the development of an infrastructure that creates a database of experiential clinical evidence.

TABLE 17-2 COMPARISON OF MODEL APPROACHES TO EVIDENCE-BASED PRACTICE		
Stetler model (Stetler, 2001)	ACE star model (Stevens, 2004)	The Iowa model of evidence-based practice to promote quality care (Titler et al., 2001)
1. Preparation 2. Validation 3. Cooperative evaluation 4. Decision making 5. Translational application 6. Evaluation	1. Discovery 2. Evidence summary 3. Translation 4. Integration 5. Evaluation	1. Select the trigger as impetus for practice (knowledge focused or practice focused) change. 2. Determine if the topic is worth pursuing for the organization and if not, pursue new trigger. 3. Determine if there is significant research base. If so, change, otherwise conduct research or seek more research. 4. If change is appropriate for practice, implement change. 5. Monitor results. 6. Disseminate results.

Meta-Analysis and the Generation of Knowledge

Systematic reviews combine results from multiple primary investigations to obtain consensus on a specific area of research. They are much more robust than a simple review of the literature that one might use to define a topic before writing a paper. The goal of a systematic review is to find and appraise all relevant literature on a topic. Studies are discarded from the review if they are not considered sound, thereby creating a reliable end result. The strength of the systematic review is its ability to corroborate findings and reach consensus. Systematic reviews show the need for more research by revealing the areas where quantitative results may be lacking or minimal. Bias may occur if the selected studies are inadequate, if all sources of evidence are not investigated, or if the publications selected are not adequately diverse (Lipp, 2005).

Meta-analysis, a more vigorous form of systematic review, uses statistical methods to combine the results of several studies (Cook, Mulrow, & Haynes, 1997). Quantitative studies are typically used. According to Glass (1976), meta-analysis is the statistical analysis of a large collection of analysis results from individual studies for the purpose of integrating the findings (p. 3). Both systematic reviews and meta-analyses require the researcher to use critical thinking in order to effectively combine and interpret the findings.

Kraft (2006) describes the documentation search strategy for meta-analysis as beginning with the identification of the studies through a search of bibliographic databases, identification of meta-analysis articles that match the search criteria, elimination of those articles that do not match the search criteria, review of the reference lists in the meta-analysis for other articles that may relate to the topic, and review of each article for quality and content. Additional sources should include unpublished works, such as conferences and dissertation abstracts, with the goal of obtaining as many relevant articles as possible. Gregson, Meal, and Avis (2002) identify the steps of a meta-analysis as (1) defining the problem, followed by protocol generation; (2) establishing study eligibility criteria, followed by literature search; (3) identifying the heterogeneity of results of studies; (4) standardizing the data and statistically combining the results; and (5) conducting sensitivity testing to determine whether the combined results are the same. The often-cited criticism of meta-analysis is that emphasis is on **quantitative studies** (those using numeric data), not **qualitative studies** (those using words and descriptions as data). Additionally, the analysis is only as good as the studies used (Gregson et al., 2002). Collection and dissemination of these meta-analysis and systematic reviews are available in paper and on the Internet, although many such databases require a subscription.

The term "open access" refers to a worldwide movement to make a library of knowledge available to anyone with Internet access. The **Open Access Initiative** came about in response to the tremendous cost of research library access. Libraries pay large fees for journal subscriptions, and the richness of library references is limited to what the budget allows. The cost of keeping current with research has caused library subscriptions to decline (Yiotis, 2005). Open access adds to the controversy, with some journals charging authors for publication of their work, which in itself may provide a financial barrier to publication in this form.

According to Suber (2004), open access refers to digital literature that is available to anyone with Internet access free of charge. There are two vehicles for open access: archives and journals. Open-access journals are generally peer reviewed and freely available. The publishers of open-access journals do not charge the reader but rather obtain funds for publishing elsewhere. Open-access journals may charge the author or depend on other forms of funding, such as donations, grants, and advertising, to publish.

The Future

Titler (2007) indicates that future priorities should include development of theoretical formulations to guide research and systematic reviews so that they may be grouped by organizational context (e.g., primary care, outpatient). Focus on other forms of research, such as qualitative research, should also be incorporated into systematic reviews.

Given the vast amounts of data, Bakken et al. (2008) identify areas of focus for health informatics in knowledge representation, data management, analysis, and predictive modeling in genomic health care and the need for policies and procedures to protect data acquisition, dissemination, privacy, security, and confidentiality as well as education in these areas. Informatics tools support professional practice, education of health care consumers, and knowledge generation. The technology is available now to incorporate evidence into reference links embedded in electronic clinical care plans. Incorporation of personalized clinical desktops to allow each clinician to have appropriate references (similar to Internet ad bot technology) provided to him or her may be possible. Time, research, and technology will tell.

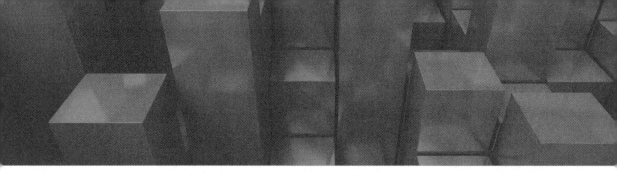

Summary

These are amazing times. Technology has taken us faster and further than we ever thought possible. Health care jobs have become more technical and more complicated. In some ways, technology has increased the margin for error. Some health care practitioners will continue to rely on little scraps of paper and nonsystematic methods to keep themselves and their patients safe. Unfortunately, individuals who become so tied to these things close their mind to new innovations. The evolving quality culture and increased patient safety concerns are dragging health care workers forward. For the benefit of our patients, health care must move forward.

Collaboration, information literacy, improved access to online libraries, research tool transparency, a common data language, organizational and informational support, and continued research are a short list of needed items to advance translational research. Repeat studies are needed to provide meaningful meta-analysis and systematic reviews. Technology advancement in the area of incorporating evidence into clinical tools must continue. Removing the barriers to knowledge-seeking behavior and providing access to evidential resources will promote knowledge and, in the end, improve patient outcomes.

In the era of EBP, health care providers must continue to think critically about their actions. What is the science behind their interventions? Health care workers must no longer do things one way just because they have always been done that way. Research the problem, use evidence-based resources, critically select electronic and non-electronic references, consolidate the research findings and combine and compare the conclusions, present the findings, and propose a solution. One will be the first to ask why and may be a key player in making change happen.

Thought-Provoking Questions

1. Reflect on copyright law and why it is needed. Suppose you determine that photographs or other images can be replicated based on your assessment of fair use but your administrative assistant refuses to photocopy them because he feels that it is copyright infringement and against company policy. Describe in detail how you would handle this situation.

2. Choose a clinical problem or topic specific to your discipline and enter the search terms at http://www.guidelines.gov. Summarize the information you found there in relation to the recommendations for practice. How are they similar to what you have learned about the topic? How are they different? If you wanted to implement the recommendations for practice, what barriers might need to be overcome?

3. The use of heparin versus saline to maintain the patency of peripheral intravenous catheters has been addressed in research for many years. The American Society of Health

System Pharmacists (2006) published a position paper advocating its support of the use of 0.9% saline in the maintenance of peripheral catheters in non-pregnant adults. It seems surprising that this position paper references articles that advocate the use of saline over heparin dating from 1991. What do you believe are some of the barriers that would have caused this delay in implementation?

Apply Your Knowledge

In this text, we have established the importance of information literacy and how it can inform practice. For this content application scenario, choose an intervention from your discipline and find at least two recent scholarly articles related to the practice intervention.

1. How does the information in these articles compare to what your text has indicated is current practice?
2. If the articles suggest a change in current practice, how does this affect clinical work flow?
3. Share your discoveries with classmates and compare and contrast EBP findings for various interventions common to your discipline.

Additional Resources

Agency for Healthcare Research and Quality
http://www.guidelines.gov
Eastern Michigan University
http://guides.emich.edu/c.php?g=217258&p=1435210
EBSCO
http://support.epnet.com/training/flash_videos/cinahl_basic/cinahl_basic.html
http://support.epnet.com/training/flash_videos/cinahl_advanced/cinahl_advanced.html

References

Agency for Healthcare Research and Quality. (2001). AHRQ profile: Quality research for quality healthcare. http://www.ahrq.gov/about/profile.htm

American Library Association. (2000). *Information literacy competency standards for higher education*. Chicago: Author.

American Society of Health System Pharmacists. (2006). ASHSP therapeutic position statement on the institutional use of 0.9% sodium chloride injection to maintain patency of peripheral indwelling intermittent infusion devices. *American Journal of Health System Pharmacy, 63,* 1273–1275.

Association of College and Research Libraries. (2000). Information literacy competency standards for higher education. http://www.ala.org/acrl/standards/informationliteracycompetency

Bakken, S. (2001). An informatics infrastructure is essential for evidence-based practice. *Journal of the American Medical Informatics Association, 8,* 199–201.

Bakken, S., Stone, P. W., & Larson, E. L. (2008). A nursing informatics research agenda for 2008–18: Contextual influences and key components. *Nursing Outlook, 56,* 206–214.

Baumann, S. (2010). The limitations of evidence-based practice. *Nursing Science Quarterly, 23*(3), 226–230.

Cochrane, A. L. (1972). *Effectiveness and efficiency: Random reflections on health services*. London: Nuffield Provincial Hospitals Trust.

Cochrane Collaboration. (2004). Bridging the gaps across the income divide: A review of the collaboration's efforts to date and recommendations for the future. http://www2.cochrane.org /colloquia/abstracts/ottawa/O-006.htm

Cook, D. J., Mulrow, C. D., & Haynes, R. B. (1997). Systematic reviews: Synthesis of best evidence for clinical decisions. *Annals of Internal Medicine, 126*(5), 376–380.

Dickersin, K., & Manheimer, E. (1998). The Cochrane Collaboration: Evaluation of health care services using systematic reviews of the results and randomized control trials. *Clinical Obstetrics and Gynecology, 41*(2), 315–331.

Estabrooks, C. A., Floyd, J. A., Scott-Findlay, S., O'Leary, K. A., & Gushta, M. (2003). Individual determinants of research utilization: A systematic review. *Journal of Advanced Nursing, 42*, 73–81.

French, P. (2002). What is the evidence on evidence-based nursing? An epistemological concern. *Journal of Advanced Nursing, 37*(3), 250–257.

Giuse, N. B., Koonce, T. Y., Jerome, R. N., Gahall, M., Sathe, N. A., & Williams, A. (2005). Evolution of a mature clinical informationist model. *Journal of the American Medical Informatics Association, 12*(3), 249–255.

Glass, G. V. (1976). Primary, secondary and meta-analysis of research. *Educational Research, 5*(10), 3–8.

Goode, C. J., & Piedalue, F. (1999). Evidence-based clinical practice. *Journal of Nursing Administration, 29*(6), 15–21.

Gregson, P. R., Meal, A. G., & Avis, M. (2002). Meta-analysis: The glass eye of evidence-based practice? *Nursing Inquiry, 9*(1), 24–30.

Heiwe, S., Kajermo, K., Lenne, R., Guidetti, S., Samuelsson, M., Andersson, I., & Wengstrom, Y. (2011). Evidence-based practice: Attitudes, knowledge and behavior among allied health care professionals. *International Journal for Quality in Healthcare, 23*(2), 198–209.

Joanna Briggs Institute. (n.d.). http://joannabriggs.org/index.html

Kirchhoff, K. T. (2004). State of the science of translational research: From demonstration projects to intervention testing. *Worldviews on Evidence-Based Nursing, 1*(Suppl. 1), S6–S12.

Kraft, M. R. (2006). Meta-analysis: A research tool. *SCI Nursing Journal, 23*(2). http://www .unitedspinal.org/publications/nursing/2006/08/27/research-corner

Lipp, A. (2005). The systematic review as an evidence-based tool for the operating room. *Association of Operating Room Nurses Journal, 81*(6), 1279–1287.

Lizarondo, L. M., Grimmer-Somers, K., Kumar, S., & Crockett, A. (2012). Does journal club membership improve research evidence uptake in different allied health disciplines: A pre-post study. *BMC Research Notes, 5*(1), 588–596.

McCaughan, D., Thompson, C., Cullum, N., Sheldon, T. A., & Thompson, D. R. (2002). Acute care nurses' perceptions of barriers to using research information in clinical decision-making. *Journal of Advanced Nursing, 39*(1), 46–60.

McKnight, M. (2006). The information seeking of on-duty critical care nurses: Evidence from participant observation and in-context interviews. *Journal of the Medical Library Association, 94*(2), 145–151.

Melnyk, B. M. (2005). Advancing evidence-based practice in clinical and academic settings. *Worldviews on Evidence-Based Nursing, 3*, 161–165.

Melnyk, B. M., Fineout-Overholt, E., Stetler, C., & Allen, J. (2005). Outcomes and implementation strategies from the first U.S. evidence-based practice leadership summit. *Worldviews on Evidence-Based Nursing, 2*(3), 113–121.

Melnyk, B. M., Fineout-Overholt, E., Stillwell, S., & Williamson, K. (2009). Igniting a spirit of inquiry: An essential foundation for evidence-based practice. *American Journal of Nursing, 109*(11), 49–52.

Melnyk, B. M., Fineout-Overholt, E., Stone, P., & Ackerman, M. (2000). Evidence-based practice: The past, the present, and recommendations for the millennium. *Pediatric Nursing, 26*(1), 77–80.

National Guideline Clearinghouse. (2015). http://www.guideline.gov

National Institutes of Health. (2009). Re-engineering the clinical research enterprise. http://commonfund.nih.gov/clinicalresearch/overviewtranslational.asp

O'Neill, T., Jinks, C., & Ong, B. N. (2007). Decision-making regarding total knee replacement surgery: A qualitative meta-synthesis. *BMC Health Services Research, 7*(52). http://www.pubmedcentral.nih.gov/articlerender.fcgi?artid=1854891

Polit, D. F., & Beck, T. C. (2008). *Nursing research: Generating and assessing evidence for nursing practice* (8th ed.). Philadelphia: Lippincott Williams & Wilkins.

Pravikoff, D. S., Tanner, A. B., & Pierce, S. T. (2005). Readiness of U.S. nurses for evidence-based practice. *American Journal of Nursing, 105*(9), 40–51.

Rycroft-Malone, J., Seers, K., Titchen, A., Harvey, G., Kitson, A., & McCormack, B. (2004). What counts as evidence in evidence-based practice? *Journal of Advanced Nursing, 47*(1), 81–90.

Saba, V. K., & McCormick, K. A. (2006). *Essentials of nursing informatics* (4th ed.). New York: McGraw-Hill.

Sackett, D. I., Rosenberg, W. M., Gray, J. A., Haynes, R. B., & Richardson, W. S. (1996). Evidence based medicine: What it is and what it isn't. *British Medical Journal, 312*, 71–72.

Stetler, C. B. (2001). Updating the Stetler model of research utilization to facilitate evidence-based practice. *Nursing Outlook, 49*(6), 272–279.

Stetler, C. B., Brunell, M., Giuliano, K. K., Morse, D., Prince, L., & Newell-Stokes, V. (1998). Evidence-based practice and the role of nursing leadership. *Journal of Nursing Administration, 28*(7/8), 45–53.

Stevens, K. R. (2004). *ACE star model of EBP: Knowledge transformation.* http://www.acestar.uthscsa.edu/Learn_model.htm

Suber, P. (2004). A very brief introduction to open access. http://www.earlham.edu/~peters/fos/brief.htm

Titler, M. G. (2004). Methods in translation science. *Worldviews on Evidence-Based Nursing, 1*, 38–48.

Titler, M. (2007). Translating research into practice: Models for changing clinician behavior. *American Journal of Nursing, 107*(6), 26–33.

Titler, M. G. (2010). Translation science and context. *Research Theory and Nursing Practice: An International Journal, 24*(1), 35–55.

Titler, M. G., Kleiber, C., Steelman, V., Rakel, B., Budreu, G., Everett, L., et al. (2001). The Iowa model of evidence-based practice to promote quality care. *Critical Care Nursing Clinics of North America, 13*(4), 497–509.

Woolf, S. H. (2008). The meaning of translational research and why it matters. *Journal of the American Medical Association, 299*(2), 211–213.

Yiotis, K. (2005). The Open Access Initiative: A new paradigm for scholarly communications. http://ejournals.bc.edu/ojs/index.php/ital/article/view/3378/2988

Bioinformatics, Biomedical Informatics, and Computational Biology

Dee McGonigle and Kathleen Mastrian

OBJECTIVES

1. Describe bioinformatics, biomedical informatics, and computational biology.
2. Appreciate the intertwining of bioinformatics and health care in biomedical informatics.
3. Imagine the future of health care based on genomics.

Introduction

The National Center for Biotechnology Information (NCBI, 2004) states that "biology in the 21st century is being transformed from a purely lab-based science to an information science as well" (para. 5). What must be remembered when delving into the new informatics frontier is that biological systems are information systems. Consider that DNA essentially is a storehouse of information. Unlocking that information and learning how that information is transcribed to RNA and ultimately expressed as proteins promises interesting and cutting-edge developments in understanding diseases and managing them at the molecular level. This chapter introduces the reader to the exciting world of bioinformatics and provides a beginning understanding of the frontiers unleashed by the collection, mapping, storage, and sharing of genetic data.

Key Terms
Alleles
Bioinformatics
Biomarkers
Biomedical informatics
Computational biology
Data sets
Dynamic network biomarkers
Genome
Genomics
Haplotypes
Human Genome Project
Informaticists
Molecular biomarkers
Personalized medicine
Precision medicine
Protein-based network biomarkers

Bioinformatics, Biomedical Informatics, and Computational Biology Defined

Three terms are frequently used: (1) **bioinformatics**, (2) **biomedical informatics**, and (3) **computational biology**. As terms continue to be bandied about, it is important to comprehend what they mean to understand better these evolving fields. According to the University of Texas at El Paso (2010) website, "Bioinformatics is an interdisciplinary science with a focus on data management and interpretation for complex biological phenomena that are analyzed and visualized using mathematical modeling and numerical methodologies with predictive algorithms" (para. 1). A website operated by the University of Minnesota (2010) states,

> Bioinformatics is defined here as an interdisciplinary research area that applies computer and information science to solve biological problems. However, this is not the only definition. The field is being defined (and redefined) at present, and there are probably as many definitions as there are bioinformaticians (bioinformaticists?). (para. 1)

The myriad definitions for the "moving target named bioinformatics" (University of Minnesota, 2010, para. 2) are reflected in those developed from 2000 to 2009. According to NCBI (2004), "Bioinformatics is the field of science in which biology, computer science, and information technology merge to form a single discipline. The ultimate goal of the field is to enable the discovery of new biological insights" (para. 5). Network Science (2009) believes that

> an absolute definition of bioinformatics has not been agreed upon. The first level, however, can be defined as the design and application of methods for the collection, organization, indexing, storage, and analysis of biological sequences (both nucleic acids [DNA and RNA] and proteins). The next stage of bioinformatics is the derivation of knowledge concerning the pathways, functions, and interactions of these genes (functional genomics) and proteins (proteomics). (para. 14)

Mulligen et al. (2008) wrote that "BioInformatics (BI) is a less mature scientific discipline which aims to research and develop algorithms, computational and statistical techniques which solve biological problems. Significantly, BI has experienced an exponential growth as a result of its importance to the understanding and interpretation of data generated by 'omics' technologies" (para. 6).

The complete sequencing of the human genome has led to systems biology referred to as "omics" and has elevated scientists' ability from studying one gene or protein to studying fundamental biological processes (**Box 18-1**).

The National Human Genome Research Institute (NHGRI, n.d.) tutorial on bioinformatics defines bioinformatics as "the branch of biology that is concerned with the acquisition, storage, display, and analysis of the information found in nucleic acid

---

BOX 18-1   OMICS

Kelly (2008) describes that "'ome' and 'omics' are suffixes that are derived from genome" (para. 1). National Public Radio (2010) credits botanist Hans Winkler with merging "the Greek words 'genesis' and 'soma' to describe a body of genes" (para. 1) in 1920. The term *genome* was born from this combination, and genomics arose as the study of the genome.

Kelly (2008) continues to explain,

Scientists like to append to these to any large-scale system (or really, just about anything complex), such as the collection of proteins in a cell or tissue (the proteome), the collection of metabolites (the metabolome), and the collection of RNA that's been transcribed from genes (the transcriptome). High-throughput analysis is essential considering data at the "omic" level, that is to say considering all DNA sequences, gene expression levels, or proteins at once (or, to be slightly more precise, a significant subset of them). (para. 1)

---

and protein sequence data. Computers and bioinformatics software are the tools of the trade" (para. 4). Based on these definitions, one can get a flavor for what bioinformatics entails. It is clear that the definition of bioinformatics varies and that there is no single definition that everyone agrees with at the present time.

Biomedicine applies bioinformatics to promote health. According to the website of the Ohio State University Medical Center (2010), "Biomedical informatics is the study and process of efficiently gathering, storing, managing, retrieving, analyzing, communicating, sharing, and applying biomedical information to improve the detection, prevention, and treatment of disease" (para. 2). The Vanderbilt University (2010) website suggests that

Biomedical Informatics is the interdisciplinary science of acquiring, structuring, analyzing and providing access to biomedical data, information and knowledge. As an academic discipline, biomedical informatics is grounded in the principles of computer science, information science, cognitive science, social science, and engineering, as well as the clinical and basic biological sciences. (para. 1)

Gennari (2002) stated, "Biomedical Informatics is the science underlying the acquisition, maintenance, retrieval, and application of biomedical knowledge and information to improve patient care, medical education, and health sciences research" (para. 1). He believes that "a primary feature of Biomedical and Health Informatics is its interdisciplinary nature: It connects computer science, medicine, biology and health care, and provides a synergy that goes beyond anything that researchers in any single domain can provide" (para. 3). According to Bioinformaticsweb.tk (2005), "Biomedical Informatics is an emerging discipline that has been defined as the study, invention, and implementation of structures and algorithms to improve communication, understanding and management of medical information" (para. 16). This organization then goes on to muddy the water with its description of bioinformatics:

> *Bioinformatics derives knowledge from computer analysis of biological data. These can consist of the information stored in the genetic code, but also experimental results from various sources, patient statistics, and scientific literature. Research in bioinformatics includes method development for storage, retrieval, and analysis of the data. Bioinformatics is a rapidly developing branch of biology and is highly interdisciplinary, using techniques and concepts from informatics, statistics, mathematics, chemistry, biochemistry, physics, and linguistics. It has many practical applications in different areas of biology and medicine. (para. 1)*

Biomedical informatics is a growing field, with significant applications and implications throughout the biomedical and clinical worlds. The authors believe that biomedical informatics is the application of bioinformatics to health care.

Computational biology is the action complement of bioinformatics and, therefore, biomedicine. NCBI (2004) stated,

> *Ultimately, however, all of this information must be combined to form a comprehensive picture of normal cellular activities so that researchers may study how these activities are altered in different disease states. Therefore, the field of bioinformatics has evolved such that the most pressing task now involves the analysis and interpretation of various types of data, including nucleotide and amino acid sequences, protein domains, and protein structures. The actual process of analyzing and interpreting data is referred to as computational biology. Important subdisciplines within bioinformatics and computational biology include:*
>
> - *The development and implementation of tools that enable efficient access to, and use and management of, various types of information*
> - *The development of new algorithms (mathematical formulas) and statistics with which to assess relationships among members of large data sets, such as methods to locate a gene within a sequence, predict protein structure and/or function, and cluster protein sequences into families of related sequences. (para. 6)*

In 2000, the Biomedical Information Science and Technology Initiative Consortium of the National Institutes of Health (NIH) defined bioinformatics and computational biology. Members of the consortium stated that "no definition could completely eliminate overlap with other activities or preclude variations in interpretation by different individuals and organizations" (NIH, 2000, para. 3). Ultimately, they defined bioinformatics as "research, development, or application of computational tools and approaches for expanding the use of biological, medical, behavioral or health data, including those to acquire, store, organize, archive, analyze, or visualize such data" (para. 4). The same group defined computational biology as "the development and application of data-analytical and theoretical methods, mathematical modeling and computational simulation techniques to the study of biological, behavioral, and social systems" (para. 5).

Bioinformatics tools help biomedical **informaticists** and health care personnel tackle the analysis of large data sets. The authors believe that biomedical informatics uses bioinformatics, whereas computational biology is its action complement. By using bioinformatics and computational biology to analyze and interpret intricate biological events, biomedical informaticists promote health and improve patient care. Biomedical informatics and bioinformatics may seem similar, but if one thinks of biomedical informatics as focusing on health care and patients, it helps distinguish between the two. Biomedical informaticists use bioinformatics methods to integrate large biological and medical **data sets** to facilitate understanding of the human body and its biological functioning; these efforts are geared toward improving health by defeating disease.

In an interesting article on the hot, bioinformatics industry, Ostler and Gollin (2015) reported that "the field of bioinformatics is flourishing, and strong growth is only projected to continue" (p. 76). According to Hare (2014), "The Global Bioinformatics Market was valued at USD 4,110.6 million in 2014 and is expected to grow at a CAGR of 20.4% from 2014 to 2020, to reach an estimated value of USD 12,542.4 million in 2020" (para. 1). The tools that we will need to advance our practice will continue to be developed and honed.

Why Are Bioinformatics and Biomedical Informatics So Important?

The future of health care is based on **genomics**. Bioinformatics and computational biology have provided the tools to make it possible to analyze and interpret complex biological processes. Through these developments, several projects have advanced understanding of the human **genome, haplotypes**, and the genomic changes related to disease.

In 2006, the Cancer Genome Atlas Project began (NHGRI, 2010). This "$100 million pilot will map the genomic changes in brain, lung and ovarian cancers to assess the feasibility of a full-scale effort to systematically explore the entire spectrum of genomic changes involved in every major type of human cancer" (para. 1). The goal of this project is to develop a "resource that will be used to develop new strategies for preventing, diagnosing and treating the disease" (para. 1).

The goal of the International HapMap Project (2006) is to

develop a haplotype map of the human genome, the HapMap, which will describe the common patterns of human DNA sequence variation. The HapMap is expected to be a key resource for researchers to use to find genes affecting health, disease, and responses to drugs and environmental factors. The information produced by the Project will be made freely available. (para. 1)

This international partnership of scientists has taken blood samples from clusters of related people, such as parents and children, from different international regions.

Using these samples, the researchers have been able to catalog some of the common variations in DNA and investigate inherited **alleles**. As the name implies, a haplotype map identifies a set of closely linked alleles on a chromosome that tend to be inherited together. The International HapMap Project states,

> *Most common diseases, such as diabetes, cancer, stroke, heart disease, depression, and asthma, are affected by many genes and environmental factors. Although any two unrelated people are the same at about 99.9% of their DNA sequences, the remaining 0.1% is important because it contains the genetic variants that influence how people differ in their risk of disease or their response to drugs. Discovering the DNA sequence variants that contribute to common disease risk offers one of the best opportunities for understanding the complex causes of disease in humans. (para. 3)*

A major contribution has been the **Human Genome Project** (HGP), which began in 1990 and was completed in 2003 (HGP, 2010). The U.S. Department of Energy and the NIH coordinated this program, which had the following goals:

- Identify all of the approximately 20,000–25,000 genes in human DNA
- Determine the sequences of the 3 billion chemical base pairs that make up human DNA
- Store this information in databases
- Improve tools for data analysis
- Transfer related technologies to the private sector
- Address the ethical, legal, and social issues that may arise from the project (para. 2)

According to NHGRI (n.d.),

> *It was understood that to meet the project's goals, the speed of DNA sequencing would have to increase and the cost would have to come down. Over the life of the project virtually every aspect of DNA sequencing was improved. It took the project approximately four years to sequence its first one billion bases but just four months to sequence the second billion bases. (para. 1)*

During the month of January 2003, 1.5 billion bases were sequenced. As the speed of DNA sequencing increased, the cost decreased from $10 per base in 1990 to $0.10 per base at the conclusion of the project in April 2003 (NHGRI, n.d., para. 2).

One of the most important aspects of bioinformatics is identifying genes within a long DNA sequence. Until the development of bioinformatics, the only way to locate genes along the chromosome was to study their function in the organism (in vivo) or to isolate the DNA and study it in a test tube (in vitro). Bioinformatics allows scientists to make educated guesses about where genes are located simply by analyzing sequence data using a computer (in silico) (NHGRI, n.d., para. 8).

The other major piece brought out through the HGP was the realization that ethical, legal, and social issues arise from studying human genomes. The participants in the HGP set aside a percentage of their annual budgets to research ethical, legal, and social issues (HGP, 2008). **Box 18-2** identifies some of the questions raised regarding ethical, legal, and social issues.

Even though the HGP has ended, researchers continue to improve DNA sequencing. Specifically, they continue to advance the bioinformatics and computational biology tools that are used in biomedical informatics. However, as Butte (2008) laments, "There is an absolute paucity of people trained to make use of these resources, to build the infrastructure, to ask these novel questions, and to even answer these questions" (p. 173).

These three projects are pivotal in genomics. The HGP focused on the DNA sequence from a single individual, the HapMap project focused on variation in the genome and on human populations, and the Cancer Genome Atlas Project is concerned

---

BOX 18-2   ETHICAL, LEGAL, AND SOCIAL ISSUES RAISED BY THE HUMAN GENOME PROJECT

- Who should have access to personal genetic information, and how will it be used?
- Who owns and controls genetic information?
- How does personal genetic information affect an individual and society's perceptions of that individual?
- How does genomic information affect members of minority communities?
- Do health care personnel properly counsel parents about the risks and limitations of genetic technology?
- How reliable and useful is fetal genetic testing?
- What are the larger societal issues raised by new reproductive technologies?
- How will genetic tests be evaluated and regulated for accuracy, reliability, and utility? (Currently, there is little regulation at the federal level.)
- How do we prepare health care professionals for the new genetics?
- How do we prepare the public to make informed choices?
- How do we as a society balance current scientific limitations and social risk with long-term benefits?
- Should testing be performed when no treatment is available?
- Should parents have the right to have their minor children tested for adult-onset diseases?
- Are genetic tests reliable and interpretable by the medical community?
- Do people's genes make them behave in a particular way?
- Can people always control their behavior?
- What is considered acceptable diversity?
- Where is the line between medical treatment and enhancement?
- Are genetically modified foods and other products safe to humans and the environment?
- How will these technologies affect developing nations' dependence on the West?
- Who owns genes and other pieces of DNA?
- Will patenting DNA sequences limit their accessibility and development into useful products?

Source: Human Genome Project (2008).

with how cancer affects the genomes. As a result of these seminal projects and a unique culture of data sharing previously unknown among biological researchers, molecular data and measurement tools are now publicly available. Two examples of publicly available databases are the Gene Expression Omnibus, which is maintained by the National Center for Biotechnology Information at the National Library of Medicine, and ArrayExpress, which is maintained by the European Bioinformatics Institute (Butte, 2008).

This section has provided an overview of why bioinformatics and biomedical informatics are so important, and in the past few years, great leaps and bounds have occurred. Chen et al. (2015) described what is being worked on currently and the impact this could have on the future of health care. **Biomarkers** generally refer to "individual genes, proteins or metabolites (**molecular biomarkers**)" (Chen et al., 2015, p. 298). With advances in bioinformatics technology, **protein-based network biomarkers** have been able to be studied. These biomarkers not only revealed the panel of proteins interactions but also their interactions with RNA, DNA, and other molecules:

> But both the molecular biomarkers and the protein-based network biomarkers have limitations because of their static nature. To increase the ability to make early diagnosis, identify disease-specific biomarkers and therapeutic targets, and predict patient outcome, *dynamic network biomarkers (DNBs) were created,* monitored and evaluated at different stages and time-points of the disease, based on non-linear dynamical theory and complex network theory. DNBs differ from molecular biomarkers and network biomarkers to describe and identify disease progress situations and interactions rather than the static nature and approach. (Chen et al., 2015, p. 298)

The promise of DNBs lies in the fact that they can help us uncover disease-specific biomarkers that we can map to compute and diagnose pre-disease circumstances and conditions:

> It is more than new nomenclature, although every molecular biomarker is embedded in a molecular network and this network will show dynamic properties over time. The common objective of developing biomarkers, network biomarkers and DNB is to discover disease-specific biomarker or a panel of biomarkers for monitoring disease occurrence, progression or treatment. (Wu, Chen, & Wang, 2014, para. 8)

As new researchers with both biology and computational expertise emerge, bioinformatics and computational biology projects will continue to contribute new insights into disease mechanisms and therapeutic interventions.

What Does the Future Hold?

It will take many more years of researching and applying bioinformatics and computational biology before the information in the human genome is understood in detail. Because these applications have the ability to allow one to analyze and interpret complex biological processes, researchers are on the path to understanding the etiology of disease and of treatment interventions at the molecular level.

Consider a typical day on any clinical unit. The advanced practice nurse who wants to prescribe a drug for a patient begins by reviewing the patient's genetic test results. The advanced practice nurse knows that this information must be assessed before prescribing so that a drug that will treat the patient's illness successfully without producing harmful side effects can be selected. The patient will receive only the medication that he or she needs and one that is designed to interfere with or enhance the specific molecular processes that are the signature for the patient's particular health challenge. The advances that bioinformatics and biomedical informatics promise will dramatically impact health care delivery as it is known. As explained by Rajappa, Sharma, and Saxena (2004),

> *Understanding molecular mechanisms lead to better classification of disease and better management. A drop of blood from a hypertensive patient gives gene expression profile by cDNA microarray analysis. It may reveal SNPs [single nucleotide polymorphisms] related to hypertension and others which predispose a patient to diabetes mellitus or myocardial infarction and the clinician can determine which drugs are beneficial and which are harmful. This scenario has a whale of difference from the current "trial and error" method of matching a patient with antihypertensives. (p. 128)*

We continue to advance our capabilities in **personalized medicine**. The U.S. Food and Drug Administration (FDA) (2015) stated,

> *The term "personalized medicine" is often described as providing "the right patient with the right drug at the right dose at the right time." More broadly, personalized medicine (also known as **precision medicine**) may be thought of as the tailoring of medical treatment to the individual characteristics, needs, and preferences of a patient during all stages of care, including prevention, diagnosis, treatment, and follow-up. (para. 1)*

The FDA is working with researchers, health care professionals, and those who are developing and producing drugs, biologics, and medical devices in order to comprehend and adjust to the promise of personalized medicine. According to Chen and Wei (2015), "Personalized medicine has become a hot topic ascribed to the development of Human Genome Project. And currently, bioinformatics methodology plays an essential role in personal drug design" (p. 341). As health care professionals, we must always consider how the advances in personalized medicine impact our provision of care and how we can take advantage of personalized medicine for our patients.

Health care professionals can be involved in bioinformatics in many ways, including as researchers helping to map molecular processes and as educators and advocates helping patients and families understand these complex biological processes.

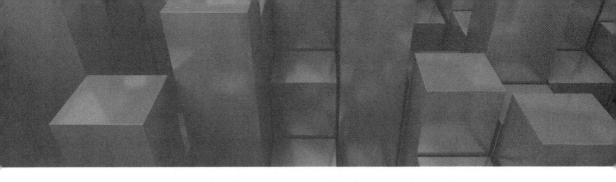

Summary

The focus of this text is on health informatics, but one can clearly see the connection between biomedical informatics and health informatics. The discipline of bioinformatics and its use in biomedical informatics epitomize the integration of computer science, information science, computational biology, and health care. These new applications deal with the resources, devices, strategies, and methods needed to optimize the acquisition, processing, storage, retrieval, generation, and use of information in health and biomedicine. Biomedicine and its applications of bioinformatics support and manage all health care behaviors. They affect how clinicians deliver health care to the infirmed, prevent disease, promote health, conduct research, and provide formal education for entry-level practitioners and continuing education for those who are currently practicing. The field of biomedical informatics—that is, bioinformatics capabilities coupled with health care—includes informatics and computational biology algorithms and tools and clinical guidelines. This knowledge can be applied to the areas of nursing, pharmacy, laboratory, dentistry, medicine, and public health. Those in the health care professions know that their practice is intertwined with the management and processing of information, including the new knowledge being generated by biomedical informatics.

On the biomedical side of informatics, one must be cognizant of the fact that medical data typically are extracted from personal, confidential, and legally protected medical records. The protection of human subjects must be paramount and all ethical, legal, and social issues must be addressed.

Biomedical informatics provides knowledge about the effects of DNA disparities among individuals. Being able to study human genomes and biological processing at the molecular level will revolutionize how conditions are diagnosed and care is provided. It is helping to prevent disease. If one can better understand an organism's biological processes and genetic coding, one can better prevent or treat medical conditions. Clinical care as it is known will change; it will become genomics based.

Thought-Provoking Questions

1. After reading this chapter, you know that the study of genomics is helping clinicians to understand better the interaction between genes and the environment. This new information and knowledge will continue to help clinicians find ways to improve health and prevent disease. How do you envision patient care will change based on genomics in 10 years, 20 years, or 50 years in the future?

2. Review the ethical, social, and legal issues resulting from the Human Genome Project presented in Box 18-2. Prepare a similar list of questions regarding these issues to apply to the public health databases being developed for health information exchanges. Can you appreciate how such questions are widely applicable to protecting information gathered from human subjects?

Apply Your Knowledge

Consider the important information you learned in this chapter related to bioinformatics.

1. Individually reflect on bioinformatics as a new frontier. How would you explain this term to your patients? Now compare and contrast your explanations.
2. Choose a health challenge (disease entity) commonly seen in your practice. Search the scholarly literature for how the underlying disease may be related to bioinformatics, proteomics, or computational biology. Based on what you have uncovered in the literature, is there an area in the treatment of this disease that may lend itself to precision medicine principles? How will the application of precision medicine for this health challenge affect practice in your discipline in the future?

References

Bioinformaticsweb.tk. (2005). Bioinformatics resource portal: Bioinformatics definition. http:// bioinformaticsweb.net/definition.html

Butte, A. (2008). Translational bioinformatics: Coming of age. *Journal of the American Medical Informatics Association*, *15*(6), 709–714.

Chen, H., Zhu, Z., Zhu, Y., Wang, J., Mei, Y., & Cheng, Y. (2015). Pathway mapping and development of disease-specific biomarkers: Protein-based network biomarkers. *Journal of Cellular and Molecular Medicine*, *19*(2), 297–314.

Chen, Q., & Wei, D. (2015). Human cytochrome P450 and personalized medicine. *Advances in Experimental Medicine and Biology*, *827*, 341–351.

Gennari, J. (2002). Biomedical informatics defined. http://faculty.washington.edu/gennari /MedicalInformaticsDef.html

Hare, G. (2014). Finances: Analysis and opinion: Global bioinformatics market will reach USD 12,542.2 million in 2020. http://www.finances.com/analyses-and-opinions/analysis -opinions/49771-global-bioinformatics-market-will-reach-usd-12542-4-million-2020.htm

Human Genome Project. (2008). Human Genome Project information: Ethical, legal, and social issues. http://www.ornl.gov/sci/techresources/Human_Genome/elsi/elsi.shtml

Human Genome Project. (2010). Human Genome Project information. http://www.ornl.gov/sci /techresources/Human_Genome/home.shtml

International HapMap Project. (2006). About the International HapMap Project. http://hapmap .ncbi.nlm.nih.gov/abouthapmap.html

Kelly, R. (2008). What are "omics" technologies? http://www.reagank.com/2007/03/what_are _omics_technologies.php

Mulligen, E., Cases, M., Hettne, K., Molero, E., Weeber, M., Robertson, K., et al. (2008). Training multidisciplinary biomedical informatics students: Three years of experience. *Journal of the American Medical Informatics Association*, *15*(2), 246–254. http://www.ncbi.nlm.nih.gov /pmc/articles/PMC2274784/?tool=pubmed

National Center for Biotechnology Information. (2004). Bioinformatics. https://web.archive.org/web/20130901174154/http://www.ncbi.nlm.nih.gov/About/primer/bioinformatics.html

National Human Genome Research Institute. (2010). 2006: The Cancer Genome Atlas (TCGA) Project started. http://www.genome.gov/25520505

National Human Genome Research Institute. (n.d.). NHGRI: Understanding the Human Genome Project CD-ROM: Mining the genome using bioinformatics (tutorial). http://www.genome.gov/19519278#al-5

National Institutes of Health. (2000). NIH working definition of bioinformatics and computational biology. http://www.bisti.nih.gov/docs/CompuBioDef.pdf

National Public Radio. (2010). Where the word *genome* came from. http://www.npr.org/templates/story/story.php?storyId=128410577

Network Science. (2009). Terms and definitions in bioinformatics. http://www.netsci.org/Science/Bioinform/terms.html

Ohio State University Medical Center. (2010). College of Medicine, School of Biomedical Science: Biomedical informatics. https://web.archive.org/web/20120308121755/http://biomed.osu.edu/bmi/index.cfm

Ostler, T., & Gollin, M. (2015). Legal and regulatory update: Which types of bioinformatics inventions are eligible for patent protection? *Journal of Commercial Biotechnology*, *21*(2), 76–82.

Rajappa, M., Sharma, A., & Saxena, A. (2004). Bioinformatics and its implications in clinical medicine: A review. *International Medical Journal*, *11*(2), 125–129.

University of Minnesota. (2010). What is bioinformatics? https://web.archive.org/web/20120605125223/http://www.binf.umn.edu/about/whatsbinf.php

University of Texas at El Paso. (2010). College of Science: Bioinformatics. https://web.archive.org/web/20121017124201/http://bioinformatics.utep.edu

U.S. Food and Drug Administration. (2015). Personalized Medicine: FDA's unique role and responsibilities in personalized medicine. http://www.fda.gov/ScienceResearch/SpecialTopics/PersonalizedMedicine/default.htm

Vanderbilt University. (2010). Department of Biomedical Informatics. https://medschool.vanderbilt.edu/dbmi

Wu, X., Chen, L., & Wang, X. (2014). Network biomarkers, interaction networks and dynamical network biomarkers in respiratory diseases. **Clinical and Translational Medicine**, *3*. http://www.clintransmed.com/content/3/1/16

Section V

Practice in the Future

You might wonder why we are ending this text with a section on caring in the future. The authors believe that health care professionals are taught to care and hone their ability to care for patients as they practice; however, in light of technologies that can sometimes be disruptive, caring can become compromised or lost. We want to refocus professionals on the art of caring, enhancing the science of practice using informatics tools.

We challenge you to reflect on what you know and what you are learning and to think of where you are going in relation to your own practice and health informatics (HI) knowledge. Just as our professional and personal lives overlap at times, so do our social and professional informatics and networking experiences. We cannot assume that what we do or use in our personal lives is appropriate or even useful in our professional practice. This section begins with a chapter (*The Art of Delivering Patient-Centered Care in Technology-Laden Environments*) that considers the heart of what health care professionals do—caring.

The final chapter, *Generating and Managing Organizational Knowledge*, refocuses what you have learned about the many facets of HI and the interfacing of knowledge workers and technology. The Foundation of Knowledge model provides a framework for examining the dynamic interrelationships among data, information, and knowledge used to meet the needs of health care delivery systems, organizations, patients, and health care professionals. The importance of knowledge management in health care is emphasized by taking this one last opportunity to ensure that the reader understands and appreciates the value of knowledge management in the health care professions and the role that technology has in knowledge acquisition, knowledge generation, knowledge dissemination, and knowledge processing.

HI entails the synthesis of disciplinary science, information science, computer science, and cognitive science to manage and enhance health care data, information, knowledge, and wisdom for the dual betterment of patient care and the health care professions. After reading the first four sections of this book, you should have a good idea of the current state of the science of HI. Now this final section challenges you to think about the future. Each reader should envision his or her current practice setting and the HI applications he or she uses. What will come next? What should come next?

The material within this text is placed within the context of the Foundation of Knowledge model (**Figure V-1**) to meet the needs of health care delivery systems, organizations, patients, and health care professionals. The first chapter in this text, *Informatics, Disciplinary Science, and the Foundation of Knowledge Model*, provided a thorough overview of the Foundation of Knowledge model—a framework that embraces knowledge so that readers can develop the wisdom necessary to apply what they have learned. Wisdom is the application of knowledge to an appropriate situation. In professional practice, one expects action or actions directed by wisdom. Wisdom uses knowledge and experience to heighten common sense and insight, allowing one to exercise sound judgment in practical matters. Wisdom is developed through knowledge, experience, insight, and reflection. Wisdom is sometimes thought of as the highest form of

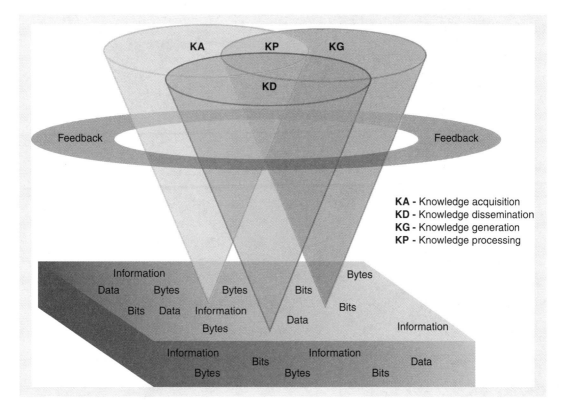

Figure V-1 Foundation of Knowledge Model
Source: Designed by Alicia Mastrian.

common sense resulting from accumulated knowledge or erudition (deep, thorough learning) or enlightenment (education that results in understanding and the dissemination of knowledge). Wisdom is the ability to apply valuable and viable knowledge, experience, understanding, and insight while being prudent and sensible. Knowledge and wisdom are not synonymous. Knowledge abounds with others' thoughts and information, whereas wisdom is focused on one's own mind and the synthesis of one's own experience, insight, understanding, and knowledge.

Reflect on the model while reading through this final section. You are challenged to ask, "How can I use my wisdom to help create the theories, tools, and knowledge of the future that will improve patient care and advance my profession?"

The Art of Delivering Patient-Centered Care in Technology-Laden Environments

Kathleen Mastrian and Dee McGonigle

OBJECTIVES

1. Explore caring theories as they apply to the art of practice.
2. Acknowledge the potential disruption of technology to the therapeutic provider–patient relationship.
3. Define presence and caring presence.
4. Formulate strategies to enhance caring presence.

Introduction

Providing health care is hard work. Depending on the site of practice, it can be both physically and mentally taxing. Health care professionals are masters at multitasking—that is, performing several caring functions simultaneously during a patient encounter. Some interventions are readily apparent and easily described, such as collecting vital signs data and assessing gait, while others are less visible yet equally important, such as interpreting the vital signs data, generating knowledge about the patient's situation, and then using that knowledge to inform practice. Equally invisible yet important to the therapeutic caring environment are the little things that professionals, say, project, and do in the caring episode. In this chapter, we pause to reflect on the art of caring. We emphasize the need to preserve this central and unique function of health care delivery and suggest ways

Key Terms
Active listening
Bracketing
Caring
Caritas processes
Centering
Presence

that health care professionals can ensure that the caring functions do not become a lost art as technologies are introduced into patient care environments.

Health care professionals are knowledge workers. Knowledge workers are those who work with information and generate information and knowledge as a product. Health care professionals ethically apply knowledge acquired through education, research, and practice to provide services and interventions to patients to maintain, enhance, or restore their health and acquire, process, generate, and disseminate knowledge to advance their respective professions. Caring functions, such as therapeutic communication, listening, touch, and mindfulness, are an integral part of professional practice, as they also help patients maintain, enhance, or restore their health. While the new technologies such as smart pumps, NAVA ventilation technology, virtual rehabilitation technologies, electronic health records (EHRs), and smartphones being introduced into our practice environments are designed to increase efficiency, promote safety, and streamline our work, we need to ask the following: To what extent do these technologies disrupt the professional—patient caring encounter? How can we continue to care effectively for our patients and promote a healing environment while incorporating the advantages and efficiencies that technologies provide?

Caring Theories

Let us begin our exploration of **caring** as a concept with the work of Jean Watson. Although she is a nurse and wrote extensively about caring in the nursing profession, the concepts of caring she describes are widely applicable to all professional—patient encounters as we all seek to provide services and interventions to patients to maintain, enhance, or restore their health. As Watson and Woodward (2010) described,

> *The Theory of Human Caring was developed between 1975 and 1979 while I was teaching at the University of Colorado. I tried to make explicit that nursing's values, knowledge, and practices of human caring were geared toward subjective inner healing processes and the life world of the experiencing person. This required unique caring—healing arts and a framework called "carative factors," which complemented conventional medicine but stood in stark contrast to "curative factors." (p. 352)*

It is important to remember that Watson developed her theory during a time when the nursing profession was struggling to define itself and identify the unique contributions of nursing to patient care. In the theory of human caring, Watson defined caring as "healing consciousness and intentionality to care and promote healing" and caring consciousness as "energy within the human—environmental field of a caring moment" (Watson & Woodward, 2010, p. 353). Think about the use of the word *energy* in these definitions and pause to appreciate the level of cognitive energy that professionals expend as they care for patients. Health care is hard work!

Watson further described the evolution of her theory from the original 10 carative factors to what she now calls **caritas processes**. As her work expands, she is recognizing the need for "love and caring to come together for a new form of deep transpersonal caring." In the evolving theory, she has emphasized that the "relationship between love and caring connotes inner healing for self and others" (Watson & Woodward, 2010, p. 353). The 10 caritas processes enumerated by Watson are summarized here:

1. The practice of loving kindness and equanimity within the context of caring consciousness
2. Being authentically present and enabling and sustaining the deep belief system and subjective life world of self and one being cared for
3. Cultivation of one's own spiritual practices and transpersonal self, going beyond ego self, opening to others with sensitivity and compassion
4. Developing and sustaining a helping—trusting, authentic caring relationship
5. Being present to, and supportive of, the expression of positive and negative feelings as a connection with deeper spirit of self and the one being cared for
6. Creative use of self and all ways of knowing as part of the caring process; to engage in artistry of caring—healing practices
7. Engaging in genuine teaching—learning experience that attends to unity of being and meaning, attempting to stay within others' frames of reference
8. Creating a healing environment at all levels (a physical and nonphysical, subtle environment of energy and consciousness, whereby wholeness, beauty, comfort, dignity, and peace are potentiated)
9. Assisting with basic needs, with an intentional caring consciousness, administering "human care essentials," which potentiate alignment of mind—body—spirit, wholeness, and unity of being in all aspects of care, tending to both embodied spirit and evolving spiritual emergence
10. Opening and attending to spiritual—mysterious and existential dimensions of one's own life—death; soul care for self and the one being cared for (Watson & Woodward, 2010, p. 355)

Think about a recent patient encounter. Were you fully present in the moment and conscious of the individual and his or her uniqueness? Did you smile and greet the patient by name and acknowledge visitors? Did you attentively listen to the concerns of the patient and family and offer them the opportunity to ask questions? Did you explain what you were doing with and for the patient, and why? Conversely, did you carry your tablet into the room, focus your attention on the screen, and talk at the screen as you clicked on the drop-down menus to document the patient encounter? Did the tablet create a barrier between you, the patient, and the patient's family? Did you depend solely on monitoring technologies to create your interpretation of the patient's experience? We must remember that "technology, however, does not take into consideration the specific symptom presentation unique to the person experiencing the illness" (O'Keefe-McCarthy, 2009, p. 792). Patient-centered care is another way of describing the need for practitioners to focus on the subjective experience of patients with health challenges. Liberati et al. (2015) define patient centeredness as "a collective achievement that is negotiated between patients and multiple health providers, comprising of social practices and relationships that are woven together through the material and immaterial resources available in specific organizational contexts" (p. 47). They suggest that a focus on patient-centered care may have three specific outcomes:

- Patients can provide their subjective experience as an input to improve several, often undermined aspects of health care delivery.
- Care providers might develop their capacity for reflexivity, which could improve their understanding of the implications of their actions.
- Patients and practitioners can thus provide insights into the overall health organization on how to innovate processes and facilities to better respond to local needs.

We will examine reflection on practice in more detail later in the chapter.

Central to the caritas processes described by Watson and the discussion about technology-mediated care by O'Keefe-McCarthy is the concept of a caring presence. Strategies for developing and enhancing caring presence are discussed in the latter part of this chapter.

The humanistic nursing theory developed by Paterson and Zderad also offers some insight into the less visible aspects of providing care (Kleiman, 2010). These authors suggested that the basis of nursing is the response to the call for help in solving health-related concerns:

> This call, a foundational concept of humanistic nursing, can be heard where nursing is offered, coming to our attention as a subtle murmur of pain, sorrow, anxiety, desperation, joy, laughter, even silence, that expresses the state-of-being of the protagonists in the drama of health-care delivery, our patients and ourselves. (Kleiman, 2010, p. 338)

We suggest that the concepts described here are equally applicable to all health care professionals. We hear the call for help and respond with our entire being. Our knowledge, experiences, ethics, and competencies shape the interaction with our patients:

> In humanistic nursing we say that each person is perceived as existing "all-at-once." In the process of interacting with patients, nurses interweave professional identity, education, intuition, and experiences, with all their other life experiences, creating their own tapestry which unfolds during their responses. (Kleiman, 2010, pp. 341–342)

This description of patient interaction easily applies to all health care professional—patient interactions. Pause to reflect on how you create your own tapestry during patient interactions.

Health care requires conscious awareness of self and the uniqueness of each of our patients. It requires emotional energy expenditure as we seek to find ways to meet the calls of our patients. We need to be aware of the potential for inadvertently dehumanizing the patient experience in our technology-laden practice environments. According to Kleiman (2010), "The context of Humanistic Nursing Theory is humans. The basic question it asks of nursing practice is: Is this particular intersubjective—transactional nursing event humanizing or dehumanizing?" (p. 349). We can ask the same question in each of our professions. We must be fully present and self-aware in every patient encounter, seeking to deliver exactly what is needed in every situation. Yes, health care is hard work, but when we are able to respond with our whole being, we may find that our patients and families are more satisfied with the care we provide and that we also experience personal satisfaction and find joy in our profession.

Presence

Presence is the act of being there and being with our patients—fully focusing on their needs. "Presence is an interpersonal process that is characterized by sensitivity, holism, intimacy, vulnerability and adaptation to unique circumstances" (Finfgeld-Connett, 2008, p. 528). Penque and Snyder (2010) defined three types of presence: physical presence, full presence, and transcendent presence. A health care professional who is physically present is largely competent in carrying out care, efficient with interventions, but inattentive to communication and nonverbal cues projected by the patient and family. When fully present, a professional will greet the patient by name, communicate appropriately with the patient, and pay attention to what is being said and not said during the encounter. When health care professionals practice transcendent presence, they will first center themselves, clearing their mind of all potential distractions, and then use the patient's name and gentle touch to convey interest and responsiveness while carrying out the necessary physical interventions.

Strategies for Enhancing Caring Presence

Health care is hard work. Our patients have complex problems and needs. They may be scared, angry, resistant to change, or happily oblivious to the extent of their health challenges. We, too, have complex personal lives with many competing roles and issues that consume our energies. Our workplace may be short-staffed, resulting in care assignments that stretch us to our maximum. We may be struggling to learn to use the new technologies that are introduced nearly daily into our practice environments. As a result, we may feel disorganized, tired, angry, and emotionally spent.

We need to take care of ourselves first so that we can be effective in our patient and family care. Caring for ourselves involves conscious attention to our health and health practices. Do we eat a balanced diet, get appropriate exercise, and get enough sleep? Do we have strategies to manage stress appropriately, and do we have adequate social support? "Just as surgical instruments are washed and sterilized before being used for another procedure, professionals who are instruments of healing must identify therapies that will ensure the cleansing of self so as to provide a personal energy field and space that facilitates healing for self and patients" (Leonard & Towey, 2010, p. 26).

As part of a "concepts of health" course, students are asked to develop a personal health plan and journal periodically during the semester about their ability to stick to the plan. Here is an example of a simple plan: "I will increase my intake of fruit and vegetables and walk outside for 30 minutes at least three times per week." As the students reflect on their ability to stick to the plan in the journal, caring for self is brought into conscious awareness. This simple self-reflective practice may be just the boost that is needed for a professional to commit to self-awareness and self-care on a long-term basis.

One additional strategy that we share with students is a breathing/meditative exercise from tai-chi, qi gong, called the five-element breathing sequence. This meditative exercise, which can be performed in less than 10 minutes and can be very energizing and stress reducing, is described in **Box 19-1**.

The simplest and perhaps most effective strategy we can use to help us be fully present to our patients is to pause to take a few deep breaths to calm ourselves and clear the clutter from our minds before we address each patient. It also helps to repeat the patient's name silently a time or two before we begin the encounter. This practice, known as **centering**, enables the professional to "be available with the whole self and be open to the personal and care needs of the patient" (Penque & Snyder, 2010, p. 40).

BOX 19-1 TAI-CHI QI GONG, FIVE-ELEMENT BREATHING SEQUENCE

1. Stand with your feet shoulder-width apart. Relax your arms and shoulders.
2. Inhale slowly as you straighten and then move both arms slightly back and then up with palms facing up (as though you are gathering a giant ball of energy). Stretch to your full height as you inhale.
3. Exhale slowly as you press both palms down in front of you with hands slightly cupped and thumbs and index fingers nearly touching. Bend your knees slightly to sink down as you exhale.
4. Turn your hands over (palms up) just below the waist, and inhale slowly as you raise your hands in front of you, to chest height. Straighten your legs as you inhale. (Imagine lifting a ball of energy.)
5. Exhale slowly and extend the arms directly in front of you, chest high, and fan your hands open to release the energy in front of your chest. Bend the knees slightly to sink down as you exhale.
6. Inhale slowly, with palms facing you, to gather the energy back toward your chest. Straighten your legs as you inhale.
7. Press both arms straight out at shoulder height as you exhale. Pretend you are pushing on walls located on either side of you. Continue the exhalation as you bring your arms in front of you. Bend your knees slightly to sink down as you exhale.
8. Inhale slowly as you gather the energy to your chest. Straighten your legs as you inhale and stretch to your full height.
9. Exhale slowly as you raise your arms above your head to set the energy free. Bend your knees slightly to sink down as you exhale.
10. Transition your hands to the beginning to repeat the sequence by inhaling as you bring your hands halfway down and exhaling the rest of the way. (You can also end here by bringing your palms together in closure, first inhaling and then exhaling as you slowly move your hands down in front of you.)

Source: Visit the following website for a demonstration of the five-element breathing: http://www.youtube.com/watch?v=KtVCCLIkcKg.

When we are with a patient, we need to be certain that our mind is fully engaged in the interaction with this patient for the moment. We must be fully attentive to the patient, be both physically and mentally present, meet the patient where he or she is emotionally, listen actively to what the patient is saying, focus on the nonverbal cues the patient is projecting, touch the patient gently and reassuringly, and demonstrate acceptance (Penque & Snyder, 2010; Zerwekh, 2006).

A related and similar concept for practicing presence, **bracketing**, is described in humanistic caring theory. Consider, for example, that an occupational therapist experienced in providing therapy to elders after a stroke will have expectations and preconceived ideas about what he or she will find in a patient situation. These expectations may not allow us to really "see" the whole patient and his or her experience of the illness. "Bracketing prepares the inquirer to enter the uncharted world of the other without expectations and preconceived ideas" (Kleiman, 2010, p. 343). We need to come to know our patients both intuitively and scientifically. Our technologies provide an objective view of the patient, and the professional synthesizes this view with his or her own perspective that is based on the experience, education, and intuition as applied to the patient's situation. This is the essence of caring.

One of the first skills we were taught in our basic professional education programs was **active listening**. We were taught to get down to the same level of the patient, make eye contact, touch gently (if culturally acceptable), listen attentively and nod appropriately, restate and clarify what we heard, ask questions to seek additional information, listen for feelings that are not being explicitly stated, and use silence to encourage the patient to think and provide additional information to us (Watanuki, Tracy, & Lindquist, 2010; Zerwekh, 2006). These communication skills are fundamental to caring. When was the last time you sat in a chair next to a patient to get to the same level as the patient? Even a brief sit next to the patient can communicate volumes about your availability and willingness to listen, and it certainly feels good to get off of your feet for a moment. We also need to think carefully about the potential barriers to active listening that technology might present. For example, what are some of the ways that these caring presence skills could be adapted for use in a telehealth encounter? What are the challenges of communicating at a distance, yet being fully present for the patient?

Finfgeld-Connett (2008) suggests that relationship-centered care promotes beneficent practice that "results in enhanced mental and physical well-being in patients" and "also results in professional satisfaction and growth" (p. 528). Let us all strive for beneficent practice that atones for the potential disruptions to the therapeutic provider—patient relationship that our use of technology produces.

Reflective Practice

As professionals, we should be constantly mindful of the need for practice improvement. Zande, Baart, and Vosman (2014) discuss ethical sensitivity as a type of practical wisdom. Ethical sensitivity is integral to high-quality care and clinical decision making. They advocate for reflection on practice:

> *Taking daily practice of care as point of entry for reflection is a way to discern both explicit moral knowledge and tacit moral knowing. Nurses and other professionals can contribute to improvement on quality of care by creating opportunities to reflect on daily ethical concerns in an inter-professional team. (p. 75)*

Liberati et al. (2015) also advocate for the use of reflection to help professionals "observe their work from a different perspective. . . . Such an exploration may help providers to generate insights on how healthcare services, processes, and facilities could be modified to better respond to patients' needs" (p. 49).

One way to focus on our practice is to engage in reflective journaling. In the concepts of health course, we ask students to complete a reflective practice assignment over a 6-week period. Students are directed to review concepts of caring presence and active listening and to commit to consciously using a strategy for 6 weeks. At 3 and 6 weeks, they are asked to complete the following reflective journal entry:

1. *Write a brief description* of the presence and therapeutic communication approaches you tried in your practice for the last 3 weeks. Provide specific examples of patient situations in which you tried the approach.
2. *Reflect* on the following: What did you do well?
   - Which behaviors and skills do you need to improve?
   - How did you feel about the experience as it was happening? Did you plan thoroughly?
   - Did you achieve your objectives?
   - Which aspects of planning do you need to improve?
   - How will this experience affect your future practice?
3. Which personal professional development needs have you identified after reflecting on your performance? Which strategies will you use to address these needs?

Our students frequently report that they enjoy this experience and that the exercise helps to remind them why they were originally attracted to the profession. They describe experiences where they felt an authentic connection to the patient. They also report that after 6 weeks of consciously practicing the strategy, it becomes a part of their daily practice. Centering is the most frequent strategy that the students choose to practice.

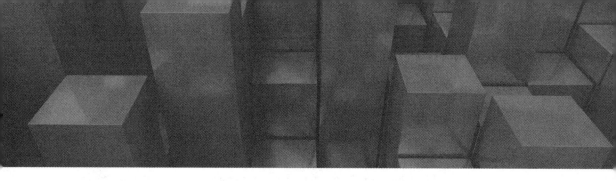

Summary

Effective practice relies on information and communication technologies that receive inputs from professionals as well as all of the patient care technologies. Computers, handheld devices, monitors, and other health care technologies are essential health care tools. Therefore, the professional must have the ability to implement, monitor, and evaluate all of this equipment based on its inputs and outputs. The increased demands on the health care professional make it easy to lose sight of the patient amid all of these technologies. Health care professionals must attend to the monitors, devices, and other gadgets to receive information; often, it is easy to forget the patient is at the core of our care.

We hope that this brief overview of caring presence prompts you to be more mindful of your practice and that you, too, will commit to employing strategies that enhance your caring presence in all patient encounters. We do not want our patients to feel that we are more focused on the machines that they are connected to or the technology that we bring with us to the patient encounter. Yes, technology is great and it does help us collect meaningful data and generate knowledge about our patient situations, but equally important is the need to collect the human-to-human data that become available only when we step away from the technology and interact authentically with our patients.

Thought-Provoking Questions

1. Examine each of the 10 caritas processes developed by Watson. Describe an example of a patient encounter that demonstrates the use of each caritas process.
2. Reflect on your personal health. Are you a role model for your patients? Which aspects of your personal health do you need to improve? Which strategies will you adopt to improve your health?
3. Choose a caring presence strategy to implement in your practice and use the reflective journal template provided in the chapter to reflect on your practice.

Apply Your Knowledge

As you embark on your professional journey, you will have some patient encounters that are less satisfactory than others. Sometimes, sharing these situations with other developing professionals provides insights that one may not realize alone. This activity is easily accomplished in an electronic discussion forum.

1. Perform a self-assessment of your practice and summarize a clinical situation in which you were unhappy with your practice. Describe the situation, specify the area of your discomfort, and suggest what you would do differently if confronted with a similar situation. Limit your discussion to 250 words.

2. Post your summary to an e-discussion forum.
3. Post your formal analysis of the submissions by your classmates, answering the question, "What common clinical knowledge issues and themes emerge from the situations?" Limit your individual analysis to 250 words.
4. What types of informatics tools might provide you with a similar opportunity for dialoging with peers for collective wisdom once you are a practicing professional? What guidelines for these professional dialogs need to be imposed?

Additional Resources

Five-Element Breathing
http://www.youtube.com/watch?v=KtVCCLlkcKg

References

Finfgeld-Connett, D. (2008). Qualitative convergence of three nursing concepts: Art of nursing, presence and caring. *Journal of Advanced Nursing, 63*(5), 527–534.

Kleiman, S. (2010). Josephine Paterson and Loretta Zderad's humanistic nursing theory. In M. Parker & M. Smith (Eds.), *Nursing theories and nursing practice* (3rd ed., pp. 337–350). Philadelphia: F. A. Davis.

Leonard, B., & Towey, S. (2010). Self as healer. In M. Snyder & R. Lindquist (Eds.), *Complementary and alternative therapies in nursing* (6th ed., pp. 25–34). New York: Springer.

Liberati, E. G., Gorli, M., Moja, L., Galuppo, L., Ripamonti, S., & Scaratti, G. (2015). Exploring the practice of patient centered care: The role of ethnography and reflexivity. *Social Science and Medicine, 127*, 13345–13352.

O'Keefe-McCarthy, S. (2009). Technologically-mediated nursing care: The impact on moral agency. *Nursing Ethics, 16*(6), 786–796.

Penque, S., & Snyder, M. (2010). Presence. In M. Snyder & R. Lindquist (Eds.), *Complementary and alternative therapies in nursing* (6th ed., pp. 35–46). New York: Springer.

Watanuki, S., Tracy, M. F., & Lindquist, R. (2010). Active Listening. In M. Snyder & R. Lindquist (Eds.), *Complementary and alternative therapies in nursing* (6th ed., pp. 47–59) New York: Springer.

Watson, J., & Woodward, T. (2010). Jean Watson's theory of human caring. In M. Parker & M. Smith (Eds.), *Nursing theories and nursing practice* (3rd ed., pp. 351–368). Philadelphia: F. A. Davis.

Zande, M., Baart, A., & Vosman, F. (2014). Ethical sensitivity in practice: Finding tacit moral knowing. *Journal of Advanced Nursing, 70*(1), 68–76.

Zerwekh, J. (2006). Connecting and caring presence. In *Nursing care at the end of life: Palliative care for patients and families* (pp. 113–130). Philadelphia: F. A. Davis.

Generating and Managing Organizational Knowledge

Dee McGonigle and Kathleen Mastrian

OBJECTIVES

1. Assess health care as knowledge-intensive professions.
2. Explore the contribution of health informatics to the foundation of knowledge.

Introduction

Throughout this text, the reader has learned about the many facets of **health informatics** (HI) and the interfacing of knowledge workers and technology. The Foundation of Knowledge model (**Figure 20-1**) has provided a framework for examining the dynamic interrelationships among **data**, **information**, and **knowledge** used to meet the needs of health care delivery systems, organizations, patients, and health care professionals. The importance of knowledge management in health care is emphasized by taking this one last opportunity to ensure that the reader understands and appreciates the value of knowledge management in the health care professions and the role that technology has in knowledge acquisition, knowledge generation, knowledge dissemination, and knowledge processing.

Key Terms
Codify
Data
Health informatics
Information
Information technology
Knowledge
Knowledge acquisition
Knowledge dissemination
Knowledge domain process
Knowledge generation
Knowledge management systems
Knowledge repositories
Knowledge workers

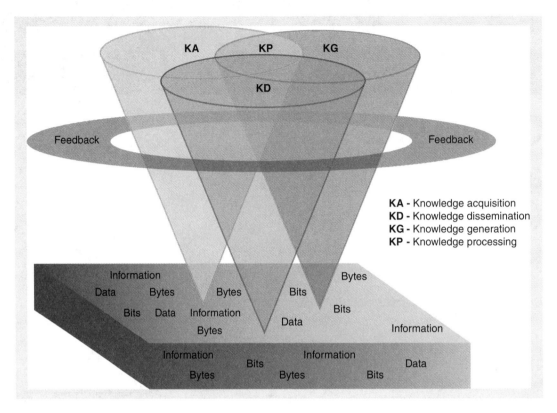

Figure 20-1 Foundation of Knowledge Model
Source: Designed by Alicia Mastrian.

Foundation of Knowledge Model Revisited

A review of the Foundation of Knowledge model that provides a framework for the development of this text is useful. At its base, the model has bits, bytes (computer terms for chunks of information), data, and information in a random representation. Growing out of the base are separate cones of light that expand as they reflect upward and represent **knowledge acquisition**, **knowledge generation**, and **knowledge dissemination**. At the intersection of the cones and forming a new cone is knowledge processing. Encircling and cutting through the knowledge cones is feedback, which acts on and may transform any or all aspects of knowledge represented by the cones.

Now imagine the model as a dynamic figure with the cones of light and the feedback rotating and interacting rather than remaining static. Knowledge acquisition, knowledge generation, knowledge dissemination, knowledge processing, and feedback are constantly evolving for health care scientists. The transparent effect of the cones is deliberate and is intended to suggest that as knowledge grows and expands, its use becomes more transparent; that is, the user is not even consciously aware of which aspect of knowledge he or she is using at any given moment during her or his practice.

If you are an experienced professional, think back to when you were a novice. Did you feel like all you had in your head were bits of data and information that did not form any type of cohesive whole? As the model depicts, the processing of knowledge as an individual in professional practice begins a bit later (imagine a timeline applied vertically), with early experiences on the bottom and expertise growing as the processing of knowledge kicks in. Early on in your education, conscious attention is focused mainly on knowledge acquisition, and learners depend on their instructors and others to process, generate, and disseminate knowledge. As learners become more comfortable with their disciplinary science, they begin to take over some of the other knowledge functions. However, to keep up with the explosion of information in your discipline and in health care, one must continue to rely on the knowledge generation and dissemination of others. In this sense, health care professionals are committed to lifelong learning and the use of knowledge in their disciplinary practice. For knowledge workers, information is their primary resource, and when one deals with information, it is done in overlapping phases. That is, the health care professional is continually acquiring, processing or assimilating, retaining, and using this information to generate and disseminate knowledge. However, it is not a sequential phasing; instead, there is a constant gleaning of data and information from the environment, with the data and information massaged into knowledge bases so that they can be applied and shared (disseminated).

Knowledge may be thought of as either explicit or tacit. Explicit knowledge is the knowledge that one can convey in letters, words, and numbers. It can be exchanged or shared in the form of data, manuals, product specifications, principles, policies, theories, and the like. We can disseminate and share this knowledge publicly or on the record and scientifically or methodically. A practice model or theory that is well developed and easily explained and understood is an example of explicit knowledge. Tacit knowledge, in contrast, is individualized and highly personal or private, including one's values or emotions. Knowing intuitively when and how to care is an example of tacit knowledge. This type of knowledge is difficult to convey, transmit, or share with others because it consists of one's own insights or slant on things, perceptions, intuitions, sense, hunches, or gut feelings. Tacit knowledge reflects skills and beliefs, which is why it is difficult to explain or communicate it to others. Farr and Cressey (2015) used grounded theory methodology to study how professionals perceive the quality of their performance and found that intangible, tacit knowledge was just as important to the perception of quality of performance as were more standardized rational measures of quality based on organizational policy. "This paper illuminates the importance of the tacit, intangible and relational dimensions of quality in actual practice. Staff values and personal and professional standards are core to understanding how quality is co-produced in service interactions. Professional experience, tacit clinical knowledge, personal standards and

values, and conversations with patients and families all contributed to how staff understood and assessed the quality of their work in everyday practice" (p. 8).

How students and health care professionals learn is directly affected by their practice
experiences within their own personal frame of reference. The quality of practice decision making is directly related to experience and knowledge. Knowledge is situational.
Explicit and tacit knowledge are used to conduct assessments, plan interventions, and
evaluate actions for each individual patient. **Knowledge management systems** (KMSs)
must blend these knowledge needs and provide knowledge bases and decision support
systems to inform professional decision making. Each person processes and assimilates
knowledge in a unique way influenced by his or her unique perspective.

Knowledge Use in Practice

One way to capture and codify tacit knowledge is to engage in reflection and reflective
practice. Schutz (2007) believes that reflection is both a way of learning about practice
and a basis for changing practice. One must engage in reflective practice because this
approach can enable a practitioner to find a means in which to put this personal or
experiential knowledge into words and to find a way of considering why the situation
turned out as it did and whether future practice might be different (p. 27).

Some health care organizations are encouraging reflective practice to codify tacit
knowledge and thus to build an organization's knowledge base. Sharing experiences
in a Practice Council is one means to encourage collaboration and knowledge sharing
among professionals. Joining a listserv or a community of practice is another example
of collaboration to build knowledge. Watson (2007) describes knowledge audits, narra-
tives, and storytelling as means of surfacing tacit knowledge and assessing the knowledge resources within an organization. He describes the use of **information technology**
(IT) tools for knowledge management in an organization, such as intranets, extranets
(shared intranets among several like organizations), knowledge directories, blogs, and
wikis. Recent research suggests that organizations that embrace and encourage knowledge transfer among workers not only sustain and build professional competence and
organizational engagement but also enhance the quality of the work life for professionals (Leiter, Day, Harvie, & Shaughnessy, 2007).

According to Gent (2007), there are three types of **knowledge workers**: (1) knowledge consumers, (2) knowledge brokers, and (3) knowledge generators. This breakdown
of knowledge workers is not mutually exclusive; instead, people transition between
these states as their situations and experience, education, and knowledge change:

- Knowledge consumers are mainly users of knowledge who do not have the
  expertise to provide the knowledge they need for themselves. New professionals or students can be thought of as knowledge consumers who use the
  knowledge of experienced professionals or who search information systems for
  the knowledge necessary to apply to their practice. As responsible knowledge
  consumers, they must also question and challenge what is known to help them
  learn and understand. Their questioning and challenging facilitate critical
  thinking and the development of new knowledge.

- Knowledge brokers know where to find information and knowledge; they generate some knowledge but are known mainly for their ability to find what is needed. More experienced professionals become knowledge brokers out of necessity, needing to know.
- Knowledge generators are the "primary sources of new knowledge" (Gent, 2007, para. 2). They include researchers and discipline experts—the people who know. They are able to answer questions, craft theories, find solutions to patient problems or concerns, and innovate as part of their practice.

Dixon (2012) blogged about knowledge work and knowledge workers and provides these insights:

- Knowledge workers, need to acquire new knowledge every 4 to 5 years, or else they become obsolete (para. 4).
- Knowledge work is invisible, interdependent, and constantly changing (para. 5).
- Knowledge workers, whether they are scientists, engineers, marketers, accountants, or administrators, must continuously read the situation in front of them and then, based on that interpretation, determine the appropriate next action to take (para. 5).
- Knowledge workers view their knowledge as their personal possession. The knowledge they possess is in their minds so when they leave the organization, the means of production leaves with them (para. 6).

The health care industry, the health care professions, and patients all benefit as professionals develop intellectual capital by gaining insight into the discipline science and its enactment: practice. HI applications of databases, knowledge management systems, and repositories where this knowledge can be analyzed and reused facilitate this process, enabling knowledge to be disseminated and reused.

To be able to enhance the acquisition, processing, generation, dissemination, and reuse of knowledge, professionals must **codify**, or be able to articulate knowledge structures, so that they can be captured within the KMSs. According to Markus (2001), an early and prolific writer about organizational knowledge management,

Synthesis of evidence from a wide variety of sources suggests four distinct types of knowledge reuse situations according to the knowledge reuser and the purpose of knowledge reuse. The types involve shared work producers, who produce knowledge they later reuse; shared work practitioners, who reuse each other's knowledge contributions; expertise-seeking novices; and secondary knowledge miners. Each type of knowledge reuser has different requirements for knowledge repositories. (para. 1)

Markus (2001) referred to **knowledge repositories** as "organizational memory systems" (para. 1). These memory systems gained popularity among help desk personnel who could access and reuse the knowledge of solutions when clients sought help for similar problems. Health care is an arena in which KMSs or knowledge repositories are clearly valuable. Capturing the explicit and tacit forms of knowledge is paramount to truly harness professional knowledge. As knowledge repositories evolve to enhance sharing and repurposing of knowledge, other professionals will be able to easily access, process, evaluate, reuse, generate, and disseminate knowledge.

Consider the retirement of a health care professional who has worked in a system for 40 years. What types of uncaptured, uncodified, tacit knowledge walk out the door on the day of the retirement? Can you appreciate the value of a well-constructed knowledge repository? Interestingly, Dixon (2012) suggested that supervisors need to first recognize and acknowledge the tacit knowledge of seasoned professionals and find ways to make them feel valued by the organization. Using seasoned professionals as mentors to new professionals is a good way to help them surface tacit knowledge and share their wisdom.

This text uses the Foundation of Knowledge model reflecting that knowledge is power, and for that reason, professionals focus on information as a key resource. The application of the model was described in each section of the text to help the reader understand and appreciate the foundation of knowledge in HI. Health care professionals are knowledge workers, working with information and generating information and knowledge as a product. They are knowledge acquirers, providing convenient and efficient means of capturing and storing knowledge. They are knowledge users, individuals or groups who benefit from valuable, viable knowledge. Professionals are also knowledge engineers, designing, developing, implementing, and maintaining knowledge. They are knowledge managers, capturing and processing collective expertise and distributing it where it can create the largest benefit. They are knowledge developers or generators, changing and evolving knowledge based on the tasks at hand and information available.

Disciplinary science is dependent on knowledge generation, and HI should facilitate the generation of knowledge and support translational research, where we attempt to bridge the gap between what we know (research) and what we do (practice). In this text, it has been established that HI is a vital tool for professional decision making, especially when one is able to demonstrate how health care professionals structure and process information.

As the HITECH Act has been implemented, the use of electronic health records (EHRs) has become more common in the United States. Such records must be designed to enhance patient outcomes through content enrichment and improved caregiver decision making. As bioinformatics and computational biology continue to evolve, their integration into the EHR is inevitable. Health informaticists must facilitate the inclusion of computational tools and algorithms to help handle the collection, organization, analysis, processing, presentation, and dissemination of biological data to help address biological questions and unravel biological mysteries. It is imperative that current research strategies, such as those used to search for biomarkers, and new pharmacologic treatments be included in the EHR. In this bioinformatics era, one must be able to delineate biomarkers and have the necessary alerts, follow-ups, and reminders built into the system to make all caregivers aware of the bioinformatics information, such as the analysis of genes causing hypertension, cardiovascular disease, and diabetes. Bioinformatics and computational biology will complement all of the current methods and aid in the analysis of populations and tracking of selected diseases' progression. Consequently, health informaticists must be proactive in the development of policies and ethically based solutions to safeguard the genetic data contained in EHRs, manage the patient care implications of bioinformatics, and wisely use computational biology in this bioinformatics era.

A paradigm shift is occurring from health care facility–owned, machine-based computing to off-site, vendor-owned, cloud computing. Web browser–based login accessible data, software, and hardware could link systems together and reduce costs. Hospitals with shrinking budgets and extreme IT needs are exploring the successes in other industries, such as Amazon's S3. As providers strive to implement potent EHRs, they are looking for cloud-based models that will offer the necessary functionality without having to assume the burden associated with all of the hardware, software, application, and storage issues. However, in the face of the HITECH Act and its associated penalties, numerous challenges must be overcome to realize the benefits of this approach. The advantages and disadvantages of cloud computing must be fully explored in light of the challenges faced by both health care providers as they strive to maintain security while relinquishing control and the vendors that are responsible for developing and maintaining this new cloud-based EHR environment.

HI can also be used to facilitate nursing administration and managerial studies of the work of health care professionals. Numerous opportunities for data mining in HI have been described. Some larger health care systems store all of the clinical information from their affiliated hospitals and clinics in a central data warehouse. General data scans and analyses looking for patterns may, for example, suggest a trend toward better outcomes for patients with a specific diagnosis, such as ventilator associated pneumonia in one of the affiliate hospitals. Does the data mined from the EHR point to specific interventions by respiratory therapists or dieticians that are effective in managing ventilator-associated pneumonia? The identification of such a trend clearly begs for further analyses. A researcher or administrator could ask, "Which factors contribute to these better outcomes, and how can these be put into practice across the system?" Other research studies might focus on assessing the effectiveness of strategic planning and organizational goal setting or studying work flow, communication processes, and interprofessional collaboration in an organization.

Managing Knowledge Across Disciplines

Interprofessional collaboration is emerging as a key to better-quality outcomes for patients. This collaboration is supported by EHRs and other technologies that facilitate communication among health professionals. Stichler (2014), in a discussion of collaboration on the design of health care facilities, describes interprofessional collaboration as "magic at the intersection"; that is, "true interprofessional practice intersects and positive outcomes can be achieved as a result of the synergy that occurs among different professionals who come together with a common purpose and goal" (p. 10). Her words can also be applied to interprofessional collaboration in patient situations. Consider the ways that HI tools and technologies can help ensure that the perspectives of all professionals are heard and valued to create this "magic at the intersection."

Another way for professionals to share perspectives and knowledge on patient situations is the HUDDLE method described in a review of the literature by Glymph et al. (2015). HUDDLE stands for "health care, utilizing, deliberate, discussion, linking, events." As they describe,

> The huddle is a team-building tool that increases effective communication among healthcare providers. It is a quick meeting of healthcare members to share information. This brief meeting or huddle takes place at the start of the workday. It is also a time where groups plan for contingencies, express concerns, address conflicts, or reassign resources. (p. 184)

Can you think of ways that the HUDDLE could be facilitated electronically in the future? Research studies aimed at advancing the state of the science of HI are becoming more common as the benefits of a robust HI system for managing knowledge are recognized. We will explore a few here. Rochefort, Buckeridge, and Forster (2015) explored the use of an algorithm to mine the EHR for the detection of three key adverse events (AEs)—hospital-acquired pneumonia, catheter-associated bloodstream infections, and in-hospital falls. Prior to their work, the hospitals used discharge diagnostic codes for adverse event detection, which they believed resulted in both under- and overestimation of adverse events. Their algorithm was designed to be more comprehensive and mine a combination of various types of data in the EHR. "To move this field forward, as well as to maximize the accuracy of AE detection, there is a need for comprehensive automated AE detection algorithms that integrate the information from all the available data sources (e.g., microbiology and laboratory results, free-text radiology reports and progress notes and electronic vital signs)" (para. 10). Evans, Yeung, Markoulakis, and Guilcher (2014) studied the use of an online community of practice to promote the creation and sharing of knowledge related to manual therapies among physiotherapists. They demonstrated that the community-of-practice approach promoted a social learning environment with a strong component of engagement, sharing, and co-creation of knowledge applicable to practice. Brown et al. (2013) demonstrated the use of a wiki platform to promote international collaboration for developing and maintaining evidence-based nutrition guidelines for adults with head and neck cancers. During the 4-month monitoring process, they reported over 2,000 page views from 33 different countries. Key to this process was the opportunity for international stakeholder feedback that was used to modify and update the practice guidelines. They conclude that "the use of this technology is expected to continue to rise as the advantages of maintaining a live current document for optimal clinical practice are realized" (p. 189). We invite you to search your discipline-specific literature for other examples of the use of information technologies to generate, share, and manage professionally knowledge.

Knowledge management and transfer in health care organizations are likely to be studied in greater depth as understanding of professional knowledge increases and processes to capture and codify it improve. The Foundation of Knowledge model is not perfect, and others have developed models of knowledge that are more complex. For example, Evans and Alleyne (2009) constructed the **knowledge domain process** (KDP) model to represent knowledge construction and dissemination in an organization. Yet they caution,

> *the KDP model, like all models, is an abstraction aimed at making complex systems more easily understood. While the model presents knowledge processes in a structured and simplified form, the nature and structure of the processes themselves may be open to debate. (p. 148)*

In the future, there will be many more attempts to capture, represent, and explain knowledge processes in professional practice. It is hoped that the reader is convinced that for the health care profession to evolve, knowledge must be dynamically generated, disseminated, and assimilated. This ever-changing interplay means that as knowledge is generated, disseminated, and assimilated, new questions about the impact of HI that will help new knowledge be generated, assimilated, and so on will arise. The assimilation of new knowledge in a profession is a multifaceted approach of individual perception, challenges, and collective thought applied to the disciplinary practice.

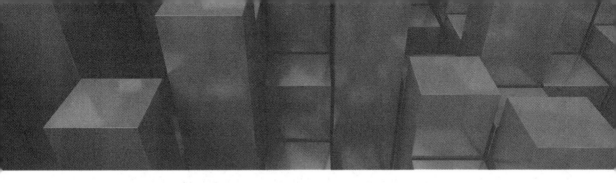

Summary

As a result of reading this text, you should have a deeper understanding of knowledge and informatics as well as the power they have to inform the science of your discipline. It is hoped that you also gained valuable insights into the core principles of HI. The future is exciting. The present chapter should motivate you to continue to learn more and perhaps delve into the science of HI in a research role specific to your discipline. Readers are invited to become active participants in molding the future of health informatics science.

Thought-Provoking Questions

Become informatics savvy and ask yourself the following questions.

1. How can I apply the knowledge I gain from my practice setting to benefit my patients and enhance my practice?
2. How can I help my colleagues and patients understand and use the current technology that is available?
3. How can I use my wisdom to help create the theories, tools, and knowledge of the future?

Apply Your Knowledge

Pause to reflect once again on disciplinary science and the foundation of knowledge in your practice. Health care professionals must be aware of knowledge management principles and the ways that technology supports and assists knowledge acquisition, generation, processing, and dissemination in people and organizations. We must realize that as knowledge workers, we need to commit to a philosophy of continuous learning in order to keep pace in the knowledge era. We must learn to use technology tools to help us continuously refine and add to our knowledge foundation. Throughout the text, we have provided you with information from journal articles reflecting the state of the science for each of the topics covered. I hope that you realize the value of information literacy to health care informatics and will commit to searching the professional journals for scholarly articles to inform your practice. There is no need to "reinvent the wheel" when you are faced with a new challenge in your practice. Check out what others have to say about the topic in professional journals and in communities of practice. As knowledge workers, we can no longer rely on what has been; we must commit to continuous improvement informed by knowledge.

1. Choose one of the new technologies that support knowledge management in an organization and discuss why this would be a good choice to support knowledge management in your organization.
2. Compare your answer with those of others in the class. Which of the technologies chosen has the most potential for use?

References

Brown, T., Findlay, M., Dincklage, J., Davidson, W., Hill, J., Isenring, E., et al. (2013). Using a wiki platform to promote guidelines internationally and maintain their currency: Evidence-based guidelines for the nutritional management of adult patients with head and neck cancer. *Journal of Human Nutrition and Dietetics, 26*(2), 182–190.

Dixon, N. (2012). Conversation matters. http://www.nancydixonblog.com/2012/10/improving-knowledge-worker-productivity.html

Evans, M., & Alleyne, J. (2009). The concept of knowledge in KM: A knowledge domain process model applied to inter-professional care. *Knowledge and Process Management, 16*(4), 147.

Evans, C., Yeung, E., Markoulakis, R., & Guilcher, S. (2014). An online community of practice to support evidence-based physiotherapy practice in manual therapy. *Journal of Continuing Education in the Health Professions, 34*(4), 215–223.

Farr, M., & Cressey, P. (2015). Understanding staff perspectives of quality in practice in healthcare. *BMC Health Services Research, 15*(1), 1–11.

Gent, A. (2007). Three types of knowledge workers. http://incrediblydull.blogspot.com/2007/10/three-types-of-knowledge-workers.html

Glymph, D. C., Olenick, M., Barbera, S., Brown, E. L., Prestianni, L., et al (2015). Healthcare utilizing deliberate discussion linking events (HUDDLE): A systematic review. *AANA Journal, 83*(3), 183–188.

Leiter, M., Day, A., Harvie, P., & Shaughnessy, K. (2007). Personal and organizational knowledge transfer: Implications for worklife engagement. *Human Relations, 60*(2), 259–283.

Markus, M. (2001). Toward a theory of knowledge reuse: Types of knowledge reuse situations and factors in reuse success. *Journal of Management Information Systems, 18*(1), 57–94.

Rochefort, C. M., Buckeridge, D. L., & Forster, A. J. (2015). Accuracy of using automated methods for detecting adverse events from electronic health record data: A research protocol. *Implementation Science, 10*(1), 150–165.

Schutz, S. (2007). Reflection and reflective practice. *Community Practitioner, 80*(9), 26–29.

Stichler, J. F. (2014). Interprofessional practice: Magic at the intersection. *Health Environments Research and Design Journal, 7*(3), 9–12.

Watson, M. (2007). Knowledge management in health and social care. *Journal of Integrated Care, 15*(1), 27–33.

Allied Health Professional Organizations

Contributed by Craig McGonigle

DENTAL HYGIENISTS						
Name	Acronym	Website	Address	Phone	E-Mail Contact	Other Information
International Federation of Dental Hygienists	IFDH	http://www.ifdh.org			Yvonne.Buunk@mondhygienisten.nl	Represent 77,000 dental hygienists
American Dental Hygienists' Association	ADHA	http://www.adha.org	444 North Michigan Ave., Suite 3400, Chicago, IL 60611312-440-8900 member.services@adha.net	312-440-8900	member.services@adha.net	
National Dental Hygienists' Association	NDHA	http://www.ndhaonline.org	P.O. Box 22463, Tampa, FL 33622		forNDHA@aol.com	https://www.ipfw.edu/departments/chhs/depts/dental/hygiene/links
American Dental Assistants Association	ADAA	http://www.adaausa.org	140 N. Bloomingdale Rd., Bloomingdale, IL 60108-1017	630-994-4247	jaykasper@sfainc.biz	

DIAGNOSTIC MEDICAL SONOGRAPHERS						
Name	Acronym	Website	Address	Phone	E-Mail Contact	Other Information
American Registry for Diagnostic Medical Sonographers	ARDMS	http://www.ardms.org		800-541-9754, ext. 3	Other@ARDMS.org	90,000 members
Society of Diagnostic Medical Sonography	SDMS	http://www.sdms.org	2745 Dallas Pkwy., Suite 350, Plano, TX 75093	214-473-8057; 800-229-9506	Complete list of e-mail addresses http://www.sdms.org/about/staff.asp	
Joint Review Committee on Education in Diagnostic Medical Sonography	JRC-DMS	http://www.jrcdms.org	6021 University Blvd, Suite 500, Ellicott City, MD 21043	443-973-3251		
American Registry of Radiologic Technologists	ARRT	http://www.arrt.org	1255 Northland Dr, St. Paul, MN 55120	651-687-0048		
American Society of Radiologic Technologists	ASRT	http://www.asrt.org	15000 Central Ave. SE, Albuquerque, NM 87123	800-444-2778; 505-298-4500	memberservices@asrt.org	List of other organizations: http://www.theagapecenter.com/Organizations/Specialties/Ultrasound.htm

DIETITIANS

Name	Acronym	Website	Address	Phone	E-Mail Contact	Other Information
International Confederation of Dietetic Associations	ICDA	http://www .internationaldietetics.org	ICDA Secretary, c/o Dietitians of Canada, 480 University Ave., Suite 604, Toronto, ON M5G 1V2, Canada	01-416-596-0857	ICDA@internationaldietetics .org	Members in over 40 countries; 160,000 members
Dietitians of Canada	DC	http://www.dietitians.ca	Same as above	Same as above	contactus@dietitians.ca	
Association of UK Dietitians	BDA	http://www.bda.uk.com	5th Floor, Charles House, 148/9 Great Charles St., Queensway, Birmingham B3 3HT, United Kingdom	44-121-200-8080	info@bda.uk.com	
Dietitians Association of Australia	DAA	http://daa.asn.au	n/a	02-6163-5200	nationaloffice@daa.asn.au	
Academy of Nutrition and Dietetics	AND	http://www.eatright.org	120 South Riverside Plaza, Suite 2000, Chicago, IL 60606	800-877-1600	List of e-mail addresses: http://www .eatrightfoundation.org /Foundation/content .aspx?id=6442483522	75,000 members
American Nutrition Association	ANA	http:// americannutritionassociation .org	n/a	n/a	Link to contact form: http:// americannutritionassociation .org/contact	
National Organization of Blacks in Dietetics and Nutrition	NOBIDAN	http://www.nobidan.org	n/a	n/a	Link to contact form: http:// www.nobidan.org/pub /contact_us.cfm	
National Association of Nutrition Professionals	NANP	http://www.nanp.org	n/a	n/a	info@nanp.org	

MEDICAL TECHNOLOGISTS

Name	Acronym	Website	Address	Phone	E-Mail Contact	Other Information
American Medical Technologists	AMT	http://www .americanmedtech .org	10700 W. Higgins Rd., Suite 150, Rosemont, IL 60018	847-823-5169	mail@americanmedtech .org	
Advanced medical Technology Association	AdvaMed	http://advamed.org	701 Pennsylvania Ave. NW, Suite 800, Washington, DC 20004	202-783-8700	info@advamed.org	
American Society for Clinical Laboratory Science	ASCLS	http://www.ascls.org	n/a	n/a	Link for contact form: http://www.ascls.org /contact-the-american -society-for-clinical -laboratory-science	

OCCUPATIONAL THERAPISTS

Name	Acronym	Website	Address	Phone	E-Mail Contact	Other Information
Canadian Association of Occupational Therapy	CAOT	http://www.caot.ca	100-34 Colonnade Rd., Ottawa, ON K2E 7J6, Canada	613-523-2268; 1-800-434-2268	advertising@caot.ca	
American Occupational Therapy Foundation	AOTF	http://www.aotf.org	4720 Montgomery Ln., Suite 202, Bethesda, MD 20814	240-292-1079	aotf@aotf.org	
Canadian Occupational Health Nurses Association	COHNA	http://cohna-aciist.ca	n/a	n/a	info@cohna-aciist.ca	
British Association of Occupational Therapists	BAOT	http://www.cot.co.uk	106-114 Borough High St., Southwark, London SE1 1LB, United Kingdom	020-7357-6480	reception@cot.co.uk	
Canadian Occupational Therapy Foundation	COTF	http://www.cotfcanada.org	n/a	n/a	skamble@cotfcanada.org; amcdonald@cotfcanada.org	Link to many occupational therapy sites: http://www.theagapecenter.com/Organizations/Specialties/Occupational-Therapy.htm

Organization	Abbr.	Website	Address	Phone	Email
Israeli Society of Occupational Therapy	ISOT	http://www.isot.org.il (will be published in English soon)	n/a	n/a	info@isot.org.il
Council of Occupational Therapists for the European Countries	COETEC	http://www.cotec-europe.org	n/a	n/a	info@cotec-europe.org
Occupational Therapy New Zealand	OTNZ	http://www.otnz.co.nz	93 Boulcott St., Wellington 6143, New Zealand	644-473-6510	nzaot@nzaot.com
World Federation of Occupational Therapists	WFOT	http://www.wfot.org	P.O. Box 30, Forrestfield, WA, Australia 6058	Fax: 618-9453-9746	admin@wfot.org.au
American Occupational Therapy Association	AOTA	http://www.aota.org	4720 Montgomery Ln., Suite 200, Bethesda, MD 20814	301-652-6611	praota@aota.org

PHYSICAL THERAPISTS

Name	Acronym	Website	Address	Phone	E-Mail Contact	Other Information
American Physical Therapy Association	APTA	http://www.apta.org	1111 North Fairfax St., Alexandria, VA 22314	800-999-2782; 703-684-2782	nationalgoverance @apta.org	90,000+ members
World Confederation for Physical Therapy	WCPT	http://www.wcpt.org	11 Belgrave Rd., London SW1V 1RB, United Kingdom	44-(0)20-7931-6465	info@wcpt.org	350,000 members through 160 member organizations
American Academy of Physical Therapy	AAPT	http://www.aaptnet .org	P.O. Box 347343, Cleveland, OH 44134	888-717-2278	greenhoward .consulting @gmail.com; jimmieflythejr @yahoo.com	Helping minorities interesting in pursuing physical therapy
Irish Society of Chartered Physiotherapists	ISCP	http://www.iscp.ie	Royal College of Surgeons, St. Stephens's Green, Dublin 2, Ireland	353-1-402-21-48	info@iscp.ie	
Malta Association of Physiotherapists	MAP	http://www .physiomalta.com	6A (5th Floor), Highrise, Triq L' Imradd, Ta' Xbiex, Malta, XBX 1150	356-21312417	secretariat @physiomalta.com	

RADIOGRAPHERS

Name	Acronym	Website	Address	Phone	E-Mail Contact	Other Information
American Registry of Radiologic Technologists	ARRT	http://www.arrt.org	1255 Northland Dr., St. Paul, MN 55120	651-687-0048	n/a	
American Board of Nuclear Medicine	ABNM	http://www.abnm.org	4555 Forest Park Blvd., Suite 119, St. Louis, MO 63108	314-367-2225	abnm@abnm.org	
American Association for Women Radiologists	AAWR	http://www.aawr.org	1891 Preston White Dr., Reston, VA 20191	703-476-7650	info@aawr.org	
American Academy of Oral and Maxillofacial Radiology	AAOMR	http://www.aaomr.org	n/a	n/a	Link to contact form: http://www.aaomr.org/general/?type=CONTACT	
American Nuclear Society	ANS	http://www.ans.org	555 North Kensington Ave., La Grange Park, IL 60526	800-323-3044; 703-352-6611	Tmarc@ans.org	
Society or Thoracic Radiology	STR	http://thoracicrad.org	c/o Matrix meetings, Inc., 1202 1/2 Seventh St. NW, Suite 209, Rochester, MN 55901	507-288-5620	str@thoracicrad.org	
Society of Skeletal Radiology	SSR	https://skeletalrad.org	2575 Northwest Pkwy, Elgin, IL 60124	847-752-6249	admin@skeletalrad.org	
Society of Abdominal Radiology	SAR	http://www.abdominalradiology.org	c/o International Meeting Managers, Inc., 4550 Post Oak Pl., Suite 342, Houston, TX 77027	713-965-0566	admin@abdominalradiology.org	
Society for Radiation Oncology Administrators	SROA	http://www.sroa.org	5272 River R., Suite 630, Bethesda, MD 20816	301-718-6510	info@sroa.org	

RESPIRATORY THERAPISTS

Name	Acronym	Website	Address	Phone	E-Mail Contact	Other Information
National Association for Medical Direction of Respiratory Care	NAMDRC	https://www.namdrc.org	8618 Westwood Center Dr., Suite 210, Vienna, VA 22182	703-752-4359	execoffice@namdrc.org	
International Association of Respiratory Therapists	IART	http://iaresp.com	410 Park Ave., 15th Floor, New York, NY 10022	631-650-2499	Link to contact form: http://iaresp.com/contact.php	
American Association for Respiratory Care	AARC	http://www.aarc.org	9425 N. MacArthur Blvd., Suite 100, Irving, TX 75063	972-243-2272	info@aarc.org	
Canadian Society of Respiratory Therapists	CSRT	http://www.csrt.com	201-2460 Lancaster Rd., Ottawa, ON K1B 4S5, Canada	800-267-3422; 613-731-3164	Link to contact form: http://www.csrt.com/contact/?rq=contact	
International Society for Respiratory Protection	ISRP	http://www.isrp.com	ASRP, Private Bag 1001, Mona Vale, NSW 2103, Australia	61-(0)2-9910-7500	info@isrp.com	

SPEECH LANGUAGE PATHOLOGISTS

Name	Acronym	Website	Address	Phone	E-Mail Contact	Other Information
American Speech-Language-Hearing Association	ASHA	http://www.asha.org		800-638-8255	Link to contact form: http://www.asha.org/Forms/Contact-ASHA	This seems to be the main site for everything. Here is a link to all of their partners: http://www.asha.org/members/international/intl_assoc
National Black Association for Speech-Language and Hearing	NBASLH	http://www.nbaslh.org				

Emerging Health Care Technologies by Discipline

Contributed by Craig McGonigle

Dental hygienists

- http://www.rdhmag.com/articles/print/volume-32/volume-12/features/trends-in-dental-hygiene.html
- http://www.dentistryiq.com/articles/2013/10/transforming-dental.html
- http://www.dentalbuzz.com

Diagnostic medical sonographers

- http://www.sdms.org/members/news/NewsWave/NW-April-2010.pdf
- http://www.sdms.org/members/news/NewsWave/NW-March-2010.pdf

Dietitians

- http://www.todaysdietitian.com/trends_archive.shtml
- https://www1.cfnc.org/Plan/For_A_Career/Career_Cluster_Profile/Cluster_Article.aspx?articleId=jXEcNxV085RwY1rgTtnWagXAP3DPAXXAP3DPAX&cId=BufXemcmHBSoBjt9hbo0XAP2BPAXwXAP3DPAXXAP3DPAX&sectionId=3

Medical technologists

- http://blog.capterra.com/top-5-medical-technology-trends-2015
- http://www.mdtmag.com/blogs/2014/12/5-trends-medical-technology-2015

Occupational therapists

- https://www1.cfnc.org/Plan/For_A_Career/Career_Cluster_Profile/Cluster _Article.aspx?articleId=10hEsM9Fvs5UeiAXAP2BPAXmDXCbgXAP3DPAXX AP3DPAX&cId=BufXemcmHBSoBjt9hbo0XAP2BPAXwXAP3DPAXXAP3DP AX&sectionId=3
- http://www.caot.ca/default.asp?pageid=291

Physical therapists

- http://www.supplementalhealthcare.com/blog/2013/4-physical-therapy -technologies-improving-patient-care
- http://www.rehabpub.com/2015/01/7-predictions-pt-2015
- http://www.ptaguide.org/top-trends-physical-therapy
- http://www.slideshare.net/Healthstartup/hsu5-topic-presentationfinal
- http://www.nova.edu/chcs/news/google-glass.html

Radiographers

- https://accrualnet.cancer.gov/sites/accrualnet.cancer.gov/files/conversation _files/Vining_ViSion_Spectrum20(8).pdf
- http://www.itnonline.com/article/new-trends-and-technology-radiology-0
- http://www.radiologytoday.net/archive/rt1011p26.shtml

Respiratory therapists

- http://www.draeger.com/sites/enus_us/Pages/Hospital/The-Future-Of -Respiratory-Care.aspx
- http://www.ncbi.nlm.nih.gov/pubmed/10315290

Speech-language pathologists

- http://www.asha.org/Careers/Market-Trends
- http://blog.asha.org/2011/05/26/technologys-emerging-frontier-in-speech -language-pathology-part-1

Abbreviations

3D	Three-dimensional
ABC	Alternative billing codes
ADT	Admission, discharge, and transfer system
AHRQ	Agency for Healthcare Research and Quality
AI	Artificial intelligence
ALA	American Library Association
Alt	Alternate key on the computer keyboard
ALU	Arithmetic logic unit
ANSI	American National Standards Institute
API	Application programming interface
ARG	Augmented-reality game
ARRA	American Recovery and Reinvestment Act
b	Bit
B	Byte
BCMA	Bar Code Medication Administration
BI	Bioinformatics
BIOS	Basic input/output system
bit/s or bps	Bits per second
BMP	Bitmap image
BRFSS	Behavioral Risk Factor Surveillance System
CAI	Computer-assisted instruction
CASE	Computer-aided software engineering
CBIS	Computer-based information system
CD	Compact disk
CD-R	Compact disk—recordable
CD-ROM	Compact disk—read-only memory
CD-RW	Compact disk—recordable and rewritable
CDC	Centers for Disease Control and Prevention
CDS/CDSS	Clinical decision support/clinical decision support system
CHI	Consolidated health informatics
CI	Cognitive informatics
CINAHL	Cumulative Index to Nursing and Allied Health Literature
CIO	Chief information officer
CIS	Clinical information systems
CMIS	Case management information system
CMP	Civil monetary penalties
CMS	Centers for Medicare and Medicaid Services; course management system; content management system
CNPII	Committee for Nursing Practice Information Infrastructure

COPD	Chronic obstructive pulmonary disease
CPGs	Clinical practice guidelines
CPOE	Computerized physician order entry; computer-based provider order entry
CPU	Central processing unit
CRA	Community risk assessment
CRT	Cathode ray tube
CSS	Cascading style sheets
CTA	Cognitive task analysis
CTO	Chief technical officer; chief technology officer
Ctrl	Control key on the computer keyboard
CWA	Cognitive work analysis
DBMS	Database management system
DHR	Digital health record
DNB	Dynamic network biomarkers
DRAM	Dynamic random-access memory
DSDM	Dynamic system development method
DSS	Decision support system
DVD	Digital versatile disk; digital video disk
DVD-R	Digital video disk—recordable
DVD-RW	Digital video disk—recordable and rewritable
DW	Data warehouse
EB	Exabyte
EBP	Evidence-based practice
EDI	Electronic data interchange
EEPROM	Electronically erasable programmable read-only memory
EHR	Electronic health record
ELSI	Ethical, legal, and social issues
EMR	Electronic medical record
EPROM	Erasable programmable read-only memory
ERD	Entity—relationship diagram
ERIC	Education Resources Information Center
ESC	Escape key
ESLI	Ethical, social, and legal implications
F key	Function key on the computer keyboard
F/OSS or FOSS	Free/open-source software
FHIE	Federal Health Information Exchange
FMEA	Failure modes and effects analysis
FPROM	Field programmable read-only memory
FPU	Floating-point unit
GB	Gigabyte
GHz	Gigahertz
GLBA	Gramm-Leach-Bliley Act
GUI	Graphical user interface
HCI	Human—computer interaction
HCT	Human—computer technology
HGP	Human Genome Project
HHA	Home Health Agency

HIE	Health information exchange
HIPAA	Health Insurance Portability and Accountability Act
HIS	Hospital information system
HIT	Health information technology
HITECH	Health Information Technology for Economic and Clinical Health Act
HL7	Health Level 7
HMIS	Health management information system
HMO	Health maintenance organization
HTI	Human—technology interaction
HTML	Hypertext Markup Language
I/O	Input/output
ICNP	International Classification of Nursing Practice
IDE	Integrated drive electronics
IEEE	Institute of Electrical and Electronics Engineers
IHIE	Indiana Health Information Exchange
IM	Instant message
IP	Internet Protocol
IS	Information system
ISO	International Standards Organization or International Organization for Standardization
IT	Information technology
KB	Kilobyte
KMS	Knowledge management system
LAN	Local area network
LCD	Liquid crystal display
LOS	Length of stay
LTC	Long-term care
MAN	Metropolitan area network
MB	Megabyte
MCIS	Managed care information system
MHDC	Massachusetts Health Data Consortium
MHz	Megahertz
MMIS	Medicaid management information systems
MMORPG or simply MMO	Massive multiplayer online role-playing game
Modem	Modulator—demodulator
MOO	Object-oriented MUD
Moodle	Modular Object-Oriented Dynamic Learning Environment
MoSCoW	Must have, Should have, Could have, and Would have
MP3	MPEG-1 Audio Layer-3
MPEG	Moving Picture Experts Group
MPI	Master patient index
MRI	Magnetic resonance imaging
NCPHI	National Center for Public Health Informatics
NGC	National Guideline Clearinghouse
NGI	Next-generation Internet
NHANES	National Health and Nutrition Examination Survey
NHII	National Health Information Infrastructure
NHIN	National Health Information Network

NHQR	National Healthcare Quality Report
NIST	National Institute of Standards and Technology
NLS	National language support
NPC	Nonplayer character
NPI	National provider identifier
OASIS	Outcomes and Assessment Information Set
OCR	Office of Civil Rights
ONC	Office of the National Coordinator for Health Information Technology
OS	Operating system
OSI	Open systems interconnection
OWL	Web ontology language
PACS	Picture archiving and communication system
PADS	Planned accelerated discharge protocols
PB	Petabyte
PBL	Problem-based learning
PC	Personal computer
PCA	Patient-controlled analgesia
PCI	Peripheral component interconnection
PCIS	Patient care information system
PDA	Personal data assistant; personal digital assistant
PERS	Personal emergency response system
PHI	Protected health information; public health informatics
PHR	Personal health record
POSIX	Portable Operating System Interface for Unix
PPS	Prospective payment system
PROM	Programmable read-only memory
PrtSc or Prnt Scrn	Print screen key
PS/2	Personal System/2
PT/INR	Prothrombin time/international normalized ratio
QA	Quality assurance
RAD	Rapid application development
RAM	Random-access memory
RATS	Readiness assessment tests
RDBMS	Relational database management system
RDF	Resource description framework
RFI	Radio-frequency identifier
RFID	Radio-frequency identification
RHIO	Regional health information organization
RIS	Radiology information system
ROM	Read-only memory
RSS	Really simple syndication
RSVP	Rapid Syndromic Validation Project
RU	Research utilization
SCSI	Small Computer System Interface
SDLC	Systems development life cycle
SDO	Standards developing organization
SDRAM	Synchronous dynamic random-access memory

SGML	Standard Generalized Markup Language
SNOMED CT	Systematic Nomenclature of Medical Clinical Terms
SOX	Sarbanes-Oxley Act
SQL	Structured English Query Language
TB	Terabyte
TCP	Transmission Control Protocol
TELOS	Technological and systems, economic, legal, operational, and schedule feasibility
TPO	Treatment payment operations
URL	Uniform resource locator
USB	Universal serial bus
VoIP	Voice-over-Internet Protocol
VR	Virtual reality
W3C	World Wide Web Consortium
WAN	Wide area network
WWW	World Wide Web
XML	Extensible Markup Language
YB	Yottabyte
YRBSS	Youth Risk Behavior Surveillance System
ZB	Zettabyte

Glossary

Access The ability to examine, explore, or retrieve data and information from an information system or a computer program.

Acceptable use A corporate policy that defines the types of activities that are acceptable on the corporate computer network, identifies the activities that are not acceptable, and specifies the consequences for violations.

Acquisition The act of acquiring; to locate and hold. We acquire data and information.

Active listening A therapeutic communication technique in which the health care professional employs conscious attention to what a patient is saying, reflects back feelings and phrases, and asks questions to clarify meaning.

Acuity system System that calculates the care requirements for individual patients based on severity of illness, specialized equipment and technology needed, and intensity of clinical interventions.

Administrative processes The processes used by administration, such as the electronic scheduling, billing, and claims management systems including electronic scheduling for inpatient and outpatient visits and procedures, electronic insurance eligibility validation, claim authorization and prior approval, identification of possible research study participants, and drug recall support.

Admission, discharge, and transfer (ADT) system A system that provides the backbone structure for the other types of clinical and business systems; it contains the groundwork for the other types of health care information systems because it includes the patient's name, medical record number, visit or account number, and demographic information, such as age, sex, home address, and contact information. It is the central source for collecting this type of patient information and communicating it to the other types of health care information systems, including clinical and business systems.

Agency for Healthcare Research and Quality (AHRQ) An agency within the U.S. Department of Health and Human Services that supports health services research initiatives.

Alarm fatigue Multiple false alarms by smart technology that cause workers to ignore or respond slowly to them.

Alerts Warnings or additional information provided to clinicians to help with decision making; the action of the clinician or system triggers the generation of an alert. Also known as triggers.

Algorithm Step-by-step procedure for problem solving or calculating; a set of rules for problem solving. In data mining, it defines the parameters of the data mining model; it is the recipe or method with which the data mining model is developed.

Allele One member of a pair or series of genes that occupy a specific position on a specific chromosome.

Alternatives Choices between two or more options.

American Library Association (ALA) A U.S.-based organization that promotes libraries and library education internationally.

American National Standards Institute (ANSI) An organization dedicated to promoting consensus on norms and guidelines related to the assessment of health agencies.

American Recovery and Reinvestment Act (ARRA) An economic stimulus package enacted in February 2009 that was intended to create jobs and promote investment and consumer spending during the recession. This act has also been referred to as the Stimulus or Recovery Act. There was a push for widespread adoption of health information technology, and Title XIII of ARRA was given a subtitle: Health Information Technology for Economic and Clinical Health (HITECH) Act. Through this act, health care organizations can qualify for financial incentives based on the level of meaningful use achieved; the HITECH Act specifically incentivizes health organizations and providers to become meaningful users.

Analysis Separating a whole into its elements or component parts; examination of a concept or phenomena, its elements, and their relations.

Antiprinciplism Theory that emerged with the expansive technological changes in recent years and the tremendous rise in ethical dilemmas accompanying these changes. Opponents of principlism include those who claim that its principles do not represent a theoretical approach and those who claim that its principles are too far removed from the concrete particularities of everyday human existence; the principles are too conceptual, intangible, or abstract; or the principles disregard or do not take into account a person's psychological factors, personality, life history, sexual orientation, religious, ethnic, and cultural background.

Antivirus software A computer program that is designed to recognize and neutralize computer viruses—that is, malicious codes that replicate over and over and eventually take over the computer's memory and interfere with its normal functioning.

App Software used on a smartphone or other mobile device.

Application The implementation software of a computer system. This software allows users to complete tasks such as word processing, developing presentations, and managing data.

Application Programming Interface (API) Processes used for building software applications.

Arithmetic logic unit (ALU) Essential building block of the central processing unit of a computer that digitally performs arithmetic and logical functions.

Artificial intelligence (AI) The field that deals with the conception, development, and implementation of informatics tools based on intelligent technologies. This field attempts to capture the complex processes of human thought and intelligence.

Asynchronous That which is not synchronous; not in real time or does not occur or exist at the same time, not having the same period or time frame. Learning anywhere and at any time using Internet and World Wide Web software tools (e.g., course management systems, e-mail, electronic bulletin boards, webpages) as the principal delivery mechanisms for instruction.

Attribute Quality or characteristic; field or element of an entity in a database.

Audiopod Utility to download podcasts.

Authentication Processes to serve to authenticate or prove who is accessing the system.

Autonomy The right of an individual to choose for himself or herself.

Avatar Image on the Internet that represents the user in virtual communities or other interactions on the Internet; three-dimensional or two-dimensional image representing a user on the Internet.

Bagging The use of voting and averaging in predictive data mining to synthesize the predictions from many models or methods or for using the same type of a model on different data; it deals with the unpredictability of results when complex models are used to data mine small data sets.

Bar-code medication administration (BCMA) A system using bar-code technology affixed to the medication, the patient ID bracelet, and the caregiver ID badge to support the five rights of medication administration.

Basic input/output system (BIOS) Also called binary input/output system, basic integrated operating system, or built-in operating system. A system that resides or is embedded on a chip that recognizes and controls a computer's devices. Any program, operation, or device that transfers data to or from a computer and to or from a peripheral device.

Behavioral Risk Factor Surveillance System (BRFSS) An assessment system initially designed to collect information on the movement of mentally impaired persons from state-operated facilities into community settings. The assessments have since been expanded to include other populations and are designed to determine the effectiveness of programs in meeting the health care needs of at-risk populations.

Beneficence Actions performed that contribute to the welfare of others.

Big data Voluminous amounts of data sets that are difficult to process using typical data processing; huge amounts of semistructured and unstructured data that are unwieldy to manage within relational databases. Unstructured big data residing in text files represent more than 75% of an organization's data.

Binary system System used by computers; a numeric system that uses two symbols: 0 and 1.

Bioethics The study and formulation of health care ethics. Bioethics takes on relevant ethical problems experienced by health care providers in the provision of care to individuals and groups.

Bioinformatics (BI) The application of computer science, information science, and cognitive science principles to biological systems, especially in the human genome field of study; an interdisciplinary science that applies computer and information sciences to solve biological problems.

Biomarkers Individual genes, proteins, or metabolites that reveal the panel of proteins interactions but also their interactions with RNA, DNA, and other molecules.

Biomedical informatics Interdisciplinary science of acquiring, structuring, analyzing, and providing access to biomedical data, information, and knowledge to improve the detection, prevention, and treatment of disease.

Biometrics Study of processes or means to uniquely recognize individual users (humans) based on one or more intrinsic physical or behavioral attributes or characteristics. Authentication devices that recognize thumb prints, retinal patterns, or facial patterns are available. Depending on the level of security needed, organizations will commonly use a combination of these types of authentication.

Bioterrorism The use of pathogens or other potentially harmful biological agents to sicken or kill members of a targeted population. Informatics database applications are used to track strategic indicators, such as emergency room visits, disease case reports, frequency and type of lab testing ordered by physicians and/or nurse practitioners, missed work, and over-the-counter medication purchases, that may indicate an outbreak that can be attributed to bioterrorism.

Bit (b) Unit of measurement that holds one binary digit: 0 or 1. The smallest possible chunk of data memory used in computer processing, making up the binary system of the computer.

Blended An approach to education that combines traditional face-to-face instruction with technology-based (online) instruction. *See also* hybrid.

Blog Interactive, online weblog. Typically a combination of what is happening on the Web as well as what is happening in the blogger's or creator's life. A blog is as unique as the blogger or person creating it. Thought of as a diary and guide.

Boosting Increasing the power of models by weighting the combinations of predictions from those models to create a predicted classification; an iterative process using voting or averaging to combine the different classifiers.

Bracketing The process of setting aside preconceived notions or expectations in the patient encounter to allow the caregiver to assess the patient's individual and unique response to the health challenge.

Brain The central information processing unit of humans. An organ that controls the central nervous system and is responsible for cognition and the interpretation, processing, and reaction to sensory input.

Browser Software used to locate and display webpages. Also known as a Web browser or Internet browser.

Brushing A technique whereby the user manually chooses specific data points or observations or subsets of data on an interactive data display; these data can be visualized in two-dimensional or three-dimensional surfaces as scatter plots. Also known as graphical exploratory data analysis.

Brute force attack A technique where software creates many possible combinations of characters in an attempt to guess passwords to gain access to a network or a computer.

Building block Basic element or part of health informatics, such as information science, computer science, cognitive science, and disciplinary science.

Bus Subsystem that transfers data between a computer's internal components or between computers.

Byte (B) Unit of memory equal to 8 bits or eight informational storage units, which represents one keystroke (e.g., any push of a key on a keyboard, such as pressing the space bar, a lowercase "a," or an uppercase "T"). It is considered the best way to indicate computer memory or storage capacity.

Cache memory Smaller and faster memory storage used by a computer's central processing unit to store copies of frequently used data in main memory.

Care ethics An ethical approach to solving moral dilemmas encountered in health care that is based on relationships and a caring attitude toward others.

Care plan A set of guidelines that outline the course of treatment and the recommended interventions that will achieve optimal results.

Caring The nontechnical aspects of interventions that communicate acceptance and concern for a patient.

Caritas processes Interventions that communicate loving concern for the unique humanity of every patient.

Case management information system (CMIS) Computer programs and information management tools that interact to support and facilitate the practice of case managers.

Casuist approach An approach to ethical decision making that grew out of the concern for more concrete methods of examining ethical dilemmas. Casuistry is a case-based ethical reasoning method that analyzes the facts of a case in a sound, logical, and ordered or structured manner. The facts are compared to the decisions arising out of consensus in previous paradigmatic or model cases.

Centering The act of taking a moment to clear one's mind of clutter and focus one's attention exclusively on a patient prior to engaging in a therapeutic encounter.

Centers for Disease Control and Prevention (CDC) An agency of the U.S. Department of Health and Human Services that works to protect public health and safety related to disease control and prevention.

Centers for Medicare and Medicaid Services (CMS) The largest health insurer in the United States, particularly for home health care services, and for the elderly, for health care services.

Central processing unit (CPU) Processors that execute computer programs, thought of as the brain controlling the functioning of the computer; the computer component that actually executes, calculates, and processes the binary computer code instigated by the operating system and other applications on the computer. It serves as the command center that directs the actions of all other components of the computer and manages both incoming and outgoing data.

Central stations Multifunctional telehealth care platforms for receiving, retrieving, and/or displaying patients' vital signs and other information transmitted from telecommunications-ready medical devices.

Certified EHR technology An electronic health record (EHR) that meets specific governmental standards for the type of record involved, either an ambulatory EHR used by office-based health care practitioners or an inpatient EHR used by hospitals. The specific standards to be met are set forth in federal regulations.

Chief information officer (CIO) Person involved with the information technology infrastructure of an organization. This role is sometimes called chief knowledge officer.

Chief technology officer or chief technical officer (CTO) Person focused on organizationally based scientific and technical issues and responsible for technological research and development as part of the organization's products and services.

Chronic disease Long-term disease, such as congestive heart failure, diabetes, and respiratory ailments.

Civil monetary penalties (CMP) Fines laid out by the Social Security Act, which the Secretary of Health and Human Services can assess for many types of noncompliant conduct.

Classification The technique of dividing a data set into mutually exclusive groups.

Classification and regression trees (CART) A decision tree method that is used for sorting or classifying a data set. A set of rules that can be applied to a new data set that has not been classified; the set of rules is designed to predict which records will have a specified outcome.

Clinical database A collection of related patient records stored in a computer system using software that permits a person or program to query the data to extract needed patient information.

Clinical decision support (CDS) A computer-based program designed to assist clinicians in making clinical decisions by filtering or integrating vast amounts of information and providing suggestions for clinical intervention. May also be called a clinical decision support system (CDSS).

Clinical documentation system Array or collection of applications and functionality; an amalgamation of systems, medical equipment, and technologies working together that are committed or dedicated to collecting, storing, and manipulating health care data and information and providing secure access to interdisciplinary clinicians navigating the continuum of client care. Designed to collect patient data in realtime and to enhance care by putting data at the clinician's fingertips and enabling decision making where it needs to occur—at the bedside. Also known as clinical information system (CIS).

Clinical guidelines Recommendations that serve as a guide to decisions and provide criteria for specific practice areas.

Clinical information system (CIS) Array or collection of applications and functionality; an amalgamation of systems, medical equipment, and technologies working together that are committed or dedicated to collecting, storing, and manipulating health care data and information and providing secure access to interdisciplinary clinicians navigating the continuum of client care. Designed to collect patient data in realtime and to enhance care by putting data at the clinician's fingertips and enabling decision making where it needs to occur—at the bedside. Also known as clinical documentation system.

Clinical practice guidelines Informal or formal rules or guiding principles that a health care provider uses when determining diagnostic tests and treatment strategies for individual patients. In the electronic health record, they are included in a variety of ways such as prompts, pop-ups, and text messages.

Clinical transformation The complete alteration of the clinical environment; widespread change accompanies transformational activities, and clinical transformation implies that the manner in which work is carried out and the outcomes achieved are completely different from the prior state, which is not always true in the case of simply implementing technology. Technology can be used to launch or in conjunction with a clinical transformation initiative; however, the implementation of technology alone is not justifiably transformational ability. Therefore, this term should be used cautiously to describe redesign efforts.

Cloud computing Web browser—based login-accessible data, software, and hardware; could link systems together and reduce costs.

Codify To classify, reduce to code, or articulate.

Cognitive informatics (CI) Field of study made up of the disciplines of neuroscience, linguistics, artificial intelligence, and psychology. This multidisciplinary study of cognition and information sciences investigates human information-processing mechanisms and processes and their engineering applications in computing.

Cognitive science Interdisciplinary field that studies the mind, intelligence, and behavior from an information-processing perspective.

Cognitive task analysis (CTA) Examination of the nature of a task by breaking it down into its component parts and identifying the performers' thought processes.

Cognitive walkthrough A technique used to evaluate a computer interface or a software program by breaking down and explaining the steps that a user will take to accomplish a task.

Cognitive work analysis (CWA) A multifaceted analytic procedure developed specifically for the analysis of complex, high-technology work domains.

Collaboration The sharing of ideas and experiences for the purposes of mutual understanding and learning.

Column Field or attribute of an entity in a database.

Communication science Area of concentration or discipline that studies human communication.

Communication software Technology programs used to transmit messages via e-mail, telephonically, paging, broadcast (such as MP3), and Internet (such as instant messaging, Voice-over-Internet Protocol, or listservs).

Communication system Collection of individual communications networks and transmission systems. In health care, it includes call light systems, wireless phones, pagers, e-mail, instant messaging, and any other devices or networks that clinicians use to communicate with patients, families, other professionals, and internal and external resources.

Community risk assessment (CRA) A comprehensive examination of a community to identify factors that potentially affect the health of the members of that community. Often used in public health program planning.

Compact disk—read-only memory (CD-ROM) Disk that can hold approximately 700 megabytes of data accessible by a computer.

Compact disk—recordable (CD-R) Compact disk that can be used once for recording.

Compact disk—rewritable (CD-RW) Compact disk that can be recorded onto many times.

Compatibility The ability to work with each other or other devices or systems, such as software that works with a computer.

Competency A statement or description of goals, skills, or behaviors to be achieved.

Compliance Conforming or performing in an acceptable manner; correctly following the rules.

Computational biology The action complement of bioinformatics and, therefore, biomedicine; it is the actual process of analyzing and interpreting data.

Computer A machine that stores and executes programs; a machine with peripheral hardware and software to carry out selected programming.

Computer-aided software engineering (CASE) Systematic application of computer software tools and techniques to facilitate engineering practice.

Computer-assisted instruction (CAI) Any instruction that is aided by the use of a computer.

Computer based That which uses the computer to interact; the computer is the base tool.

Computer-based information system (CBIS) Combinations of hardware, software, and telecommunications networks that people build and use to collect, create, and distribute useful data, typically in organizational settings.

Computer science Branch of engineering (application of science) that studies the theoretical foundations of information and computation and their implementation and application in computer systems; the study of storage/memory, conversion and transformation, and transfer or transmission of information in machines—that is, computers—through both algorithms and practical implementation problems. Algorithms are detailed, unambiguous action sequences in the design, efficiency, and application of computer systems, whereas practical implementation problems deal with the software and hardware.

Computerized physician (provider) order entry (CPOE) system A system that automates the way that orders have traditionally been initiated for patients. Clinicians place orders within these systems instead of using traditional handwritten transcription onto paper. These systems provide major safeguards by ensuring that physician orders are legible and complete, thereby providing a level of patient safety that was historically missing with paper-based orders. They provide decision support and automated alert functionality that was previously unavailable with paper-based orders.

Conferencing software Electronic communications system or software that supports and facilitates two or more people meeting for discussion. High-end systems offer telepresence (a lifelike experience allowing people to feel as if they were present in person—it would be as though the health care professional were physically there with the patient—so people can work, learn, and play in person over the Internet or have an effect at a remote location).

Confidentiality The mandate that all personal information be safeguarded by ensuring that access is limited to only those who are authorized to view that information.

Connected health A model of health care delivery using technology to provide services including information and education.

Connectionism A component of cognitive science that uses computer modeling through artificial neural networks to try to explain human intellectual abilities.

Connectivity Ability to hook up to the electronic resources necessary to meet the user's needs. The ability to use computer networks to link to people and resources. The unbiased transmission or transport of Internet Protocol packets between two end points.

Consequences Outcomes or products resulting from one's decision choices.

Consolidated Health Informatics (CHI) A collaborative effort to adopt health information interoperability standards, particularly health vocabulary and messaging standards, for implementation in federal government systems.

Context of care The setting, services, patient, environment, and professional and social interactions surrounding the delivery of patient interventions.

Continuing education Course work or training completed after achievement of a baccalaureate degree, often for the purpose of recertification.

Copyright A legal term used by many governments around the world that gives the inventor or designer of an original product sole or exclusive rights to that product for a limited time; the same laws that cover physical books, artwork, and other creative material are still applicable in the digital world.

Core business system System that enhances administrative tasks within health care organizations. Unlike clinical information systems, whose aim is to provide direct patient care, these systems support the management of health care within an organization. They provide the framework for reimbursement, support of best practices, quality control, and resource allocation. There are four common types of core business systems: (1) admission, discharge, and transfer; (2) financial; (3) acuity; and (4) scheduling systems.

Courage The strength to face difficulty.

Course management system (CMS) Software system designed for both faculty and students that supports educational episodes, including tools for grading, learner assessment, content presentation/interaction, and communication. These systems provide for the support of learning activities throughout course delivery; proprietary examples include ANGEL, Blackboard, WebCT, Learning Space, and eCollege.

Covered entity A health care provider that conducts certain transactions in electronic form (a "covered health care provider"), a health care clearinghouse, or a health plan that electronically transmits any health information in connection with transactions (billing and payment for services or insurance coverage) for which the U.S. Department of Health and Human Services has adopted standards; identified in the Administrative Simplification regulations.

Creativity software Programs that support and facilitate innovation and creativity (an intellectual process relating to the creation or generation of new ideas, concepts, or new relationships between currently existing ideas or concepts); they allow users to focus or concentrate more on creating new things in today's digital age and less on the mechanics or workings of how they are created or developed.

Crowdsourcing Information generated by individuals on social media.

Cumulative Index to Nursing and Allied Health Literature (CINAHL) A comprehensive nursing and allied health literature database.

Data Raw facts that lack meaning.

Data dictionary Software that contains a listing of tables and their details, including field names, validation settings, and data types.

Data file A collection of related records.

Data mart Collection of data focusing on a specific topic or organizational unit or department created to facilitate management personnel making strategic business decisions. Could be as small as one database or larger, such as a compilation of databases; generally smaller than a data warehouse.

Data mining A process of utilizing software to sort through data so as to discover patterns and ascertain or establish relationships. This process may help to discover or uncover previously unidentified relationships among the data in a database.

Data set Collection of interrelated data.

Data warehouse (DW) An extremely large database or repository that stores all of an organization's or institution's data and makes this data available for data mining. A combination of an institution's many different databases that provides management personnel flexible access to the data.

Database A collection of related records stored in a computer system using software that permits a person or program to query the data so as to extract needed information; it may consist of one or more related data files or tables.

Database management system (DBMS) Software programs and the hardware used to create and manage data.

Decision making Output of cognition; outcome of our intellectual processing.

Decision support Recommendations for interventions based on computerized care protocols. The decision support recommendations may include such items as additional screenings, medication interactions, or drug and dosage monitoring.

Decision tree A set of decisions represented in a tree-shaped pattern; the decisions produce the rules for the classification of a data set.

Degradation Loss of quality; for example, in telecommunications, it is the loss of quality in the electronic signal.

Desktop Computer's interface that resembles the top of a desk, where the user keeps things he or she wants to access quickly, such as paper clips, pens, and paper. On the computer's desktop, the user can customize the look and feel to have easy access to the programs, folders, and files on the hard drive that the individual uses the most.

Digital divide The gap between those who have and those who do not have access to online information.

Digital video disk (DVD) Optical disk storage format that can generally hold or store more than six times the amount of data that a compact disk can.

Digital video disk—recordable (DVD-R) Disk on which a user can record once.

Digital video disk—rewritable (DVD-RW) Disk on which a user can record many times.

Data—information—knowledge—wisdom (DIKW) paradigm A paradigm used as the basis of informatics.

Dissemination A thoughtful, intentional, goal-oriented communication of specific, useful information or knowledge.

Distance education Education provided from a remote location.

DMAIC (define, measure, analyze, improve, control) The steps contained in a data driven process improvement procedure for organizations; typically associated with Six Sigma.

Document To capture and save information for later use.

Domain name A series of alphanumeric characters that forms part of the Internet address or URL (e.g., psu.edu denotes Penn State's address).

Drill-down A means of viewing data warehouse information by going down to lower levels of the database to focus on information that is pertinent to the user's needs at the moment.

Duty One's feeling of being bound or obligated to carry out specific tasks or roles based on one's rank or position.

Dynamic network biomarkers (DNBs) DNBs are created, monitored, and evaluated at different stages and time points of the disease based on nonlinear dynamical theory and complex network theory. DNBs differ from molecular biomarkers and network biomarkers to describe and identify disease progress situations and interactions rather than the static nature approach. The promise of DNBs lies in the fact that they can help us uncover disease-specific biomarkers that we can map to compute and diagnose pre-disease circumstances and conditions.

Dynamic random-access memory (DRAM) Type of RAM chip requiring less space to store the same amount on a similar static RAM (SRAM) chip; however, DRAM requires more power than SRAM because DRAM needs to keep its charge by constantly refreshing.

Dynamic system development method (DSDM) An agile software development strategy based on the rapid application development model, which is iterative and used in the system development life cycle and project management.

E-brochure Electronic brochure. Patient education material that is typically tied to an agency website and may include such information as descriptions of diseases and their management, medication information, or where to get assistance with a health care issue.

E-health Health care initiatives and practice supported by electronic or digital media. The most typical use is in patient and family education where information is communicated electronically.

e-Health Initiative Initiative developed to address the growing need for managing health information and to promote technology as a means of improving health information exchange, health literacy, and health care delivery; an organization dedicated to the use of information technology to improve health through education, advocacy, and research (https://www.ehidc.org/).

E-learning Electronic learning or learning that is facilitated by electronic means such as computers and the Internet. E-learning, online, and Web-based education have caused a significant shift in student—teacher relationships in health care professional education.

E-mail Electronic mail. To compose, send, receive, and store messages in electronic communication systems.

E-mail client Program that manages e-mail functions.

Earcons Auditory tones that are combined to represent relationships among data elements, such as the relationship of systolic blood pressure to diastolic blood pressure; auditory tone that indicates an event on an electronic system, such as receiving a text message or e-mail.

Educational Resources Information Center (ERIC) A comprehensive educational resources database. An international database of educational literature.

Electronic communication Any exchange of information that is transmitted electronically.

Electronic health record (EHR) A computer-based data warehouse or repository of information regarding the health status of a client that is replacing the former paper-based medical record; it is the systematic documentation of a client's health status and health care in a secured digital format, meaning that it can be processed, stored, transmitted, and accessed by authorized interdisciplinary professionals for the purpose of supporting efficient, high-quality health care across the client's health care continuum. Also known as electronic medical record.

Electronic mailing list Automatic mailing list server such as listserv that sends an e-mail addressed to the list to everyone who has subscribed to the list automatically. Similar to an electronic bulletin board or news forum.

Electronically erasable programmable read-only memory (EEPROM) A nonvolatile storage chip used in computers and other devices to store small amounts of volatile data (e.g., calibration tables or device configuration).

Empiricism Knowledge that is derived from our experiences or senses.

Empowerment Promotion of self-actualization; achievement of power or control over one's own life.

End users Target users or consumers of software and computer technology. Software or computing applications should be designed for the end user, the person who will ultimately be using them.

Enterprise integration Electronically linking health care providers, health plans, government, and other interested parties to facilitate electronic exchange and use of health information among all stakeholders.

Entity *See* covered entity.

Entity—relationship diagram (ERD) Diagram that specifies the relationships among the entities in the database. Sometimes the implied relationships are apparent based on the entities' definitions; however, all relationships should be specified as to how items relate to one another. There are typically three relationships: one to one, one to many, and many to many.

Epidemiology The field of study identifying things that come on the people. Incidence, prevalence, and control of disease. Case finding.

Epistemology Study of the nature and origin of knowledge; what it means to know.

Electronic protected health information See protected health information.

Electronically Erasable programmable read-only memory (EEPROM) Type of computer memory chip that retains its data when its power supply is switched off and can be erased with ultraviolet light.

Ergonomics In the United States, this term is used to describe the physical characteristics of equipment—for example, the optimal fit of a scissors to a human hand. In Europe, it is synonymous with human factors—that is, the interaction of humans with physical attributes of equipment or the interaction of humans and the arrangement of equipment in the work environment.

Ethical decision making The process of making informed choices about ethical dilemmas based on a set of standards differentiating right from wrong. The decision making reflects an understanding of the principles and standards of ethical decision making as well as philosophical approaches to ethical decision making. It requires a systematic framework for addressing the complex and often controversial moral questions.

Ethical dilemma A difficult choice or issue that requires the application of standards or principles to solve. Issues that challenge us ethically.

Ethical, social, and legal implications (ESLI) Consideration and understanding of the ethical, social, or legal connections or aspects of an issue that relate to a moral question of right and wrong.

Ethicist Expert in the arbitrary, ambiguous, and ungrounded judgments of other people. Ethicists know that they make the best decision they can based on the situation and stakeholders at hand.

Ethics A process of systematically examining varying viewpoints related to moral questions of right and wrong.

Eudaemonistic A system of ethical evaluation that involves consideration of which actions lead to being an excellent and happy person.

Events Occurrences that might be significant to other objects in a system or to external agents; for example, creating a laboratory request is an example of a health care event in a laboratory application. An event is defined and could be a triggering event for the task or work flow; a task or work flow can have several triggering events.

Evidence Artifacts, productions, attestations, or other examples that demonstrate an individual's knowledge, skills, or valued attributes.

Evidence-based practice (EBP) Health care professional practice that is informed by research-generated evidence of best practices.

Exabyte (EB) One quintillion bytes of computer memory.

Execute To carry out software's or a program's instructions.

Exploratory data analysis (EDA) Approach or philosophy that uses mainly graphical techniques to gain insight into a data set. It identifies the most important variables. Conducted during the exploratory phase, EDA provides guidance into the complexity or general nature of the various models that should be considered for implementation during pattern discovery.

Extensibility System design feature that allows for future expansion without the need for changes to the basic infrastructure.

Face-to-face Most widely used teaching method among educators, where the teacher and the learners meet together in one location at the same time.

Failure modes and effects analysis (FMEA) A systematic evaluation of a process to determine how and why it failed to produce the desired results.

Fair use Doctrine that permits the limited use of original works without the copyright holder's permission; an example would be quoting or citing an author in a scholarly manuscript.

Federal Health Information Exchange (FHIE) A federal information technology health care initiative that enables the secure electronic one-way exchange of patient medical information from the Department of Defense's legacy health information system, the Composite Health Care System, for all separated service members to the Veterans Affairs VistA Computerized Patient Record System. The point of care in veterans' affairs.

Feedback Input in the form of opinions about or reactions to something such as shared knowledge. In an information system, feedback refers to information from the system that is used to make modifications in the input, processing actions, or outputs.

Fidelity The extent to which a simulation mimics the processes of a real environment.

Field Column or attribute of an entity in a database.

Field study Study in which end users evaluate a prototype in the actual work setting prior to its general release. Also called field test, alpha test, or beta test.

Financial system System used to manage the expenses and revenues accrued while providing health care. The finance, auditing, and accounting departments within an organization most commonly use financial systems. These systems determine the direction for maintenance and growth for a given facility. Financial systems often interface to share information with materials management, staffing, and billing systems to balance the financial impact of these resources within an organization. These systems report the fiscal outcomes so that these outcomes can be tracked against the organizational goals of an institution. Financial systems are one of the major decision-making factors as health care institutions prepare their fiscal budgets. They often play a pivotal role in determining the strategic direction for an organization.

Firewall A tool commonly used by organizations to protect their corporate networks when they are attached to the Internet. A firewall can be hardware, software, or a combination of the two. It examines all incoming messages or traffic to the network. The firewall can be set up to allow only messages from known senders into the corporate network; it can also be set up to look at outgoing information from the corporate network.

FireWire Apple Computer's version of a high-performance serial bus used to connect devices to a computer.

Firmware Hardware and software programs or data written onto ROM, PROM, and EPROM.

Flash drive Small, removable storage device.

Flash memory Special type of EEPROM that can be erased and reprogrammed in blocks instead of one byte at a time. Many modern PCs have their BIOS stored on a flash memory chip so that it can easily be updated if necessary.

Foundation of Knowledge model A model proposing that humans are organic information systems constantly acquiring, processing, generating, and disseminating information or knowledge in both their professional and their personal lives. The organizing framework of this text.

Genome A body of genes. Hans Winkler is credited with merging *genesis* and *soma* (*genome*) to create this term.

Genomics The study of the genome.

Gigabyte (GB) Unit of measure used to express bytes of data storage and capability in computer systems; 1 gigabyte equals 1,000 megabytes.

Gigahertz (GHz) Unit of measure used to express speed and power of some components such as the microprocessor; 1 gigahertz equals 1,000 megahertz.

Good Favorable outcome in ethics.

Google Glass A wearable computer from Google that can take pictures, play video, and display text messages without anyone else knowing.

Gramm-Leach-Bliley Act (GLBA) Federal legislation in the United States that controls how financial institutions handle the private information they collect from individuals.

Graphical user interface (GUI) Software that provides a user-friendly desktop metaphor interface that is made up of the input and output devices as well as icons that represent files, programs, actions, and processes.

Graphics card A board that plugs into a personal computer to give it display capabilities.

Gray gap A term used to reflect the age disparities in computer connectivity; there are fewer persons older than age 65 who use computer technology than members of younger age-groups.

Gulf of evaluation The gap between knowing one's intention (goal) and knowing the effects of one's actions.

Gulf of execution The gap between knowing what one wants to have happen (the goal) and knowing what to do to bring it about (the means to achieve the goal).

Hacker Computer-savvy individual most commonly thought of as a malicious person who hacks or breaks through security to steal or alter data and information; can also be any of a group of computer aficionados who band together in clubs and organizations or who use their skills as a hobby.

Half-life of knowledge The time span from when knowledge is gained to when it becomes obsolete.

Haplotype Set of closely linked alleles on a chromosome that tends to be inherited together.

Hard disk Magnetic disk that stores electronic data.

Hard drive Permanent data storage area that holds the data, information, documents, and programs saved on the computer, even when the computer is shut off. The actual physical body of the computer and its components.

Hardware Physical or tangible parts of the computer. Computer parts that one can touch and that are involved in the performance or function of the computer, such as the keyboard and monitor.

Harm Physical or mental injury or damage. Unfavorable outcome in ethics.

Health disparities The health status differences between different groups of people, especially minorities and nonminorities; the gaps between the health status of minorities and nonminorities in the United States are ongoing even with the advances in technology and health care practices.

Health informatics (HI) A specialty that integrates concepts from a disciplinary science, computer science, information science, and cognitive science to manage and communicate data, information, knowledge, and wisdom in the delivery of health care.

Health information Data that has been interpreted regarding the state of one's level of wellness or illness; Information that is related to health and well-being of a person, especially information related to therapeutic (care) interactions between people and health care providers.

Health information exchange (HIE) Organization that prepares and organizes people and resources to manage health care information electronically across organizations within a community or region.

Health Information Portability and Accountability Act (HIPAA) Law signed by President Bill Clinton in 1996 addressing the need for standards to regulate and safeguard health information and making provisions for health insurance coverage for employed persons who change jobs.

Health information technology (HIT) Hardware, software, integrated technologies or related licenses, intellectual property, upgrades, or packaged solutions sold as services that are designed for or support the use by health care entities or patients for the electronic creation, maintenance, access, or exchange of health information.

Health Information Technology for Economic and Clinical Health (HITECH) Act Title XIII of the American Recovery and Reinvestment Act, which was enacted in February 2009. Under this act, health care organizations can qualify for financial incentives based on the level of meaningful use achieved; the HITECH Act specifically incentivizes health organizations and providers to become "meaningful users."

Health Insurance Portability and Accountability Act (HIPAA) Federal law enacted in 1996 to curtail health-care fraud and abuse, enforce standards for health information, guarantee the security and privacy of health information, and ensure health insurance portability for employed persons.

Health Level 7 (HL7) An accredited standards-developing organization that is committed to developing standard terminologies for information technology that support interoperability of health care information management systems.

Health literacy The acquisition of knowledge that promotes the ability to understand and to manage one's health.

Health management information system (HMIS) An information system that is specially intended to support and help with the planning, resource allocation, and management of health programming to make health care more effective and efficient; an information system that plans and manages health programs rather than the actual delivery of health care.

Heuristic evaluation An evaluation in which a small number of evaluators (often experts in relevant fields such as human factors or cognitive engineering) evaluate the degree to which an interface design complies with recognized usability principles (the "heuristics").

High fidelity A high level of realism generated by the equipment used in simulations.

High-hazard drug A drug known to cause significant adverse side effects when administered inappropriately; a drug subject to frequent administration errors.

HONcode One of the two most common symbols that power users look for to identify trusted health sites.

Hospital information system (HIS) An information system intended to manage the clinical, financial, and administrative needs of the hospital; refers to the paper-based as well as computer-based information processing that manages the functional aspects (administrative, financial, and clinical) of a hospital.

Human—computer interaction (HCI) The study of how people use computers and software applications and the ways that computers influence people.

Human—computer interface The hardware and software through which the user interacts with the computer.

Human factors Characteristics of people that influence the ways in which they interact with technology.

Human factors engineering Recognizing the limitations of human performance and developing products to overcome these limitations.

Human Genome Project (HGP) A 13-year project designed to identify all of the 20,000 to 25,000 genes in human DNA, determine the sequences of 3 billion chemical base pairs in human DNA, create databases to store this information, and address the resultant ethical, legal, and social issues.

Human mental workload The stress or work imposed on the mind by interacting with technologies.

Human—technology interaction (HTI) How users interact with technology. The study of that interaction.

Human—technology interface The hardware and software through which the user interacts with any technology (e.g., computers, patient monitors, telephone).

Hybrid A descriptor for individual courses in which instruction is delivered using multiple formats such as online, face-to-face, print based, or audio or videoconference (e.g., PicTel).

Hypertext Clickable words that allow users to access another document at a remote location.

Indiana Health Information Exchange (IHIE) A collaborative effort among institutions in Indiana to provide high-quality patient care and enhance the safety and efficiency of health care.

Informaticist A person with specialized training or certification in informatics; one who is a specialist in using technology to manage health data and information.

Informatics A field that integrates a specialty's science, computer science, cognitive science, and information science to manage and communicate data, information, knowledge, and wisdom in a specialty's practice.

Information Data that are interpreted, organized, or structured. Data processed using knowledge or data made functional through the application of knowledge.

Information Age Period at the end of the 20th century, when information was easily accessible using computers, networks, and the Internet.

Information literacy Recognizing when information is needed and having the ability to locate, evaluate, and effectively use the needed information. An intellectual framework for finding, understanding, evaluating, and using information.

Information science The science of information, studying the application and usage of information and knowledge in organizations and the interfacings or interaction between people, organizations, and information systems. An extensive, interdisciplinary science that integrates features from cognitive science, communication science, computer science, library science, and social sciences.

Information system (IS) The manual and/or automated components of a system of users or people, recorded data, and actions used to process the data into information for a user, group of users, or an organization.

Information technology (IT) Use of hardware, software, services, and supporting infrastructure to manage and deliver information using voice, data, and video or the use of technologies from computing, electronics, and telecommunications to process and distribute information in digital and other forms. Anything related to computing technology, such as networking, hardware, software, the Internet, or the people who work with these technologies. Many hospitals have such departments for managing the computers, networks, and other technical areas of the health care industry.

Input Data and information entered into a computer system.

Input devices Hardware and software used to enter data and information into a computer.

Instant message (IM) Form of real-time communication between two or more people based on typed text conveyed via computers connected over a network.

Integrated drive electronics (IDE) Technology where the drive controller is located on the drive itself instead of being a separate controller connected to the motherboard of a computer.

Integration Assimilating or combining to make whole; in computer terminology, the process through which different technologies—software and hardware components—are synchronized and combined to make a functional and structural system.

Integrity Quality and accuracy. Employees need to have confidence that the information they are provided is, in fact, true. To accomplish this, organizations need clear policies to clarify how data are actually input, to determine who has the authorization to change such data, and to track how and when data are changed.

Intelligence Mental ability to think logically, reason, prepare, ideate, assess alternative solutions to problems, problem solve by choosing a proposed solution, think abstractly, comprehend and grasp ideas, understand and use language, and learn.

Interactions Interfacing with users, commonly using tasks or notifications.

Interactive technologies Technologies that promote or support user communication with other persons (e.g., e-mail) or technologies that depend on a user response (e.g., games).

Interdisciplinary collaboration Members of various disciplines in a health care organization, who work together, each contributing unique knowledge to problem-solving or management of patient care situations.

Interface Mechanism or a system used by separate things to interact. For example, if one wants to change a CD in a CD player, one could use a remote; the human user is not related to the CD player but can interact with it using the remote control. Therefore, the remote control becomes the interface that enables that person to tell the CD player which CD to play.

International Organization for Standardization (ISO) An international network supporting collaboration among the standards-developing agencies of numerous countries for the development of consistent standards in a multitude of industries to support a global economy. ISO is best known in the technology industries for the ISO 9000 standards. *See* International Standards Organization.

Internet A global system of computer networks whose connectivity promotes worldwide communications via computers.

Internet2 A nonprofit consortium that develops and deploys advanced network applications and technologies for education and high-speed data transfer purposes. Led by 212 universities, it is also known as University Corporation for Advanced Internet Development.

Internet browser Software used to locate and display webpages. Also known as Web browser or browser.

Interoperability Ability of various systems and organizations to work together to exchange information.

Interprofessional collaboration Various health care professionals, each contributing unique knowledge, working together to problem-solve or manage patient care situations.

Intranet A computer network that is contained within an enterprise and that has restricted access; it has the look and feel of the Internet and often provides links to the Internet. The purpose of an intranet varies but can include provision of employee and departmental

directories, policies and procedures, internal and external resources, schedules, and updates on programs and business. The benefits are browsing capabilities and the ability to maintain contact information and phone numbers in a central location, with easy dissemination.

Intrusion detection devices Both hardware and software that allow an organization to monitor who is using its network and which files that user has accessed.

Intrusion detection system Method of security that uses both hardware and software detection devices as a system that can be set up to monitor a single computer or an entire network. Corporations must diligently monitor for unauthorized access of their networks.

Intuition A way of acquiring knowledge that cannot be obtained by inference, deduction, observation, reason, analysis, or experience.

Iowa model A model that facilitates the translation of research evidence into clinical practice. Also known as the Iowa model of evidence-based practice.

iPod The name given to a family of portable MP3 players from Apple Computer.

Iteration Replication and refinement of a method until it meets a goal or provides the desired result; each repetition is referred to as an iteration.

Jump drive Small, removable storage device.

Justice Fairness. Treatment of everyone in the same way.

Key field Within each database record, one of the fields identified as the primary key. It contains a code, name, number, or other bit of information that acts as a unique identifier for that record. In a health care system, for example, a patient is assigned a patient number or ID that is unique for that patient.

Keyboard Set of keys resembling an actual typewriter that permits the user to input data into a computer.

Know—do gap Situation that exists because solutions to global health problems are available but are not implemented in a timely fashion because of the lack of access to important health information. The Internet connections in developing countries are widely scattered, for example, and may not be efficient or sufficient for viewing health care information.

Knowledge The awareness and understanding of a set of information and ways that information can be made useful to support a specific task or arrive at a decision; abounds with others' thoughts and information. Information that is synthesized so that relationships are identified and formalized. Understanding that comes through a process of interaction or experience with the world around us. Information that has judgment applied to it or meaning extracted from it. Processed information that helps to clarify or explain some portion of our environment or world that we can use as a basis for action or on which we can act. Internal process of thinking or cognition. External process of testing, senses, observation, and interacting.

Knowledge acquisition The act of getting knowledge.

Knowledge brokers People who know where to find information and knowledge. They generate some knowledge but are mainly known for their ability to find what is needed.

Knowledge consumers Users of knowledge who do not have the expertise to provide the knowledge they need for themselves.

Knowledge discovery and data mining Using special analytics tools to aggregate data and uncover new understandings about that data.

Knowledge discovery in data A process of utilizing software to sort through data so as to discover patterns and ascertain or establish relationships. This process may help to discover or uncover previously unidentified relationships among the data in a database. Also known as data mining.

Knowledge discovery in databases A process of utilizing software to sort through data stored in a database to discover patterns and ascertain or establish previously unidentified relationships among the data in a database.

Knowledge dissemination Distribution and sharing of knowledge.

Knowledge domain process (KDP) model A model that represents knowledge construction and dissemination in an organization.

Knowledge exchange The product of collaboration when sharing an understanding of information promotes learning to make better decisions in the future.

Knowledge generation The creation of new knowledge by changing and evolving knowledge based on one's experience, education, and input from others.

Knowledge generators Health care researchers and experts—the people who know; they are able to answer questions, craft theories, find solutions to health problems or concerns, and innovate practice.

Knowledge management system (KMS) A repository of information that contains the latest collective expertise based on experience and research. The knowledge is

typically stored in a computerized system that promotes easy access for use.

Knowledge processing The activity or process of gathering or collecting, perceiving, analyzing, synthesizing, saving or storing, manipulating, conveying, and transmitting knowledge.

Knowledge repositories Collections of information made available to an organization's workers to support and inform their work.

Knowledge users Individuals or groups who benefit from valuable, viable knowledge.

Knowledge workers Those who work with information and generate information and knowledge as a product.

Laboratory information system A system that reports on blood, body fluid, and tissue samples along with biological specimens that are collected at the bedside and received in a central laboratory. These systems provide clinicians with reference ranges for tests indicating high, low, or normal values so that they can make care decisions. Often the laboratory system provides result information directing clinicians toward the next course of action within a treatment regimen.

Laptop Portable battery-powered computer that the user can take with him or her. Also known as a notebook.

Lean An organizational process where the focus is on value, safety, and optimal outcomes.

Length of stay (LOS) The duration of a single episode of hospitalization where the inpatient days are calculated by subtracting the day of submission from the day of discharge.

Liberty The independence from controlling influences.

Library science An interdisciplinary science that integrates law, applied science, and the humanities to study issues and topics related to libraries (collection, organization, preservation, archiving, and dissemination of information resources).

Logic A system of thinking that uses principles of inference and reasoned ideas to govern action.

Machine learning A subset of artificial intelligence that permits computers to learn either inductively or deductively. Inductive machine learning is the process of reasoning and making generalizations or extracting patterns and rules from huge data sets—that is, reasoning from a large number of examples to a general rule. Deductive machine learning moves from premises that are assumed true to conclusions that must be true if the premises are true.

Main memory A computer's internal memory.

Mainframe An extremely high-performance computer that is smaller than a supercomputer, used for high-volume, processor-intensive computing. Computers used by some large businesses and/or for scientific processing purposes.

Malicious code Software that includes spyware, viruses, worms, and Trojan horses with the intent of destroying or overtaking computer processing.

Malicious insider An insider or employee who sabotages or adds malicious code or hacks into systems to cause damage or to steal data and information.

Malware Malicious software; an evil, malicious program that infects a device and is intended to steal information, take control, irritate, damage, or destroy data, information, or the device.

Managed care information system An information system that crosses organizational boundaries so that data can be obtained at any and all of the patient areas; these information systems make it possible for health care professionals to make clinical decisions while being mindful of their financial ramifications.

Mapping How environmental facts (e.g., the order of light switches or variables in a physiologic monitoring display) are accurately depicted by the information presentation.

Mask Method that a proxy server uses to protect the identity of a corporation's employees while they are surfing the World Wide Web. The proxy server keeps track of which employees are using which masks and directs the traffic appropriately.

Massachusetts Health Data Consortium (MHDC) A consortium of regional health care organizations that collects data, publishes comparative information, supports and promotes electronic standards, educates, and researches.

Master patient index A tool that identifies, compares, removes duplicate entries, combines, and cleans patient records so that they can be added to a master index; it provides a comprehensive and single view of a patient via that person's record while establishing a master index of all patients.

Meaningful use The American Recovery and Reinvestment Act of 2009 specifies three main components of meaningful use: (1) the use of a certified electronic health record (EHR) in a meaningful manner, such as e-prescribing; (2) the use of certified EHR technology for electronic exchange of health information to improve quality of health care; and (3) the use of certified EHR technology to submit clinical quality and other measures. The criteria for meaningful use will be staged in three steps. Stage 1 (2011–2012) sets the baseline for electronic data capture and information sharing. Stage 2 (2013) and Stage 3 (expected to be implemented in 2015) will continue to expand on this baseline and be developed through future rule making.

Medical home/health information exchange An information technology platform that enables the seamless exchange of important patient information among many providers in a health care system. Typically, the primary care physician (medical home) initiates the collection of patient data, coordinates the care of the patient, and helps maintain the accuracy of such data. Other care providers access the information and add to it as they provide services to patients.

Medication management devices Range of telecommunications-ready medication devices to remind or otherwise alert patients to medication compliance needs.

MEDLINE A database that contains more than 10 million records, maintained and produced by the National Library of Medicine.

Megabyte (MB) Unit of measure used to express the amount of data storage and capability in computer systems; 1 megabyte equals 1,000 kilobytes.

Megahertz (MHz) Unit of measure used to express the speed and power of some components such as the microprocessor.

Memory Data stored in digital format; generally refers to random-access memory.

Meta-analysis A form of systematic review that uses statistical methods to combine the results of several research studies.

Meta-learning Learning that combines the predictions from several data mining models with the goal of synthesizing these predicted classifications to generate a final best predicted classification; also known as stacking.

Metadata Data about data; in data mining, data contained in the data mining model that describes other data. For example, metadata would describe the patterns, trends, and relationships of the mined data.

Metrics Measurements or a set of measurements to quantify performance; they provide understanding about the performance of a process or function. Typically, within clinical technology projects, one identifies and collects specific metrics about the performance of the technology or metrics that capture the level of participation or adoption. Equally important is the need for process performance metrics. Process metrics are collected at the initial stage of a project or problem identification. Current-state metrics are then benchmarked against internal indicators. When there are no internal indicators to benchmark against, a suitable course of action is to benchmark against an external source, such as a similar business practice within a different industry.

Microprocessor Chip that integrates the processor onto one circuit, incorporating the functions of the computer's central processing unit. Microprocessors continue to evolve in terms of their processing capacity.

Microsoft Surface A windows-based personal computing device. Its light weight and functionality make it especially attractive for point of care use.

Milestones Predetermined planned occurrences that indicate the completion or achievement of a deliverable.

Mind The brain's conscious processing; encompasses thought processes, memory, imagination and creativity, emotions, perceptions, and inner drive or will.

Modeling Using technology tools to create a simulation of reality.

Modem Hardware that allows a user to send and receive information over the phone or cable lines, for example, with a computer. It enables Internet connectivity via a telephone line or cable connection through network adapters situated within the computer apparatus.

Molecular biomarkers Metabolites; advances in bioinformatics technology, protein-based network biomarkers have been able to be studied. These biomarkers not only revealed the panel of protein interactions but also their interactions with RNA, DNA, and other molecules; both molecular biomarkers and protein-based network biomarkers have limitations because of their static nature.

Monitor Computer display that allows the user to view text and graphic images.

Moral dilemma Situation for which there is no clear evidence that one of several alternatives is morally right or wrong.

Moral rights Ethical privileges.

Morals Social conventions about right and wrong human conduct that are socially constructed and tacitly agreed on as good or right.

MoSCoW Must have, Should have, Could have, and Would have; an approach where a team works with stakeholders to develop a prioritized requirements list and a development plan.

Motherboard A key foundational computer component. All other components are connected to it in some way (either via local sockets, attached directly to it, or connected via cables). The essential structures of the motherboard include the major chipset, super I/O chip, BIOS, read-only memory, bus communications pathways, and a variety of sockets that allow components to plug into it.

Mouse A small device that one can roll along or scroll to control the movement of the pointer or cursor on a display and click to search for and/or execute features.

MP3 aggregator A program that can facilitate the process of finding, subscribing to, and downloading podcasts. A commonly known aggregator is Apple Computer's iTunes, which is a free program available as a download from Apple.com. Using a program such as iTunes gives the user the ability to search for podcasts based on many criteria, including category, author, or title. iTunes provides access to audio downloads, which may be either songs or podcasts.

MPEG-1 Audio Layer-3 (MP3) Digital or electronic audio programming format.

Multidimensional database Type of database that combines data from numerous data sources and is optimized for online analytical processing applications; uses multidimensional structures to organize the data, and each data attribute is considered as a separate dimension.

Multimedia A computer-based technology that incorporates traditional forms of communication to create a seamless and interactive learning environment.

Multispatial Relating to the need for educators in the age of technology to account for both physical and virtual spaces and their relationship to the learning process.

National Center for Public Health Informatics (NCPHI) Center created in 2005 by the Centers for Disease Control and Prevention to provide leadership in the field of public health informatics.

National Guideline Clearinghouse (NGC) A comprehensive database of clinical practice guidelines developed as a result of research. The NGC website allows users to browse for clinical guidelines, view abstracts and full-text links, download full-text clinical guidelines to personal digital assistants, obtain technical reports, and compare guidelines.

National Health and Nutrition Examination Survey (NHANES) A survey sponsored by the Centers for Disease Control and Prevention that combines both questionnaires and physical examinations to collect data on the health and nutritional status of adults and children in the United States.

National Health Information Infrastructure (NHII) An initiative intended to improve the effectiveness, efficiency, and overall quality of health and health care in the United States. A comprehensive knowledge-based network of interoperable systems of clinical, public health, and personal health information that would improve decision making by making health information available when and where it is needed. The set of technologies, standards, applications, systems, values, and laws that support all facets of individual health, health care, and public health. The infrastructure is voluntary and not a centralized database of medical records or a government regulation.

National health information network An agency of the U.S. Department of Health and Human Services charged with the development of a safe, secure, interoperable health information infrastructure. Also known as the Nationwide health information network.

National Institute of Standards and Technology (NIST) A nonregulatory federal agency within the U.S. Department of Commerce that was founded in 1901; its mission is to promote U.S. innovation and industrial competitiveness by advancing measurement science, standards, and technology in ways that enhance economic security and improve the quality of life. From automated teller machines and atomic clocks to mammograms and semiconductors, innumerable products and services rely in some way on technology, measurement, and standards provided by NIST.

Nationwide Health Information Network (NHIN) An agency of the U.S. Department of Health and Human Services charged with the development of a safe, secure, interoperable health information infrastructure.

Negligence A departure from the standard of due care—prudent, reasonable care—toward others, including intentionally posing risks that are unreasonable as well as unintentionally but carelessly imposing risks.

Negligent insider An employee of a healthcare organization who imposes risks to privacy and security of the technology infrastructure by acting outside of the accepted standards for protecting information, such as writing down network passwords, leaving workstations unattended without logging off, or transferring sensitive data to unapproved storage devices.

Net generation Students used to surfing the Web and interacting online.

Network Connection of computers that can be local and/or organizationally based, joined together into a local area network, on a wider area scope (such as a city or district) using a metropolitan area network, or from an even greater distance (e.g., a whole country or continent or the Internet in general) using a wide area network configuration.

Network accessibility The ability of the network to be accessed by the right user to obtain what that person needs when he or she needs it.

Network availability The state in which network information is accessible when needed.

Network security The specific precautions taken to ensure that the integrity of a network is safe from unauthorized entry and that the data and information stored on the network are accessible only by authorized users.

Neural network A nonlinear predictive model. Such models learn by training and resembling the structure of biological neural networks. Neural networks model the neural behavior of the human brain and are a way to bridge the gap between computers and humans.

Neuroscience The study of the nervous system.

New England Health EDI Network (NEHEN) An example of an implementation model for building regional health information organizations that are functional, sustainable, and growing while reducing administrative costs.

Next-Generation Internet (NGI) A government project to develop new, faster technologies to enhance research and communication.

Nicomachean An approach to ethical thinking based on the work of Aristotle.

Nonmaleficence Doing no harm.

Nonsynchronous That which is not in realtime or does not occur or exist at the same time, having the same period or time frame. Occurring anywhere and anytime using Internet and World Wide Web software tools (e.g., course management systems, e-mail, electronic bulletin boards, and webpages) as the principal delivery mechanisms.

Object-oriented systems development A process of designing systems in sets of interacting objects allowing for changes to objects in the system when a process needs to be modified as opposed to changing the entire architecture of a system.

Office of Civil Rights (OCR) Part of the U.S. Department of Health and Human Services and responsible for enforcing the Health Insurance Portability and Accountability Act. It provides significant information and guidance to clinicians who must comply with the Privacy and Security Rules. It has been tracking complaints and investigating violations since 2003.

Office of the National Coordinator for Health Information Technology (ONC) An office within the U.S. Department of Health and Human Services that was established through the HITECH Act. The ONC is headed by the national coordinator, who is responsible for overseeing the development of a nationwide health information technology infrastructure that supports the use and exchange of information.

Office suite Software that is generally distributed together with a consistent user interface that is designed for knowledge workers and clerical personnel. These software packages can interact with each other to enhance productivity and ease of use.

One health Health care delivery approach implemented by interprofessional teams working together to improve the health of animals and humans alike to improve the collective health of a community or population.

Online Something accomplished over a distance or on the Internet while connected to or using a computer.

Online analytic processing (OLAP) A fast analysis of shared data stored in a multidimensional database that allows the user to easily and selectively extract and view data from different points of view. OLAP and data mining complement each other even though they are quite different.

Online chat Synchronous interaction with another person facilitated by an Internet connection technology.

Open Access Initiative A worldwide movement to make a library of knowledge available to anyone with Internet access.

Open-source software (OSS) Computer software where the source code is made available for use and/or modification without charge. The developers share code in the hopes that the software will evolve as others modify and improve on the base.

Open Systems Interconnection (OSI) A model of standardization for communications in a network developed to ensure that various programs would work efficiently with one another.

Operating system (OS) The most important software on any computer. It is the very first program to load on computer start-up and is fundamental for the operation of all other software as well as the computer's hardware.

Operations Jobs or tasks related to information management whereby data are input to a system and manipulated to produce an output. A series of operations constitute a process.

Order entry management A program that allows a clinician to enter medication and other care orders directly into a computer, including orders for laboratory, microbiology, pathology, radiology, nursing, and medicine; supply orders; ancillary services; and consults.

Order entry system A system that automates the way that orders are initiated for patients. Clinicians place orders within these systems instead of using traditional handwritten transcription onto paper. Such systems provide major safeguards by ensuring that physician orders are legible and complete, thereby providing a level of patient safety that was historically missing with paper-based orders. They also provide decision support and automated alert functionality that was previously unavailable with paper-based orders.

Outcome Changes, results, and/or impacts from inputting and processing.

Output Changes that exit a system and that can activate or modify processing.

Palm computer Miniature or small computer that fits in the palm of the hand.

Parallel port Interface for connecting an external device that is capable of receiving more than 1 bit at a time.

Password A code established by the user to identify himself or herself when the user enters the system. Most organizations today enforce a strong password policy. Strong password policies include using combinations of letters, numbers, and special characters, such as plus (+) signs and ampersands (&). Policies typically include the enforcement of changing passwords every 30 or 60 days.

Patient care information system (PCIS) Patient-centered information systems focused on collecting data and disseminating information related to direct care. Several of these systems have become mainstream types of systems used in health care. The four types of systems most commonly found in health care organizations include (1) clinical documentation systems, (2) pharmacy information systems, (3) laboratory information systems, and (4) radiology information systems.

Patient care support system System of components that make up each of the specialty disciplines within health care and their associated patient care information systems. The four types of systems most commonly found in health care organizations include (1) clinical documentation systems, (2) pharmacy information systems, (3) laboratory information systems, and (4) radiology information systems.

Patient centered Focused on the patient as the essential element in an interaction.

Patient-centered care Focused on the patient/person (rather than on the illness/health care professional), with patients becoming active participants in their own health care initiatives. Patients as active participants receive services designed to meet their individual needs and preferences, under the guidance and counsel of their health care professionals. Data, observations, interventions, and outcomes focused on direct patient care.

Patient engagement Encouraging patients to take responsibility for their own health, including helping them to acquire knowledge about their health challenges and ways to promote and maintain health.

Patient support The total array of tools and software that can be used to provide information and assistance to help meet the health care needs of consumers.

Payment Monetary compensation for goods or services received.

Perception The process of acquiring knowledge about the environment or situation by obtaining, interpreting, selecting, and organizing sensory information from seeing, hearing, touching, tasting, and smelling. Sensory experience foundational to formulating knowledge.

Peripheral biometric (medical) devices A variety of telecommunications-ready measurement devices, such as blood pressure cuffs and blood glucose meters, that typically use the household telephone jack to transmit patient data to a central server location. Examples of commonly used peripheral devices include a weight scale, blood pressure monitor, pulse oximeter, thermometer, glucometer, spirometer, prothrombin/international normalized ratio meter, digital camera (to capture images of wounds), and a personal digital assistant—based or telephonic self-reporting device.

Peripheral component interconnection (PCI) Mechanism for attaching peripheral devices to a motherboard via computer bus, expansion slots, or integrated circuits.

Personal computer (PC) Computer made for individual use or directly used by an end user.

Personal digital assistant (PDA) A handheld device, miniature or small computer, or palmtop that uses a pen for inputting data instead of a keyboard. Also called a handheld computer. Also known as personal digital assistive.

Personal emergency response systems Signaling devices that enable patients to access emergency and other care needs.

Personalized medicine Interventions that are tailored to specific patients based on their genetic type, individual characteristics, preferences, and needs; also known as precision medicine.

Petabyte (PB) A unit of information or computer storage equal to 1 quadrillion bytes, or 1,000 terabytes.

Pharmacy information system Information system that facilitates the ordering, managing, and dispensing of medications for a facility. It also commonly incorporates allergy and height/weight information for effective medication management; it streamlines the order entry, dispensing, verification, and authorization process for medication administration while often interfacing with clinical documentation and order entry systems so that clinicians can order and document the administration of medications and prescriptions to patients while having the benefits of decision support alerting and interaction checking.

Picture archiving and communication system (PACS) System that is designed to collect, store, and distribute medical images such as computed tomography scans, magnetic resonance images, and X-rays; it replaces traditional hard-copy films with digital media that are easy to store, retrieve, and present to clinicians. This system may be a stand-alone system, separate from the main radiology system, or it can be integrated with a radiology information system and a computer information system. The benefit of such systems is their ability to assist in diagnosis and to store vital patient care support data.

Plug and play The ability to add new devices to a computer easily without having to manually install and reconfigure the computer to accept the device.

Podcast A digital media file or collection of related files that are distributed over the Internet using syndication or subscription feeds for playback on portable media players, such as MP3 players, laptops, and personal computers; the subscription relies on RSS feeds. Online media delivery. Enhanced podcasts contain slides and pictures; vodcasts contain videos.

Policy Basic principle that guides behavior and performance and is enforced. For example, in a corporation, corporate policy would be enforced by corporate administration; the U.S. government enforces public policy.

Population health management A term adopted by health care management companies to express their goal of achieving optimal health outcomes at a reasonable cost. The management process involves data collection and trend analyses that are used to predict clinical outcomes in a group of people.

Port Interface between a computer and other devices or other computers.

Portability Ability to be transported easily. For example, users can easily take handheld computers wherever they go.

Portable Operating System Interface for Unix (POSIX) A uniform set of standards adopted by the Institute of Electrical and Electronics Engineers and the International Standards Organization that define an interface between programs and operating systems. The standardization ensures that software can be easily ported to other POSIX-compliant operating systems.

Portals Tools for organizing information from webpages into simple menus on one's desktop. A tool for patient engagement with health care providers and organizations. Also, multifunctional telehealth care platforms for receiving, retrieving, and/or displaying patients' vital signs and other information transmitted from telecommunications-ready medical devices.

Portfolio A collection of evidence used to demonstrate knowledge and skill achievement. An education portfolio provides the opportunity for a student to document a variety of sometimes unquantifiable skills, such as creativity, communication, and critical thinking.

Power supply A device that supplies electrical energy or power; the device that provides the electrical energy or power to the computer. A battery can be a source of energy or power.

Precision medicine Interventions that are tailored to specific patients based on their genetic type, individual characteristics, preferences, and needs; also known as personalized medicine.

Presence The act of being fully there and being fully with patients; exclusively focusing on patients and their unique needs.

Presentation Act of presenting or showing; typically uses presentation software in a slide show format. The most commonly used presentation software in the United States is Microsoft PowerPoint.

Primary key A field within a record (also known as the key field) that contains a code, name, number, or other bit of information that acts as a unique identifier for that record. In a health care system, for example, a patient is assigned a patient number or ID that is unique for that patient.

Principlism A foundation for ethical decision making. Principles are expansive enough to be shared by all rational individuals regardless of their background and individual beliefs.

Privacy An important issue related to personal information, about the owner or about other individuals, that focuses on sharing this information with others electronically and the mechanisms that restrict access to this personal information.

Problem based Typically refers to a type of student-centered instructional strategy where students collaboratively solve problems and reflect on their experiences.

Problem solving Cognitive process of critically thinking through a problem or issue to determine a course of action.

Process analysis Breaking down the work process into a sequential series of steps that can be examined and assessed to improve effectiveness and efficiency; explains how work takes place and gets done or how it can be done.

Process owners Those persons who directly engage in the work flow to be analyzed and redesigned and have the ultimate responsibility for the performance of the process. These individuals can speak about the intricacy of the process, including process variations from the normal. When constructing a team, it is important to include individuals who are able to contribute information about the exact current-state work flow and offer suggestions for future-state improvements.

Processing Acting on something by taking it through established procedures so as to convert it from one form to another. Examples include the processing of information into data and the processing of a credit application to get a loan.

Productivity software Programs or software that help us compose, create, or develop. An example is the Microsoft Office suite of productivity tools, which offers word processing, spreadsheet, database, presentation, and Web tools to help us complete both professional and personal tasks.

Professional development Acquisition of skills required for maintaining a specific career path or general skills offered through continuing education, including the more general skills area of personal development. It can be seen as training to keep current with changing technology and practices in a profession or as part of the concept of lifelong learning.

Professional networking Connecting with other professionals in a field with a predetermined and focused purpose as well as an identified target audience in mind.

Programmable read-only memory (PROM) Form of digital memory where the setting of each bit is locked on a chip by a fuse or antifuse. PROM is used to store programs permanently, so it is useful in applications where the programming needs to be permanent. The device cannot be erased, so it must be replaced if changes are deemed necessary in the system.

Protected health information (PHI) Any and all information about a person's health that is tied to any type of personal identification.

Protein-based network biomarkers Advances in bioinformatics technology, protein-based network biomarkers have been able to be studied. These biomarkers revealed not only the panel of proteins interactions but also their interactions with RNA, DNA, and other molecules. Both molecular biomarkers and protein-based network biomarkers have limitations because of their static nature.

Prototype Original mock-up or first model; original form that is studied, tested, and processed before duplication.

Proxy server Hardware security tool to help protect an organization against security breaches.

Psychology The field that studies the mind and behavior.

PsycINFO A comprehensive database in the field of education and psychology.

Public health The science of protecting the well-being of communities and the population through education, research, intervention, and prevention.

Public health informatics (PHI) An aspect of informatics focused on the promotion of health and disease prevention in populations and communities.

Public health interventions Actions taken to promote and secure the well-being of a population or a community.

Publishing The process of production and dissemination of information.

Qualified electronic health record An electronic record containing health-related information on an individual that consists of the individual's demographic and clinical health information, including medical history and a list of health problems, and that supports entry of physician orders. A qualified electronic health record can capture and query information relevant to health care quality and exchange electronic health information with and assimilate such information from other sources to provide support for clinical decision making.

Qualitative study A type of research design that focuses on the human experience of a phenomenon using words, concepts, language, and meanings rather than numbers to capture the essence of the subject under study. Subjective study.

Quality A level or grade of excellence; relative merit; a distinct or essential characteristic, attribute, or property.

Quantitative study Research that looks at the *what*, *where*, and *when* to provide understanding of phenomena based on quantifying data and using statistical measures; depending on the research, a study may ascertain cause-and-effect relationships. Objective study.

Query A form of questioning. A request for information; an example would be a database query.

QWERTY Name given to the typical computer keyboard layout, derived from the six letters in the first row below the numeric or number row.

Radio-frequency identification (RFID) chip An identification chip that stores information for retrieval.

Radio-frequency identifier (RFI) A reprogrammable chip that communicates with a reader to aid in identifying an object.

Radiology information system (RIS) Information system designed to schedule, report, and store information as it relates to diagnostic radiology procedures. One common feature found in most radiology systems is a picture archiving and communication system (PACS). The benefit of RISs and PACSs is their ability to assist in diagnosing complex cases and storing vital patient care support data.

Random-access memory (RAM) Volatile, temporary storage system that allows a computer's processor to access program codes and data while working on a task. RAM is lost once the system is rebooted, shut off, or loses power.

Rapid application development (RAD) A method using prototyping and reiteration to develop products faster and of superior quality.

Rapid prototyping Creation of a computer generated 3-D model of a physical part that is printed on a 3-D printer to allow for immediate testing and remodeling. These processes will be huge in the future to support 3-D printing of body parts such as joint replacements.

Rapid Syndromic Validation Project (RSVP) System where local health care professionals report cases such as influenza. Data are analyzed centrally, and the resulting information is shared with appropriate local authorities in an attempt to identify outbreaks early and prevent the spread of contagious diseases.

Rationalism An ethical position that contends that knowledge is derived from deductive reasoning and not from the senses.

Read-only memory (ROM) Essential permanent or semi-permanent, nonvolatile memory that stores saved data and is critical in the working of the computer's operating system and other activities. ROM is stored primarily in the motherboard but may also be available through the graphics card, other expansion cards, and peripherals.

Real time Human time; occurs live, with users or learners interacting at the same time.

Real-time telehealth Live interactions between two or more clinicians, usually performed with videoconferencing equipment.

Really simple syndication (RSS) A form of web feed used to publish frequently updated content in podcasts, blog entries, or even news headlines. Subscribers receive update notices whenever new content is added or a site is updated. Also known as RDF site summary (RSS 1.0 and RSS 0.90) and rich site summary (RSS 0.91).

Reasoning Way of thinking, calculating, interpreting, or introspectively rethinking or critically thinking through an issue; reflective thought to analyze or think through one's ideas and alternatives.

Record Row in a relational database representing one patient, for example; also called a tuple. Group of related fields in a database. To record or capture audio and video using specific devices.

Reflective commentary Narrative comments that focus on why an individual thinks specific evidence is important, the ways in which the individual values what he or she has learned, or why the individual thinks the evidence is important for his or her profession.

Regional health information exchange *See* health information exchange.

Relational database A database that can store and retrieve data very rapidly. "Relational" refers to how the data are stored in the database and how they are organized.

Relational database management system (RDBMS) A system that manages data using the relational model. A relational database could link a patient's table to a treatment table, for example, by a common field such as the patient ID number field.

Reporting The act of using of documents or information system outputs to convey information to stakeholders.

Reports Documents that contain data or information based on a query or investigation designed to yield customized content in relation to a situation and a user, a group of users, or an organization. Designed to inform, reports may include recommendations or suggestions based on programming and other embedded parameters.

Repository Central place where data are collected, stored, and maintained. Central location for multiple databases or files that can be distributed over a network or directly accessible to the user. Location for files and databases so that the data can be reused, analyzed, explored, or repurposed.

Research utilization (RU) The process of moving new understandings generated in research into practice.

Research validity A conclusion that can be drawn about the conduct of research based on an analysis of the research design and methods (internal validity) and the applicability of the findings to the general population (external validity).

Resource description framework (RDF) A structure of consistent semantics adopted by the World Wide Web Consortium to promote encoding, exchange, and reuse of metadata.

Results management An approach to evaluating the outcomes of a process to determine whether that process was useful or valuable.

Return on investment A measure to compare the effectiveness of an IT or equipment purchase.

Rights Privileges; include the right to privacy, confidentiality, and so on.

Risk Possibility of loss, injury, illness or death or when a person places him- or herself or others in danger; expectation that a threat may succeed and the potential damage that can occur. In health care, we assess for risks to prevent them, identify health problems arising from them, or develop priorities to deal with them.

Risk assessment Determination of risk or danger, such as assessing for risk factors related to heart disease.

Risk factor Something that increases someone's risk or susceptibility to loss, injury, illness, or death.

Role playing Situation that allows students to try on real-life scenarios by filling either prescribed or ad-libbed health care professional roles without the fear or pressure of putting another's life at risk while trying to determine the best course of action or find a solution to a fictitious patient's health issue.

Root-cause analysis Similar to failure modes and events analysis; analysis to discover why a process is faulty or produces an undesired result.

Row A record in a database; also known as a tuple.

Safety culture An organizational commitment to patient safety and the prevention of medical errors.

Sarbanes-Oxley Act (SOX) Legislation that was put in place to protect shareholders as well as the public from deceptive accounting practices in organizations.

Scenario Mock description of a situation or series of events.

Scheduling system A system designed to track resources within a facility while managing the frequency and distribution of those resources. For example, resource scheduling systems provide information about operating room utilization or availability of intensive care unit beds and other hospital beds.

Scoring The data mining process of applying a model to new data.

Second Life A proprietary virtual reality tool that allows users to create virtual communities.

Secure information Information that is protected from error, unauthorized access, and other threats that can compromise its integrity and safety.

Security Protection from danger or loss. In informatics, one must protect against unauthorized access, malicious damage, and incidental and accidental damage and enforce secure behavior and maintain security of computing, data, applications, information, and networks.

Security breach Any security violation.

Self-control Self-discipline. Strength of will.

SEMMA (sample, explore, modify, model, access) A data mining methodology where the user follows a series or prescribed steps—sample, explore, modify, model, access—to extract information from a database.

Sensor and activity-monitoring systems Systems for tracking activities of daily living of seniors and other at-risk individuals in their places of residence. Additional applications' use of sensors to detect anomalies or problems such as faucets and stoves left turned on.

Serial port An interface for connecting an external device that is capable of receiving only 1 bit at a time, such as a mouse, a modem, and some printers.

Server A computer or a group of computers that link computers together or provide services to a group of computers.

Shoulder surfing Watching over someone's back as he or she is working on a computer. This is still a major way that confidentiality is compromised.

Simulated documentation A replicated documentation system that health care professional students can use to learn how to access electronic health records and document care.

Simulation An imitation of a real-life event or circumstance; in health care professional education, the replication of a clinical scenario developed to provide an opportunity for practice in a mock situation.

Simulation scenario A virtual case situation developed in a simulation laboratory to mimic a clinical practice situation.

Simulator A mechanical or electronic device that provides an environment in which a simulation can occur. Some of these may be quite large.

Situational awareness The ability to detect, integrate, and understand critical information that leads to an overall understanding of a problem or situation.

Six Sigma/Lean Business management tactic that seeks to improve the quality of process outputs by identifying and removing the causes of imperfections (errors) and reducing inconsistency and variability in processes;

Lean and Six Sigma are a complementary combination of activities that focus on doing the right steps and actions (Lean) and doing them right the first time (Six Sigma).

Small Computer System Interface (SCSI) Set of standards for physically connecting and transferring data between computers and peripheral devices. The SCSI standards define commands, protocols, and electrical and optical interfaces. Standardization among commercial products helps to ensure that devices will interface with many different systems.

Smart pump Machine used to infuse medication that includes dose-checking technology and safeguards designed to help avert medication errors.

Smart room Patient room that is equipped with technologies to increase patient safety and improve patient care.

Smartphone A cell phone that has many personal digital assistant capabilities. Smartphones have some personal computer functionality; they have an operating system and facilitate the use of e-mail and other applications.

Social engineering The manipulation of a relationship based on one's position in an organization. For example, someone attempting to access a network may pretend to be an employee from the corporate information technology office who then simply asks for an employee's digital ID and password. Another example of social engineering is a hacker impersonating a federal government agent. After talking an employee into revealing network information, the hacker basically has an open door to enter the corporate network.

Social media Communication tools such as Twitter and Facebook that promote real-time information exchange.

Social sciences Collection of academic and scientific fields or disciplines concerned with the study of the human aspects of our world and environment.

Software Anything that can be stored electronically. Software is divided into two types: system software (includes the operating system and other software necessary for the computer to function) and application software (allows users to complete specific tasks, such as word processors, spreadsheet software, presentation software, database managers, and media players).

Sound card A computer expansion card that facilitates the input and output of audio signals to and from a computer under control of computer programs. Also known as an audio card.

Spreadsheet Text and numbers located in cells on a grid and the software necessary to process formulas and other computations, such as creating graphs and charts.

Spyware A program that may contain malicious code that may attack or attempt to "take over" a computer. Spyware may also be nonmalicious in intent and monitor the user's behavior in an attempt to gain information about the user for targeted advertising.

Stacking The process of synthesizing the predictions from several models.

Stakeholder An individual or group with the responsibility for completing a project and influencing the overall design and that is most impacted by success or failure of the system implementation.

Standard Benchmark. Criterion. Rule. Norm. Principle.

Standardized plan of care A plan that presents clinicians with treatment protocols to maximize their outcomes and support best practices.

Standards-developing organization (SDO) An organization that creates guidelines, standards, and rules to help health care entities collect, store, manipulate, dispose of, and exchange secure protected health information.

Static medium Something that cannot be updated; for example, a print-based brochure may be outdated almost as soon as it is printed.

Store-and-forward telehealth transmission An application of telehealth care in which images and other clinical data are captured and transmitted to specialist clinicians.

Structured English Query Language (SQL) (Pronounced "sequel.") A database querying language rather than a programming language. SQL is a standard language for accessing and manipulating databases. It simplifies the process of retrieving information from a database in a functional or usable form while facilitating the reorganization of data within the database.

Suicide Prevention Community Assessment Tool Risk assessment method that addresses general community information, prevention networks, and the demographics of the target population as well as community assets and risk factors.

Summary A condensed version of the original designed to highlight its major points.

Supercomputer The fastest computer; designed to run special applications that require numerous calculations.

Surveillance The act of watching for trends in health-related data for early detection of health threats.

Surveillance data system A networked computer system designed to use health-related data trends to predict the probability of an outbreak of a contagious or infectious disease or to detect morbidity and mortality trends in a geographic area as a precursor to public health planning or response.

Synchronous Realtime or occurring at the same time; having the same period or time frame. Learning anywhere and anytime in realtime using delivery modalities such as traditional face-to-face, Internet, and World Wide Web software tools (e.g., course management systems, chat, e-mail, electronic bulletin boards, audio/video communication tools).

Synchronous dynamic random-access memory (SDRAM) The most common type of dynamic random-access memory found in personal computers.

Syndromic surveillance A specialized system of data collection that seeks to detect trends in the incidence and severity of a specific disease or health-related syndrome and plan the public health response.

Synthesis Combining parts of existing material or ideas into a new entity or concept.

Systems development life cycle (SDLC) Stages involved in the life of a system, typically an information system; a model used in the project management of a system's development effort, spanning from feasibility to its demise.

Table A collection of related records in a database.

Task analysis Analytic technique that focuses on how a task must be accomplished, including detailed descriptions of task-related activities, task characteristics and complexity, and the environmental conditions required for a person to perform a given task.

Tasks Actions that are value added and necessary. For example, some tasks come about because of workarounds or for other unsubstantiated reasons. Tasks that are considered non—value added and are not necessary for the purpose of compliance or regulatory reasons should be eliminated from the future-state process.

Technology Method by which people use knowledge and tools. Knowledge used to solve problems, control and adapt to our environment, and extend human potential. Generally people use technology to refer to machines or devices such as computers and the infrastructure that supports them. For example, cell phones and planes are technologies that are tangible—one can see and touch them—but cannot see and touch the vast infrastructures supporting them, such as the wireless communications between the device (cell phone) and the cell towers and the electronic guidance used by the device (plane) to navigate the skies.

Telecommunications Broadcasting or transmitting signals over a distance from one person to another person or from one location to another location for the purpose of communication.

Telehealth Telecommunication technologies used to deliver health-related services or to connect patients and health care providers to maximize patients' health status. A relatively new term in the health care vocabulary, referring to a wide range of health services that are delivered by telecommunications-ready tools, such as the telephone, videophone, and computer.

Telehealth care Health services delivered by telecommunications-ready tools. Hardware and software tools capture patient data and transmit it via a communication hub where it is interpreted by a professional at another location. Some telehealth tools also allow for real-time interaction with patients in their homes.

Telemonitoring Remote measurement of patients' vital signs and other necessary data.

Telephony Telephone monitoring of patients at their residences by off-site health care professionals.

Teleradiology Use of telecommunications technology to electronically transmit and exchange radiographic patient images with the consultative text or radiologist reports from one location to another.

TELOS strategy An approach that provides a clear picture of the feasibility of a project; TELOS stands for "technologic and systems, economic, legal, operational, and schedule feasibility."

Terabyte (TB) A measurement term for data storage capacity. One terabyte equals 1,024 gigabytes.

Threat A harmful act, such as the deployment of a virus or illegal network penetration.

Throughput The amount of work a computer can do in a given time period; a measure of computer performance that can be used for system comparison.

Thumb drive Small, removable storage device.

Tiering Also referred to as data tiering; the process of monitoring data usage to reveal where data should be stored or warehoused. The most frequently accessed data will be housed in robust technologies for easy retrieval, while the less frequently accessed data could be placed in low-cost storage systems.

Touchscreen A display used as an input device for interacting with or relating to the display's materials or content. The user can touch or press on the designated display area to respond, execute, or request information or output.

Translational research Research that is conducted with a vision toward transforming clinical practice (translating the results into practice).

Transparent Done without conscious thought.

Treatment An intervention by a health professional designed to improve the status of a patient.

Triage The process of assessing patients who are ill or injured and determining the need for intervention based on the severity of the health issue. The practice of collecting, organizing, and prioritizing or ranking information to determine what is applicable or significant for scientific analyses, syntheses, and decision making.

Trojan horse Malicious code, capable of replicating within a computer, that is hidden in data or a program that appears to be safe.

Trust-e One of the two most common symbols that power users look for to identify trusted health sites.

Truth Fact. Certainty. Sincere action, character, and fidelity.

Tuple A record in a database; also known as a row.

Tutorial Learning materials available to the learner, who must then be self-directed to study the specific topical area presented.

Uncertainty Ambiguity. Insecurity. Vagueness.

Universal serial bus (USB) A means of connecting myriad plug-in devices, such as portable flash drives, digital cameras, MP3 players, graphics tablets, light pens, and so on, using a plug-and-play connection without rebooting the computer.

Unstructured data Data that are not contained in a database; data residing in text files, which can represent more than 75% of an organization's data; data that are not organized or that lack structure.

Usability The ease with which people can use an interface to achieve a particular goal. Issues of human performance during computer interactions for specific tasks within a particular context.

User-friendly Programs and peripherals that make it easy to interact or use computers. Design of a program to enhance the ease with which the user can utilize and maximize the productivity from computer programs.

User interface Mechanisms or systems used by people to interact with programs.

Value Relative worth of an object or action, such as aesthetic beauty or ethical value.

Veracity Right to truth.

Video adapter card A board or card that is inserted or plugged into a computer to provide display capabilities.

Videopod Self-contained system with a video transmitter.

Virtual memory The use of hard disk space on a temporary basis when the user is running many programs simultaneously. This temporary use frees up RAM to allow programs to run simultaneously and seamlessly.

Virtual reality (VR) Technology that simulates reality in a virtual medium.

Virtual world World that exists in cyberspace where people can establish avatars, purchase land, and interact with others. Emerging virtual worlds such as Second Life are changing the meaning of social networking.

Virtue A certain ideal toward which we should strive that provides for the full development of our humanity. Attitude or character trait that enables us to be and to act in ways that develop our highest potential; examples are honesty, courage, compassion, generosity, fidelity, integrity, fairness, self-control, and prudence. Like habits, virtues become characteristics of a person. The virtuous person is the ethical person.

Virtue ethics Theory that suggests individuals use power to bring about human benefit. One must consider the needs of others and the responsibility to meet those needs.

Virus Malicious code that attaches to an existing program and executes its harmful script when opened.

Voice recognition A type of software that allows the user to input data or to navigate the Web using voice commands. Voice interactivity should help to reduce the disparity associated with those who have limited keyboard or mousing skills.

Waterfall model An early systems development life cycle model that is linear in nature; when one phase ends, you move on to the next phase and do not go back, unlike in its modern counterparts that stress iterative development.

Wearable technology Devices that a person can don or put on such as articles of clothing or watches, jewelry, and other accessories. Wearable devices are being used to provide remote monitoring of physiologic parameters in care settings, including patients' own homes.

The study or practice of inventing, designing, building, or using miniature body-borne computational and sensory devices.

Web 2.0 Developing tools for social networking. The implications of the social networking technologies that are major elements of Web 2.0 will have significant impacts on the amount of information and knowledge that are generated and the ways in which they are used.

Web based Originating from the World Wide Web.

Web enhanced That which uses the World Wide Web to enhance or promote functions or tasks, such as effective learning and skill acquisition.

Web publishing The design and development of webpages that include links to digital files that are uploaded to Web servers, thereby making these files accessible to others via Web browsers.

Web quest A search of the World Wide Web for information.

Web servers Multifunctional telehealth care platforms for receiving, retrieving, and/or displaying patients' vital signs and other information transmitted from telecommunications-ready medical devices.

Webcast Media distributed over the Internet as a broadcast, which relies on streaming media technology to facilitate downloading and participation. Such broadcasts could be distributed in real time, live, or recorded for asynchronous interaction.

Webinar Web-based seminar. Web conferencing that allows a presenter to share his or her computer screen/files and collaborate with the audience; attendance is controlled by an access code.

Weblog A website that contains the contributions of single or multiple users about a particular topic or issue. Similar in nature to a threaded discussion board or a personal diary, weblogs (also known as blogs) can provide insight into the perceptions of the contributors about the topic.

Wiki Server software that allows users to create, edit, and link webpage content from any Web browser. Server software that supports hyperlinks. The simplest online database; used to develop collaborative websites.

Wisdom Knowledge applied in a practical way or translated into actions; the use of knowledge and experience to heighten common sense and insight so as to exercise sound judgment in practical matters. Sometimes thought of as the highest form of common sense, resulting from accumulated knowledge or erudition

(deep, thorough learning) or enlightenment (education that results in understanding and the dissemination of knowledge). Wisdom is the ability to apply valuable and viable knowledge, experience, understanding, and insight while being prudent and sensible. It is focused on our own minds; it is the synthesis of our experience, insight, understanding, and knowledge. Wisdom is the appropriate use of knowledge to solve human problems. It is knowing when and how to apply knowledge.

Word processing Creating documents using a word processing software package, such as Microsoft Word.

Work process *See* work flow.

Work-around A way invented by users to bypass a technology system or a policy or procedure to accomplish a task; usually indicates a poor fit of the procedure, the system, or the technology to the work flow or user. A devised way to beat a system that does not function appropriately or is not suited to the task for which it was developed.

Work flow A progression of steps (tasks, events, and interactions) that constitute a work process, involve two or more persons, and create or add value to the organization's activities. In a sequential work flow, each step depends on the occurrence of the previous step; in a parallel work flow, two or more steps can occur concurrently. The term "work flow" is sometimes used interchangeably with "process" or "process flow," particularly in the context of implementations. A sequence of connected steps in the work of a person or team of people—that is, the process or flow of work within an organization or a virtual illustration of the "real" work or steps (flow) that workers enact to complete their tasks (work). The purpose of examining and redesigning work flow is to streamline the work process by removing any unnecessary steps that do not add value or might even hinder the flow of work.

Work flow analysis Not an optional part of clinical implementations but rather a necessity for safe patient care fostered by technology. The ultimate goal of work flow analysis is not to "pave the cow path" but rather to create a future-state solution that maximizes the use of technology and eliminates non—value-added activities. Although many tools and methods can be used to accomplish work flow redesign (e.g., Six Sigma, Lean), the best method is the one that complements the organization and supports the work of clinicians.

World Wide Web (WWW) An international network of computers and servers that offers access to stored documents written in HTML code and access to graphics, audio, and video files.

Worm A form of malicious code. A self-replicating computer program that uses a network to send multiple copies of itself to other computers, subsequently tying up bandwidth and incapacitating networks.

Yottabyte (YB) A unit of information or computer storage equal to 1 septillion bytes.

Youth Risk Behavior Surveillance System (YRBSS) An epidemiologic survey conducted by the Centers for Disease Control and Protection to identify and track the most common health risk behaviors that lead to illnesses and mortality among youth.

Zero day attack Exploitation by a hacker of a software vulnerability that is initially unknown to the manufacturer. Once the attack is discovered, the software developer works to close the vulnerability.

Zettabyte (ZB) A unit of information or computer storage equal to 1 sextillion bytes.

Index

Page numbers followed by *b, f,* or *t* indicate material in boxes, figures, or tables, respectively.